Pediatric ESAP™ 2019-2020

Endocrine Society's
Pediatric Endocrine Self-Assessment Program
Questions, Answers, and Discussions

Paola A. Palma Sisto, MD, Program Chair (2017-Present)
Associate Professor
Medical College of Wisconsin
Children's Hospital of Wisconsin

Rachel I. Gafni, MD, Program Chair (2014-2017)
Bethesda, Maryland

Andrew J. Bauer, MD
Director, The Thyroid Center Children's
Hospital of Philadelphia
Associate Professor of Pediatrics
Perelman School of Medicine
University of Pennsylvania

Mark D. DeBoer, MD, MSc, MCR
Associate Professor of Pediatrics
University of Virginia School of Medicine

Alison M. Boyce, MD
Bethesda, Maryland

Cem S. Demirci, MD
Director, Type 1 Diabetes Program
Connecticut Children's Medical Center

Oscar Escobar, MD
Associate Professor
University of Pittsburgh School of
Medicine
Children's Hospital of Pittsburgh

Reema L. Habiby, MD
Associate Professor of Pediatrics
Northwestern University Feinberg School
of Medicine
Ann & Robert H. Lurie Children's Hospital
of Chicago

Oksana Lekarev, DO
Assistant Professor of Pediatrics
New York-Presbyterian Hospital
Weill Cornell Medicine

Bradley S. Miller, MD, PhD
Professor of Pediatrics
University of Minnesota Masonic
Children's Hospital

Ryan S. Miller, MD
Assistant Professor
University of Maryland School of Medicine

Ron Newfield, MD
Clinical Professor
University of California – San Diego
Rady Children's Hospital San Diego

Liuska M. Pesce, MD
Clinical Associate Professor
Pediatric Thyroid Clinic Director
Stead Family Department of Pediatrics
Division of Pediatric Endocrinology and
Diabetes
University of Iowa

Sripriya Raman, MD
Visiting Associate Professor
University of Pittsburgh School of
Medicine
Children's Hospital of Pittsburgh

Lawrence A. Silverman, MD
Goryeb Children's Hospital
Atlantic Health System

Paul S. Thornton, MD
Medical Director, Diabetes and
Endocrinology
Director, Congenital Hyperinsulinism Center
Cook Children's Medical Center

Abbie L. Young, MS, CGC, ELS(D)
Medical Editor

Endocrine Society
2055 L Street NW, Suite 600, Washington, DC 20036
1-888-ENDOCRINE • www.endocrine.org

ENDOCRINE
SOCIETY
Hormone Science to Health

ENDOCRINE SOCIETY

Hormone Science to Health

The Endocrine Society is the world's largest, oldest, and most active organization working to advance the clinical practice of endocrinology and hormone research. Founded in 1916, the Society now has more than 18,000 global members across a range of disciplines. The Society has earned an international reputation for excellence in the quality of its peer-reviewed journals, educational resources, meetings, and programs that improve public health through the practice and science of endocrinology.

Visit us at:
education.endocrine.org
endocrine.org

Other Publications:
www.endocrine.org/publications

ISBN: 978-1-879225-60-2
Library of Congress Control Number: 2019951723

On the cover: *Top left:* Pedigree of a patient with diabetes mellitus showing multiple affected family members in 3 generations; subsequent evaluation documented that the etiology of diabetes in this family was maturity-onset diabetes of the young type 3 (MODY 3) due to an *HNF1A* pathogenic variant.
Bottom left: Neck ultrasonography showing a subcentimeter right thyroid nodule with microcalcifications; after fine-needle aspiration biopsy, pathologic examination revealed multifocal papillary thyroid cancer.
Right: Brain MRI (sagittal view) documenting pituitary hyperplasia due to severe primary hypothyroidism.

The Pediatric Endocrine Self-Assessment Program (Pediatric ESAP™) is a self-study curriculum specifically designed for endocrinologists seeking a self-assessment and a broad review of pediatric endocrinology. Pediatric ESAP consists of 100 multiple-choice questions in all areas of pediatric endocrinology, diabetes, growth, and metabolism. There is extensive discussion of each correct answer and references.

The Pediatric ESAP reference book is intended primarily for consultation and self-assessment of knowledge relating to endocrinology. As a reference book, educational credits are not available upon completion of the multiple-choice questions included. For information on educational products that include educational credit, please visit endocrine.org/store.

LEARNING OBJECTIVES

Pediatric ESAP 2019-2020 will allow learners to assess their knowledge of all aspects of pediatric endocrinology.

Upon completion of this educational activity, participants will be able to:

- Recognize clinical manifestations of pediatric endocrine, growth, and metabolic disorders and select among current options for diagnosis, management, and therapy.
- Identify risk factors for endocrine and metabolic disorders in pediatric patients and develop strategies for prevention.
- Evaluate pediatric endocrine and metabolic manifestations of systemic disorders.
- Use current, evidence-based clinical guidelines and treatment recommendations to guide diagnosis and treatment of pediatric endocrine and metabolic disorders.

TARGET AUDIENCE

Pediatric ESAP is a self-study curriculum aimed at physicians seeking certification or recertification in pediatric endocrinology, program directors interested in a testing and training instrument, and clinicians seeking a self-assessment and a broad review of pediatric endocrinology.

STATEMENT OF INDEPENDENCE

The Endocrine Society has a policy of ensuring that the content and quality of this educational activity are balanced, independent, objective, and scientifically rigorous. The scientific content of this activity was developed under the supervision of the Endocrine Society's Pediatric ESAP Faculty.

DISCLOSURE POLICY

The faculty, committee members, and staff who are in position to control the content of this activity are required to disclose to the Endocrine Society and to learners any relevant financial relationship(s) of the individual or spouse/partner that have occurred within the last 12 months with any commercial interest(s) whose products or services are related to the content. Financial relationships are defined by remuneration in any amount from the commercial interest(s) in the form of grants; research support; consulting fees; salary; ownership interest (eg, stocks, stock options, or ownership interest excluding diversified mutual funds); honoraria or other payments for participation in speakers' bureaus, advisory boards, or boards of directors; or other financial benefits. The intent of this disclosure is not to prevent planners with relevant financial relationships from planning or delivering content, but rather to provide learners with information that allows them to make their own judgments of whether these financial relationships may have influenced the educational activity with regard to exposition or conclusion.

The Endocrine Society has reviewed all disclosures and resolved or managed all identified conflicts of interest, as applicable.

The faculty reported the following relevant financial relationships during the content development process for this activity: **Rachel I. Gafni, MD**, reports that the institution that employs her receives research support from Shire Pharmaceuticals. Her spouse is partner-owner of the Surgery Center of Bethesda, as well as the Orthopedics Center. **Allison M. Boyce, MD**, reports that her employer receives research support from Amgen. **Bradley S. Miller, MD, PhD**, is a consultant for and is on the Advisory Board for Abbvie, Ferring, Novo Nordisk, Pfizer, Sandoz, and Versartis. He has also received research funding from Alexion, BioMarin, Eli Lilly, Endo Pharmaceuticals, Genentech, Novo Nordisk, Tolmar, and Versartis. **Liuska Pesce, MD**, reports that her spouse is a consultant for Vidas Diagnostics. **Lawrence Silverman, MD**, is a consultant/advisor for Opko Biologics, Endo Pharmaceuticals, Novo Nordisk, and Abbvie and is a contracted researcher for Novo Nordisk and Versartis. He is also a speaker for Abbvie. **Paul S. Thornton, MD**, is an investigator for Endo Pharmaceuticals, Roche, and Ascendis.

The following faculty members reported no relevant financial relationships: **Andrew J. Bauer, MD; Mark D. DeBoer, MD, MSc, MCR; Cem S. Demirci, MD; Oscar Escobar, MD; Reema L. Habiby, MD; Oksana Lekarev, DO; Ryan S. Miller, MD; Ron Newfield, MD; Paola A. Palma Sisto, MD;** and **Sripriya Raman, MD**.

The medical editor for this program, **Abbie L. Young, MS, CGC, ELS(D)**, reported no relevant financial relationships.

The Endocrine Society staff associated with the development of this program reported no relevant financial relationships.

DISCLAIMERS

The information presented in this activity represents the opinion of the faculty and is not necessarily the official position of the Endocrine Society.

USE OF PROFESSIONAL JUDGMENT:

The educational content in this self-assessment test relates to basic principles of diagnosis and therapy and does not substitute for individual patient assessment based on the health care provider's examination of the patient and consideration of laboratory data and other factors unique to the patient. Standards in medicine change as new data become available.

DRUGS AND DOSAGES:

When prescribing medications, the physician is advised to check the product information sheet accompanying each drug to verify conditions of use and to identify any changes in drug dosage schedule or contraindications.

POLICY ON UNLABELED/OFF-LABEL USE

The Endocrine Society has determined that disclosure of unlabeled/off-label or investigational use of commercial product(s) is informative for audiences and therefore requires this information be disclosed to the learners. Uses of some pharmaceutical agents, medical devices, and other products discussed in this educational activity may not be the same as those indicated in product labeling approved by the United States Food and Drug Administration (FDA). The Endocrine Society requires that any discussions of such "off-label" uses be based on scientific research that conforms to generally accepted standards of experimental design, data collection, and data analysis. Before prescribing or recommending any therapeutic agent or device, learners should review the complete prescribing information, including indications, contraindications, warnings, precautions, and adverse events.

ACKNOWLEDGMENT OF COMMERCIAL SUPPORT

This activity is not supported by educational grant(s) or other funds from any commercial supporter.

PUBLICATION DATE: December 2018

Abbreviations

ACTH --- corticotropin
ACE inhibitor --------------- angiotensin-converting enzyme inhibitor
ALT --- alanine aminotransferase
AST -- aspartate aminotransferase
BMI --- body mass index
CNS -- central nervous system
CT -- computed tomography
DHEA --------------------------------------- dehydroepiandrosterone
DHEA-S -------------------------- dehydroepiandrosterone sulfate
DNA -- deoxyribonucleic acid
DPP-4 inhibitor --------------------- dipeptidyl-peptidase 4 inhibitor
DXA --------------------------- dual-energy x-ray absorptiometry
FDA ---------------------------------- Food and Drug Administration
FGF-23 ---------------------------------- fibroblast growth factor 23
FNA -- fine-needle aspiration
FSH ------------------------------------ follicle-stimulating hormone
GH --- growth hormone
GHRH ----------------------------- growth hormone–releasing hormone
GLP-1 receptor agonist ----- glucagonlike peptide 1 receptor agonist
GnRH ----------------------------- gonadotropin-releasing hormone
hCG ------------------------------- human chorionic gonadotropin
HDL ------------------------------------- high-density lipoprotein
HIV ---------------------------------- human immunodeficiency virus
HMG-CoA reductase inhibitor ------------ 3-hydroxy-3-methylglutaryl
    coenzyme A reductase inhibitor
IGF-1 -------------------------------------- insulinlike growth factor 1
LDL -- low-density lipoprotein
LH -- luteinizing hormone
MCV -- mean corpuscular volume
MRI ---------------------------------- magnetic resonance imaging
NPH insulin --------------------- neutral protamine Hagedorn insulin
PCSK9 inhibitor - - - - proprotein convertase subtilisin/kexin 9 inhibitor
PET ---------------------------------- positron emission tomography
PSA ------------------------------------- prostate-specific antigen
PTH --- parathyroid hormone
PTHrP ----------------------- parathyroid hormone–related protein
SGLT-2 inhibitor ---------- sodium-glucose cotransporter 2 inhibitor
SHBG ------------------------------ sex hormone–binding globulin
T_3 --- triiodothyronine
T_4 --- thyroxine
TPO antibodies ----------------------- thyroperoxidase antibodies
TRH ----------------------------- thyrotropin-releasing hormone
TRAb ---------------------------- thyrotropin-receptor antibodies
TSH --- thyrotropin
VLDL ---------------------------------- very low-density lipoprotein

PEDIATRIC ENDOCRINE SELF-ASSESSMENT PROGRAM 2019-2020

Part I

1 A 6-year-old girl presents to your clinic for evaluation of bone health after sustaining a minimally traumatic wrist fracture. She has a history of Crohn disease diagnosed at age 3 years. Her disease has been difficult to control, resulting in multiple surgical bowel resections. She has been receiving parenteral nutrition for the majority of her nutrition over the past 3 years.

Which of the following is most likely contributing to this child's bone disease?
   A. Aluminum toxicity
   B. Selenium deficiency
   C. Calcium and phosphorus deficiency
   D. Metabolic alkalosis
   E. Inadequate protein intake

2 A 14-month-old boy presents with cardiogenic shock associated with parvovirus cardiomyopathy. The toddler is started on amiodarone secondary to developing a life-threatening cardiac arrhythmia. One week later, endocrinology is consulted because of abnormal thyroid function tests showing increased TSH and free T_4 levels (*see table, time point #1*). You recommend repeating laboratory tests in 1 week, and the results are once again abnormal (*see table, 1 week later*). You decide to continue following the patient's thyroid levels without treatment, and over the next month his TSH normalizes without thyroid hormone replacement (*see table, 2 and 4 weeks later*).

Measurement	Time Point #1	1 Week Later	2 Weeks Later	4 Weeks Later
TSH (0.5-4.5 mIU/L)	15.7 mIU/L	21.0 mIU/L	8.0 mIU/L	2.9 mIU/L
Free T_4 (0.9-1.7 ng/dL [SI: 11.6-21.9 pmol/L])	2.5 ng/dL (32.2 pmol/L)	1.4 ng/dL (18.0 pmol/L)	1.4 ng/dL (18.0 pmol/L)	1.3 ng/dL (16.7 pmol/L)
Total T_3 (80-190 ng/dL [SI: 1.2-2.9 nmol/L])	...	150 ng/dL (2.3 nmol/L)	...	...
Reverse T_3 (10-24 ng/dL [SI: 0.15-0.37 nmol/L])	33.8 ng/dL (0.52 nmol/L)	...	...	...

In this patient, which of the following is the physiologic mechanism to explain the increase in TSH after initiation of amiodarone therapy?
   A. Amiodarone-induced hypothyroidism (Wolff-Chaikoff effect)
   B. Decreased renal clearance of reverse T_3
   C. Nonthyroidal illness (euthyroid sick syndrome)
   D. Amiodarone-induced decreased conversion of T_4 to T_3
   E. Amiodarone-induced activation of type III deiodinase

3 A 4-month-old girl presents for evaluation of poor growth. Her mother had normal prenatal care and the pregnancy and delivery were uneventful. The patient's birth weight was 7 lb 11 oz (3490 g), and her length was 19 in (48.2 cm). Weight gain has been steady since birth, but she has been slow to gain length. She breastfeeds every 2 hours. She occasionally goes 4 hours without a feed at night. She has normal bowel movements. Her developmental milestones are normal. Her medical history is notable for an admission to the neonatal intensive care unit at birth for mild hypoglycemia. She underwent a sepsis workup and was treated for 48 hours with antibiotics, which were discontinued after her blood cultures were negative. Her blood glucose measurements were normal off intravenous dextrose for 24 hours before discharge. Her mother's height is 64 in (162.5 cm), and her father's height is 74 in (188 cm). The patient's family history is noncontributory.

   On physical examination, her blood pressure is 94/55 mm Hg and pulse rate is 138 beats/min. Her length is 21 in (53.3 cm) (0.02% of growth percentile based on length-for-age), weight is 11.8 lb (5.38 kg) (9.6th growth percentile based on weight-for-age), and head circumference is 15.8 in (40.2 cm) (21.7th percentile). Examination findings are notable for small stature and relative excess weight. She has a prominent forehead and flat nasal bridge. She has no striae or bruising.

Laboratory test results:
  Free T$_4$ = 1.31 ng/dL (0.89-1.60 ng/dL) (SI: 16.7 pmol/L [11.5-20.6 pmol/L])
  TSH = 4.6 mIU/L (0.4-8.2 mIU/L)
  GH = 20.9 ng/mL (1.4-7.1 ng/mL) (SI: 20.9 µg/L [1.4-7.1 µg/L])
  IGF-1 = <25 ng/mL (25-109 ng/mL) (SI: <3.3 nmol/L [3.3-14.3 nmol/L])
  IGFBP-3 = 0.52 mg/L (0.7-3.6 mg/L)
  ACTH = 27 pg/mL (no reference range established for this age) (SI: 5.9 pmol/L)
  Random cortisol = 6.0 µg/dL (2.8-23.0 µg/dL) (SI: 165.5 nmol/L [77.2-634.5 nmol/L])

Which of the following tests is most likely to reveal the diagnosis?
  A. Skeletal survey
  B. 24-Hour urinary free cortisol measurement
  C. MRI of the pituitary and hypothalamus
  D. GH-binding protein measurement
  E. Karyotype analysis

4 A 16-year-old boy with a 9-year history of type 1 diabetes mellitus is referred to your diabetes clinic for a second opinion regarding his diabetes control. He was found in bed having a seizure, and his point-of-care blood glucose level was 27 mg/dL (1.5 mmol/L). After administering glucagon, his mother called 911 and emergency medical technicians brought him to the emergency department. The emergency technicians placed a line and gave him D50% glucose. On arrival, he was awake but could not explain how he got to the emergency department. His plasma glucose measurement was 216 mg/dL (12.0 mmol/L). After careful review of his history, it was discovered that he had recently increased his insulin glargine dosage by 2 units and had played pool volleyball with his friends and spent time in a hot tub after dinner. This was the first time he had a seizure or needed glucagon.

In your office 3 days later, he is well and fully recovered. He reports he has glucose levels in the range of 50 to 60 mg/dL (2.8-3.3 mmol/L) 4 to 6 times a week and that he rarely feels hypoglycemic. His hemoglobin A$_{1c}$ level today is 6.8% (51 mmol/mol).

His mother wants to know which factors most likely contributed to his recent episode of hypoglycemia associated with seizure. Which of the following was the most likely etiology?
  A. Increasing the insulin glargine dosage
  B. Relative excess insulin and exercise
  C. Loss of glucagon secretion due to loss of intra-islet insulin secretion
  D. The 4 to 6 episodes of moderate hypoglycemia the week before
  E. Hypoglycemia-associated autonomic failure

5 A 6-year-old boy and his parents present for a follow-up visit to discuss his newly diagnosed illness. His parents initially sought evaluation by his pediatrician after noting hyperactive behavior. His teachers reported that he was having difficulty concentrating in class. He also seemed to be more tired and irritable than usual. The patient was initially referred to a neurologist who obtained an MRI of the brain, which demonstrated symmetric occipital white matter lesions.

When you examine the patient, he appears well but has slight darkening of the skin, particularly at the palmar creases, and he also has a few hyperpigmented spots on his tongue and gums.

Laboratory test results (sample drawn at 8 AM):
  Cortisol = 1.9 µg/dL (5.0-21.0 µg/dL) (SI: 52.4 nmol/L [137.9-579.3 nmol/L])
  ACTH = 2120 pg/mL (6-48 pg/mL) (SI: 466.4 pmol/L [1.3-10.6 pmol/L])
  Plasma very long-chain fatty acids, elevated

Both parents are healthy. The patient's mother was adopted and does not know her family history. You plan to arrange for genetic testing and to start treatment. The mother tells you that she is pregnant and knows she is expecting a girl.

Which of the following do you tell the parents regarding the expected clinical presentation in the female sibling if she inherits the same mutation?
  A. She will remain asymptomatic
  B. She may develop neurologic manifestations but likely no adrenal manifestations
  C. She will develop both adrenal and neurologic manifestations
  D. She may develop only adrenal manifestations
  E. She will have a risk of developing an adrenal tumor in late adolescence or adulthood

6 A 6-year-old boy presents for evaluation of obesity. He was born at 38 weeks estimated gestational age with a birth weight of 6 lb 8 oz (2950 g) to a 36-year-old mother (G1P0 to 1) following a pregnancy complicated only by advanced maternal age. He had failure to thrive as an infant, but began gaining weight as a toddler despite a continued small appetite. More recently, he has become constantly focused on food but is able to be redirected. He began walking at age 22 months. He is struggling in school. Family history is unremarkable.

On physical examination, his weight is 61.6 lb (28 kg) (+3.18 SDS), and height is 41.3 in (105 cm) (−2.17 SDS). He has small eyes and red hair. Genital examination reveals a small phallus with retractile testicles and a prominent prepubic fat pad. He has small hands and feet.

Which of the following is the most likely cause of this child's obesity?
  A. Pathogenic variant in the *MC4R* gene (melanocortin 4 receptor)
  B. Maternal uniparental disomy of chromosome 15
  C. Maternal uniparental disomy of chromosome 7
  D. Pathogenic variant in the *PCSK1* gene (proprotein convertase)
  E. Methylation abnormality on chromosome 11

7 You are asked to evaluate a 14-year-old girl for concerns regarding consistent weight gain. The family reports that she started gaining excess weight at age 9 years. Menarche was at age 10 years, and she has approximately 10 menstrual periods yearly. Her growth chart is shown (*see image*).

On physical examination, she has a large dorsocervical fat pad and multiple pink striae on her abdomen.

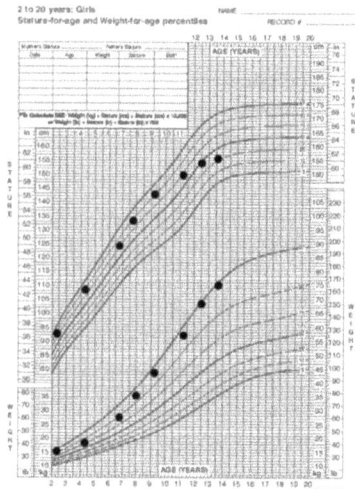

Laboratory test result:
  Urinary free cortisol = 96 µg/24 h (10-100 µg/24 h) (SI: 265.0 nmol/d [27.6-276.0 nmol/d])

Given these clinical findings, which of the following is the best next step in this patient's evaluation?
  A. Three-day dietary history
  B. Low-dose dexamethasone suppression test
  C. Dexamethasone corticotropin-releasing hormone test
  D. Adrenal CT
  E. Pituitary MRI

8 An 11-year-old girl with hypothyroidism is referred for evaluation of short stature. She was born full term, and her birth weight and length were adequate for gestational age. Her medical history is unremarkable, except for short stature and a diagnosis of hypothyroidism 1 year ago. Her parents noticed that she was shorter than her peers at the age of 5 years. They report that for the last 3 to 4 years, she has not grown well. She has had delayed teeth eruption, dry skin, and hair loss. She also always seems more tired than her peers, although her parents have attributed this to her quiet, tranquil disposition.

Last year, her pediatrician measured her TSH, which was documented to be greater than 500 mIU/L. Levothyroxine, 25 mcg daily, was prescribed and the dosage has been adjusted every 4 to 6 weeks. She is currently euthyroid on a dosage of 88 mcg daily.

On physical examination, she has normal vital signs. Her height is 50.4 in (127.9 cm) (<1st percentile; Z-score, −2.84), weight is 74 lb (33.6 kg) (29.5th percentile; Z-score, −0.54), and BMI is 18.22 kg/m^2 (54th percentile). Her height age is 7.5 years. Midparental target height is 63 in (160 cm). Her thyroid gland is mildly enlarged and firm. Both pubic hair and breast development are Tanner stage 1. She has dry skin and hair. The rest of her physical examination findings are normal. Her bone age (at a chronologic age of 11 years) is interpreted to be 8 years.

Her parents are concerned about her predicted adult height. You tell them that her final adult height will be:
- A. Normal because she has been on thyroid hormone replacement and will have catch-up growth
- B. Normal because her bone age is delayed
- C. Normal because she has not yet entered puberty
- D. Below midparental target height because she will have rapidly progressing puberty
- E. Below midparental target height because of the duration of hypothyroidism before treatment

9   You have been consulted regarding a 1-day-old female newborn (born at 37 weeks' gestation) noted to be small-for-gestational-age (birth weight, 4 lb 2 oz [1885 g]). Her weight is below the 1st percentile and length and head circumference are at the 5th percentile. She was born vaginally to a nonobese mother who had received prenatal care and reported no exposure to illegal drugs, alcohol, or cigarette smoke. The mother did not have gestational diabetes.

On physical examination, the baby appears pale. She has typical female genitalia. The rest of the examination findings are normal.

Laboratory test results (sample drawn at 24 hours of life):
Sodium = 137 mEq/L (130-145 mEq/L) (SI: 137 mmol/L [130-145 mmol/L])
Potassium = 3.7 mEq/L (3.7-5.9 mEq/L) (SI: 3.7 mmol/L [3.7-5.9 mmol/L])
Chloride = 105 mEq/L (97-108 mEq/L) (SI: 105 mmol/L [97-108 mmol/L])
Bicarbonate = 18 mEq/L (17-24 mEq/L) (SI: 18 mmol/L [17-24 mmol/L])
Serum urea nitrogen = 18 mg/dL (2-19 mg/dL) (SI: 6.4 mmol/L [0.7-6.7 mmol/L])
Creatinine = 0.7 mg/dL (0.3-1.0 mg/dL) (SI: 61.9 μmol/L [27-88 μmol/L])
Glucose = 197 mg/dL (50-90 mg/dL) (SI: 10.9 mmol/L [2.8-5.0 mmol/L])

You follow her glucose levels over the next 24 hours:
29 hours of life: 225 mg/dL (12.5 mmol/L)
33 hours of life: 307 mg/dL (17.0 mmol/L)

Which of the following is the most likely causative factor for the laboratory findings?
- A. Hypopituitarism
- B. Placental insufficiency
- C. Neonatal hyperthyroidism
- D. Insulin resistance in the liver
- E. Cortisol excess

10   A newborn girl born at 40 weeks' gestation is admitted to the neonatal intensive care unit for respiratory distress. On day 2 of life, a blood sample for newborn screening is collected. One week later, the neonatal intensive care unit is notified of a positive result and confirmatory thyroid function testing is obtained by venipuncture, which confirms congenital hypothyroidism. Thyroid ultrasonography reveals a eutopic but hypoplastic-appearing thyroid gland.

A pathogenic variant in which of the following genes most likely explains the constellation of diagnoses in this patient?

    A. *PAX8* (paired box 8)
    B. *NKX2-1* (formerly *TITF1*) (NK2 homeobox 1)
    C. *FOXE1* (formerly *TITF2*) (Forkhead box E1)
    D. *SLC5A5* (formerly *NIS*) (solute carrier family 5 member 5)
    E. *NKX2-5* (NK2 homeobox 5)

11 You are referred a 12-year-old girl with recently diagnosed Turner syndrome (confirmed 45,X/46,XX mosaicism). The question of future fertility and fertility preservation is raised.

Measurement of which of the following would be most informative to address the possibility of future fertility?

    A. Inhibin B
    B. FSH
    C. Estradiol
    D. Antimullerian hormone
    E. Follistatin

12 A 15-year-old girl presents to her pediatrician with a 2-year history of fatigue and weakness.

Laboratory test results:
    Calcium = 17.1 mg/dL (8.2-10.6 mg/dL) (SI: 4.3 mmol/L [2.1-2.7 mmol/L])
    Phosphate = 2.1 mg/dL (3.0-4.5 mg/dL) (SI: 0.7 mmol/L [1.0-1.5 mmol/L])
    Alkaline phosphatase = 4740 U/L (138-511 U/L) (SI: 79.2 μkat/L [2.3-8.5 μkat/L])
    25-Hydroxyvitamin D = 17 ng/mL (20-80 ng/mL) (SI: 42.4 nmol/L [49.9-199.7 nmol/L])
    PTH = 170 pg/mL (15-65 pg/mL) (SI: 170 ng/L [15-65 ng/L])

Radiographs reveal generalized osteopenia and 2 cystlike tumors in the posterior parietal bone and clavicle. Treatment is started with intravenous normal saline at 2.5 times maintenance rate, as well as calcitonin. A technetium-99 sestamibi scan and thoracic magnetic resonance imaging demonstrate an ectopic anterior mediastinal parathyroid adenoma, with the other parathyroid glands detected in the normal position. She undergoes surgery the following morning, and the ectopic parathyroid gland (15 × 13 × 8 mm) within the thymus is removed.

During the postoperative period, the patient develops paresthesia and muscular cramps in the lower limbs.

Laboratory test results:
    Calcium = 6.7 mg/dL (8.2-10.6 mg/dL) (SI: 1.7 mmol/L [2.1-2.7 mmol/L])
    Alkaline phosphatase = 3107 U/L (138-511 U/L) (SI: 51.9 μkat/L [2.3-8.5 μkat/L])

Which of the following is the most likely etiology of this patient's current mineral abnormalities?

    A. Insufficient secretion of PTH due to accidental removal of parathyroid glands
    B. Effects of preoperative calcitonin
    C. Insufficient gastrointestinal calcium absorption due to vitamin D deficiency
    D. Increased calcium requirements due to rapid skeletal mineralization
    E. Fluid overload from aggressive intravenous hydration

13 You are asked to evaluate a 6-year-old boy with short stature. He was born at the 50th percentile for both height and weight and his growth has slowly decelerated; his height is now at the 5th percentile and weight is at the 25th percentile. His midparental target for both is at the 50th percentile. He is otherwise a healthy child with no signs of chronic illness.

Baseline laboratory test results:

Free T$_4$ = 1.1 ng/dL (0.8-2.2 ng/dL) (SI: 14.2 pmol/L [10.30-28.32 pmol/L])

TSH = 1.29 mIU/L (0.6-5.5 mIU/L)

IGF-1 = 44 ng/mL (60-228 ng/mL) (SI: 5.8 nmol/L [7.9-29.9 nmol/L])

IGFBP-3 = 1.7 mg/L (1.5-3.4 mg/L)

IGF-2 = 407 ng/mL (334-642 ng/mL)

You perform an arginine clonidine stimulation test and obtain the following results:

Arginine

Time point	GH level
Time 0	4 ng/mL (4 µg/L)
15 min	7 ng/mL (7 µg/L)
30 min	6 ng/mL (6 µg/L)
45 min	5 ng/mL (5 µg/L)
60 min	6 ng/mL (6 µg/L)

Clonidine

Time point	GH level
Time 0	6 ng/mL (6 µg/L)
30 min	5 ng/mL (5 µg/L)
60 min	7 ng/mL (7 µg/L)
90 min	5 ng/mL (5 µg/L)

To what degree are the following factors most likely to be affected by the therapy you initiate?

Answer	Most affected	Moderately affected	Least affected
A.	IGF-1	IGFBP-3	IGF-2
B.	IGF-1	IGF-2	IGFBP-3
C.	IGF-2	IGF-1	IGFBP-3
D.	IGFBP-3	IGF-1	IGF-2
E.	IGFBP-3	IGF-2	IGF-1

14 A 13-month-old girl is brought to the local emergency department because of lethargy. She was born full term with a normal birth weight after an uncomplicated pregnancy and delivery. She breastfed normally for the first 6 months of life. After weaning off the breast at 6 months of age, she became more and more interested in drinking water. Her parents report that over time she would demand water whenever she saw them drinking it. At 12 months of age, she started waking every couple of hours overnight crying for water. Her diapers were very wet and often leaked. After obtaining water, she would fall back to sleep. About 3 weeks ago, her water-seeking behavior seemed worse and her intake of solid foods decreased. Her parents tried to limit fluids in order to increase her solid food intake. However, over the past week she has become increasingly lethargic.

When reviewing her history, her parents note she has always been slow to gain weight. There are no other family members with excessive thirst or urination.

On physical examination, her blood pressure is 103/49 mm Hg and pulse rate is 113 beats/min. Her height is 29 in (73.7 cm) (Z-score, −0.57), weight is 14.3 lb (6.5 kg) (Z-score, −4.14), BMI is 11.97 kg/m^2, and head circumference is 16.5 in (42 cm). She is irritable and very thin. Findings on neurologic examination are normal. There are no rashes. The rest of her physical examination findings are normal.

Laboratory test results:

Sodium = 162 mEq/L (134-146 mEq/L) (SI: 162 mmol/L [134-146 mmol/L])

Potassium = 4.7 mEq/L (3.7-5.5 mEq/L) (SI: 4.7 mmol/L [3.7-5.5 mmol/L])

Chloride = 130 mEq/L (98-108 mEq/L) (SI: 130 mmol/L [98-108 mmol/L])

Carbon dioxide = 21.1 mEq/L (23.0-30.0 mEq/L) (SI: 21.1 mmol/L [23.0-30.0 mmol/L])

Glucose = 92 mg/dL (70-110 mg/dL) (SI: 5.1 mmol/L [3.9-6.1 mmol/L])

Serum urea nitrogen = 36 mg/dL (5.0-15.0 mg/dL) (SI: 12.9 mmol/L [1.8-5.4 mmol/L])

Creatinine = 0.32 mg/dL (0.25-0.64 mg/dL) (SI: 28.3 μmol/L [22.1-56.6 μmol/L])

Total calcium = 10.1 mg/dL (8.8-10.8 mg/dL) (SI: 2.5 mmol/L [2.2-2.7 mmol/L])

Serum osmolality = 346 mOsm/kg (285-295 mOsm/kg) (SI: 346 mmol/kg [285-295 mmol/kg])

Urine osmolality = 140 mOsm/kg (50-1400 mOsm/kg) (SI: 140 mmol/kg [50-1400 mmol/kg])

Free T$_4$ = 1.0 ng/dL (0.92-1.99 ng/dL) (SI: 12.9 pmol/L [11.8-25.6 pmol/L])

TSH = 1.83 mIU/L (0.73-8.35 mIU/L)

IGF-1 = 52 ng/mL (56-144 ng/mL) (SI: 6.8 nmol/L [7.3-18.9 nmol/L])

IGFBP-3 = 1.0 mg/L (0.8-4.3 mg/L)

Prolactin = 3.5 ng/mL (2.0-14.0 ng/mL) (SI: 0.15 nmol/L [0.09-0.61 nmol/L])

MRI of the brain shows an absent posterior pituitary bright spot. She is admitted to the intensive care unit. Her urine output is 17 mL/kg per h. She is given subcutaneous vasopressin (1 unit/m^2) and subsequently intravenous vasopressin. There is no decrease in her urine output or change in urine osmolality.

A pathogenic variant in which of the following genes is most likely responsible for her condition?

A. *AVP* (arginine vasopressin)

B. *AVPR2* (arginine vasopressin receptor 2)

C. *AQP2* (aquaporin 2)

D. *WFS1* (wolframin ER transmembrane glycoprotein)

E. *HESX1* (HESX homeobox 1)

15 An 8-year-old boy is referred by neurosurgery because of a recently diagnosed pituitary adenoma. The child had been complaining of headaches and neck pain, for which a brain MRI was performed (*see images*). The child's height has not increased for the last 2 years, and his mother reports that he has had dry skin and constipation for the last 2 to 3 years.

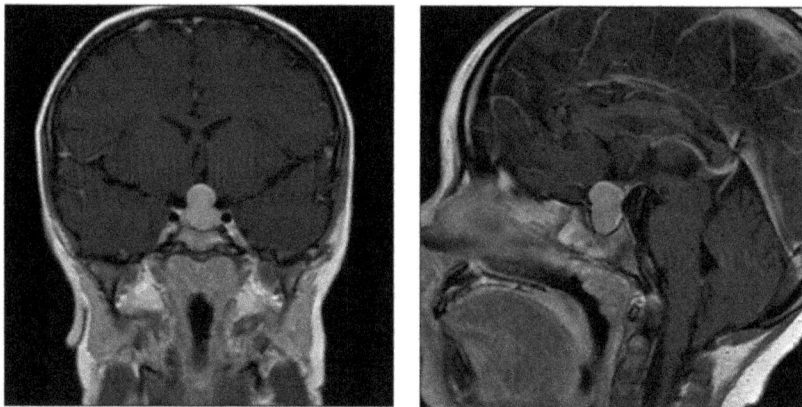

On physical examination, his height is 43.4 in (110.3 cm) (Z-score, –3.12), weight is 51 lb (23 kg) (25th percentile; Z-score, –0.675), and BMI is 19.76 kg/m^2 (94th percentile). Testicular volume is 4 mL bilaterally and pubic hair development is Tanner stage 1.

Laboratory test results:
    TSH = 2527 mIU/L (0.27-4.20 mIU/L)
    Free T$_4$ = <0.1 ng/dL (0.9-1.7 ng/dL) (SI: 1.3 pmol/L [11.6-21.9 pmol/L])
    Prolactin = 252.5 ng/mL (4.0-15.2 ng/mL) (SI: 11.0 nmol/L [0.2-0.7 nmol/L])
    Cortisol = 10 μg/dL (10-20 μg/dL) (SI: 275.9 nmol/L [275.9-551.8 nmol/L])

Which of the following is most likely to correct this patient's problem?
    A. Transsphenoidal resection
    B. Cabergoline
    C. Thyroid hormone replacement
    D. Thyroid hormone replacement and cabergoline
    E. Thyroid hormone replacement and transsphenoidal resection

16 A 1-and-6/12-year-old boy presents to the emergency department with a 24-hour history of vomiting and diarrhea. When his mother tried to wake him at 7 AM, he was difficult to arouse. He ate very poorly the previous day and aside from some sugar-free fluids, he did not eat a full meal for 24 hours. He has not urinated since 9 PM the night before.

On physical examination, his height is at the 50th percentile and his weight is at the 25th percentile. His mother notes that today's weight is 2.6 lb (1.2 kg) less than the weight recorded at his pediatrician's office 2 weeks ago.

Laboratory test results in the emergency department:
    Point-of-care glucose = 36 mg/dL (70-100 mg/dL) (SI: 2.0 mmol/L [3.9-5.6 mmol/L])
    Confirmatory plasma glucose = 40 mg/dL (SI: 2.2 mmol/L)

The emergency department physician orders a hypoglycemia panel, which subsequently (1 week later) shows the following:
    Insulin = <1 μIU/mL (2-12 μIU/mL [fasting]) (SI: 6.9 pmol/L [13.9-83.3 pmol/L])
    Cortisol = 24 μg/dL (>10 μg/dL) (SI: 662.1 nmol/L [>275.9 nmol/L])
    GH = 12 ng/mL (>7.5 ng/mL [stimulated]) (SI: 12 μg/L [>7.5 μg/L])
    Free fatty acids = 47.9 mg/dL (<11.3 mg/dL) (SI: 1.7 mmol/L [<0.4 mmol/L])
    β-Hydroxybutyrate = 26.0 mg/dL (<5.2 mg/dL) (SI: 2.5 mmol/L [<0.5 mmol/L])

In the emergency department (before the results above were available), the patient was given a 2 mL/kg bolus of D10 and then started on a drip of D10 at a glucose infusion rate of 5 mg/kg per min. An hour later, the glucose concentration was 47 mg/dL (2.6 mmol/L). Over the next 24 hours, he required a glucose infusion rate of 10 mg/kg per min to maintain a glucose level above 60 mg/dL (>3.3 mmol/L).

Endocrinology is consulted, and it is attempted to wean the dextrose. Three hours after a meal and while on a glucose infusion rate of 7 mg/kg per min (which he was on for the preceding 6 hours), his glucose value is 50 mg/dL (2.8 mmol/L) with the following critical laboratory test results:
    Plasma glucose = 48 mg/dL (70-100 mg/dL) (SI: 2.7 mmol/L [3.9-5.6 mmol/L])
    Insulin = 4 μIU/mL (2-12 μIU/mL [fasting]) (SI: 27.8 pmol/L [13.9-83.3 pmol/L])
    Free fatty acids = 5.6 mg/dL (<11.3 mg/dL) (SI: 0.2 mmol/L [<0.4 mmol/L])
    β-Hydroxybutyrate = 3.1 mg/dL (<5.2 mg/dL) (SI: 0.3 mmol/L [<0.5 mmol/L])
    Ammonia = <10 mmol/L (10-33 mmol/L)

A glucagon stimulation test is done, and his glucose rises from 45 to 107 mg/dL (2.5 to 5.9 mmol/L). Two days later, after weaning down the intravenous fluids, a protein challenge is conducted (3 hours after a standard breakfast) and the glucose levels following 1 g/kg of protein without carbohydrates are as follows:

Time	Glucose Value
0 minutes	62 mg/dL (3.4 mmol/L)
30 minutes	64 mg/dL (3.6 mmol/L)
60 minutes	58 mg/dL (3.2 mmol/L)
90 minutes	55 mg/dL (3.1 mmol/L)
120 minutes	56 mg/dL (3.1 mmol/L)
150 minutes	52 mg/dL (2.9 mmol/L)

Which of the following is the most likely diagnosis?
- A. Congenital hyperinsulinism due to glutamate dehydrogenase deficiency (*GLUD1* hyperinsulinism)
- B. Idiopathic ketotic hypoglycemia
- C. Glycogen storage disease type 0 (glycogen synthase deficiency)
- D. Congenital hyperinsulinism due to a pathogenic variant in the glucokinase gene (*GCK*)
- E. Congenital hyperinsulinism due to pathogenic variants in the K_{ATP} channel genes (*ABCC8* or *KCNJ11*)

17 You are asked to counsel the family of a 6-year-old girl with Turner syndrome (karyotype = mosaic 45,X/46, X with a marker chromosome).

In discussing the next management steps, which include potential intervention for possible gonadoblastoma risk, which of the following is the best course of action?
- A. *SRY* gene analysis
- B. Serial measurement of tumor markers
- C. Serial measurement of testosterone
- D. Serial imaging
- E. Assessment for Y-chromosome–specific markers

18 A 4-and-6/12-year-old boy presents for evaluation of tall stature. He has been growing above the 95th percentile for height since he was an infant. Birthweight was 10 lb 5 oz (4700 g). He has developmental delay requiring early intervention. His parents are of average stature with a midparental target height of 69.5 in (176.5 cm) (+0.04 SDS, 50th percentile).

On physical examination, he has a round face, heavy horizontal eyebrows, and narrow palpebral fissures. Current height is 46.9 in (119.0 cm) (+3.05 SDS), consistent with a height age of 6 and 5/12 years. Head circumference is 21.4 in (54.3 cm) (+2.5 SDS). Lower segment is 22.8 in (58 cm). Upper-to-lower segment ratio is 1.05. Bone age is 5 years. Genitalia are prepubertal (Tanner stage 1), and testes are 1 mL bilaterally. There are no unusual birthmarks. He has no evidence of hemihypertrophy, arachnodactyly, hyperflexibility, or chest wall deformity. He has mild thoracolumbar scoliosis and an umbilical hernia.

His family history is unremarkable.

Which syndrome and associated genetic alteration would cause this clinical picture?
- A. DNMT3A overgrowth syndrome; pathogenic variant in the *DNMT3A* gene (DNA methyltransferase 3 alpha)
- B. Marfan syndrome; pathogenic variant in the *FBN1* gene (fibrillin 1)
- C. Klinefelter syndrome; sex chromosome duplication (47,XXY)
- D. Beckwith-Wiedeman syndrome; pathogenic variants in imprinted genes within the chromosomal region 11p15.5, including *CDKN1C* (cyclin-dependent kinase inhibitor 1C)
- E. Homocystinuria; pathogenic variants in the *CBS* gene (cystathionine β-synthase)

19 Six months ago, a 15-year-old girl with a history of hypothyroidism secondary to chronic lymphocytic thyroiditis underwent total thyroidectomy and radioactive iodine treatment for papillary thyroid carcinoma, follicular variant (T3, N1b, M0). Thyroid hormone replacement was adjusted following treatment. For the last 2 months, she has had progressively worsening fatigue. Two weeks ago, she was evaluated in the emergency department for paresthesias in the neck, face, arms, and legs, which progressed into muscle weakness, left leg pain, and inability to move her left foot. Her primary care physician calls you and reports that the patient has left leg swelling. Evaluation obtained in the emergency department includes a normal anteroposterior and lateral x-ray of her left leg and normal Doppler flow on duplex ultrasonography of the left lower extremity without evidence of deep venous thrombosis. She has a normal basic metabolic profile and liver enzymes.

Which of the following is the best next step in this patient's evaluation?
- A. Electromyography
- B. TSH measurement
- C. Creatine kinase measurement
- D. Myositis-specific autoantibody assessment
- E. MRI of the left leg

20 You are trying to determine the next management steps for a 6-year-old girl with Turner syndrome who is taking GH therapy. As part of your decision process, you review the medical records of 2 other patients with Turner syndrome who are now 11 years old (Patients 1 and 2). At age 6 years, the patients were on the regimens shown (*see table*).

	Regimen
Patient 1	Somatotropin, 0.35 mg/kg per week Ethinyl estradiol, 0.35 mg/kg per week
Patient 2	Somatotropin, 0.35 mg/kg per week

The parents of both patients report excellent adherence, and growth charts reveal adequate linear growth over the last 5 years. At their 6-year evaluations, both patients had bone ages of 6 years.

Consider what you would predict if you assess the bone ages of these 2 patients now (at age 11 years). Compared with Patient 2's bone age, Patient 1's bone age...:
- A. Is advanced by 1.5 SD
- B. Is advanced by 1 SD
- C. Has matured at an equal pace
- D. Is delayed by 1.5 SD
- E. Is delayed by 1 SD

21 You are asked to evaluate a 6-and-2/12-year-old boy with a 6-month history of progressive pubic hair development, bilateral gynecomastia, and breast tenderness. There is no history of galactorrhea, vision changes, or headaches. The boy's parents note that he has been growing more rapidly recently and has been outgrowing his clothing more quickly than his twin brother. There is no family history of breast development in males or precocious puberty in males or females.

On physical examination, he is a well-appearing boy with no dysmorphic or cushingoid features. His blood pressure is normal. He has early Tanner stage 3 breasts, axillary wetness (but no axillary hair), and no acne. His genital examination demonstrates Tanner stage 2 pubic hair and testes measuring 1 mL bilaterally.

Bone age is advanced to 8 years.

Laboratory test results (sample drawn at 8 AM):
    17-Hydroxyprogesterone = 69 ng/dL (<91 ng/dL) (SI: 2.09 nmol/L [<2.76 nmol/L])
    Testosterone = <2.5 ng/dL (<2.5-10 ng/dL) (SI: <0.087 nmol/L [<0.087-0.35 nmol/L])
    Androstenedione = 25 ng/dL (<10-17 ng/dL) (SI: 0.87 nmol/L [0.35-0.59 nmol/L])
    DHEA-S = 52 µg/dL (13-83 µg/dL) (SI: 1.40 µmol/L [0.35-2.25 µmol/L])
    Estradiol = 36 pg/mL (5-11 pg/mL) (SI: 132.2 pmol/L [18.4-40.4 pmol/L])
    Cortisol = 12.0 µg/dL (8.0-19.0 µg/dL) (SI: 331.1 nmol/L [220.7-524.2 nmol/L])
    LH = 0.1 mIU/mL (0.02-0.30 mIU/mL) (SI: 0.1 IU/L [0.02-0.30 IU/L])
    FSH = <0.1 mIU/mL (0.26-3.00 pg/mL) (SI: 0.1 IU/L [0.26-3.00 IU/L])
    Plasma renin activity = 3.9 ng/mL per h (0.5-5.9 ng/mL per h)

Which of the following tests is most likely to provide the diagnosis?
    A. Karyotype analysis
    B. Testicular ultrasonography
    C. Adrenal CT
    D. Genetic testing for aromatase excess syndrome
    E. Prolactin measurement

22   A 16-year-old girl with polycystic ovary syndrome comes for a follow-up appointment. Over the past 2 years, she has been taking metformin, oral contraceptive pills, and a topical retinoid cream for acne. On this regimen, she has had regular menstrual periods and no progression of virilizing features. Despite weight-loss attempts, her BMI has steadily increased. Over the past 4 months, she has experienced frequent headaches. At a visit to her primary care physician 2 months ago, she had normal visual fields by confrontation; funduscopic examination revealed papilledema. Head MRI performed at that time was normal.

Laboratory test results (2 months ago):
    Prolactin, high-normal
    Free T$_4$ = 1.1 ng/dL (0.8-1.8 ng/dL) (SI: 14.2 pmol/L [10.30-23.17 pmol/L])
    TSH = 5.4 mIU/L (0.5-5.0 mIU/L)
    Urinary free cortisol, high normal

Which of the following is the most likely cause of her headaches?
    A. Obesity
    B. Prolactinoma
    C. Hypothyroidism
    D. Oral contraceptive pills
    E. Retinoid cream

23   A 6-year-old boy presents for evaluation of a thyroid nodule that has rapidly increased in size over the last 4 months. He has a history of constipation, peripheral neuropathy, bilateral clubfoot, and hypotonia. He has undergone an extensive workup by a gastroenterologist and neurologist that has not resulted in a diagnosis to explain his findings. An endocrinologist evaluated him 2 years ago for poor linear growth, although no conclusive diagnosis was made.

    Thyroid ultrasonography reveals a large, solid, hypoechoic nodule in the left lobe (*see image A*) with smooth margins, not taller-than-wide shape on transverse imaging, and with 1 hyperechoic focus (*arrow*). Also documented is a solid, hypoechoic nodule with irregular margins (*see image B*), taller-than-wide shape on transverse imaging, and several hyperechoic foci (*arrows*). There are no abnormal lymph nodes on physical examination or ultrasonography.

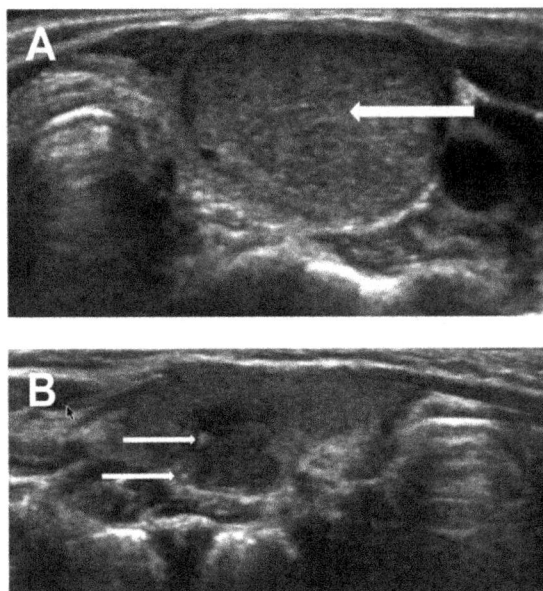

Which of the following tests is the best next step in the evaluation to determine the risk of malignancy in the nodule?

    A. Serum calcitonin measurement
    B. Thyroid uptake and scan (scintigraphy)
    C. Axial imaging of the neck (CT or MRI)
    D. Thyroglobulin measurement
    E. Lactate dehydrogenase measurement

24 A 15-year-old girl is referred for evaluation of abnormal menstrual pattern and mild acne and hirsutism. She had menarche at age 12 years, and over the last year she has had 3 menstrual cycles (the last one was 2 months ago).

On physical examination, her height is 61.8 in (157 cm) and weight is 121 lb (55 kg) (BMI = 22.3 kg/m^2). Examination findings are unremarkable, aside from mild hirsutism (Ferriman-Gallwey score = 10). Mild facial acne is also noted. There is no acanthosis nigricans. She has Tanner stage 4 breast and pubic hair development.

Laboratory test results:
    LH = 10.0 mIU/mL (0.02-12.0 mIU/mL) (SI: 10.0 IU/L [0.02-12.0 IU/L])
    FSH = 5.0 mIU/mL (1.0-11.7 mIU/mL) (SI: 5.0 IU/L [1.0-11.7 IU/L])
    Testosterone = 63 ng/dL (20-38 ng/dL) (SI: 2.2 nmol/L [0.7-1.3 nmol/L])
    DHEA-S = 250 μg/dL (44-248 μg/dL) (SI: 6.8 μmol/L [1.2-6.7 μmol/L])

Which of the following is the best next step in this patient's management?

    A. Perform pelvic ultrasonography
    B. Perform an oral glucose tolerance test with insulin levels
    C. Initiate an oral contraceptive
    D. Initiate metformin
    E. Initiate spironolactone

25 A mother brings her 4-and-5/12-year-old son to your office with concerns about possible early puberty. He has neurofibromatosis type 1, an optic chiasm glioma, and a history of renovascular hypertension. His mother first noted that he had pubic hair 6 months ago. He has also developed some acne, and she thinks that his penis has grown larger. He has a voracious appetite. Since angioplasty for renovascular hypertension, he has gained 20 lb (9.1 kg). His midparental target height is 70 in (177.8 cm). His father also has neurofibromatosis type 1. Both parents had normal timing of puberty.

On physical examination, his blood pressure is 116/52 mm Hg and pulse rate is 97 beats/min. His height is 45.28 in (115 cm) (98.8th percentile), and weight is 57 lb (25.9 kg) (99.7th percentile) (BMI = 19.58 kg/m^2 [99.7th percentile]). He is a tall, overweight boy with scattered café-au-lait macules over his trunk, legs, and arms. There is axillary and inguinal freckling. There are a few comedones on his face. He has mild acanthosis nigricans on his neck. Genitals are Tanner stage 3, pubic hair is Tanner stage 2, and testicular volume is 6 to 8 mL bilaterally. Findings on neurologic examination are normal.

Laboratory test results:
Free T$_4$ = 1.15 ng/dL (0.96-1.77 ng/dL) (SI: 14.8 pmol/L [12.4-22.8 pmol/L])
TSH = 5.57 mIU/L (0.70-5.97 mIU/L)
IGF-1 = 446 ng/mL (54-178 ng/mL) (SI: 58.4 nmol/L [7.1-23.3 nmol/L])
IGFBP-3 = 6.84 mg/L (1.0-5.2 mg/L)
LH = 2.65 mIU/mL (0.07-0.30 mIU/mL) (SI: 2.65 IU/L [0.07-0.30 IU/L])
Testosterone = 165 ng/dL (<10 ng/dL) (SI: 5.7 nmol/L [<0.3 nmol/L])
Hemoglobin A$_{1c}$ = 5.6% (4.1%-5.8%) (38 mmol/mol [21-40 mmol/mol])

Bone age is determined to be 7 years.

For which of the following endocrine disorders is this child at increased risk?
A. GH excess, central precocious puberty, hyperthyroidism, obesity/insulin resistance
B. GH deficiency, central precocious puberty, hypothyroidism, diabetes insipidus
C. GH excess, central precocious puberty, prolactinoma, obesity/insulin resistance
D. Pheochromocytoma, short stature, TSH deficiency, Cushing syndrome
E. GH excess, GH deficiency, central precocious puberty, obesity/insulin resistance

26 A 15-year-old girl with irregular menstrual cycles comes for a follow-up appointment. In clinic today, her weight is 160.5 lb (73 kg) (93rd percentile), and BMI is 28.5 kg/m^2 (96th percentile). Her waist circumference is 31.3 in (79.5 cm) (75th percentile), and waist-to-hip ratio is 0.78 (normal range for normal-weight women, <0.80; normal for overweight women, 0.80-0.84; normal for obese women, <0.85).

On the basis of current knowledge of body composition and her anthropometric measures, you would anticipate which of the following?
A. Below normal amount of total fat for age and height
B. Below normal amount of muscle for height
C. Below normal amount of bone mineral content for height
D. Higher proportion of subcutaneous fat than visceral fat
E. The presence of nonalcoholic fatty liver disease

27 A 6-year-old boy presents for evaluation of short stature. He was born at 40 weeks estimated gestational age with a birth weight of 6 lb 8 oz (2848 g) following an uncomplicated pregnancy.
On physical examination, his height is 41 in (104 cm) (−2.38 SDS) and weight is 39.5 lb (18 kg) (−1.19 SDS). Head circumference is normal. Arm span is 39.4 in (100 cm). There is no bowing of the limbs. The rest of the examination findings are normal.
His mother's height is 57 in (144.8 cm) (−2.53 SDS), and his father's height is 69.5 in (176.5 cm) (+0.04 SDS).

Which of the following is the most likely cause of this child's short stature?
A. Inactivating mutation in the *NPR2* gene
B. Inactivating mutation in the *FGFR3* gene
C. Pathogenic variants in the *RMRP* gene
D. Pathogenic variants in the *ARSB* gene
E. Pathogenic variants in the *COL10A1* gene

28 An 11-year-old girl who was diagnosed with Graves disease 1 month ago comes for a second opinion. She initially presented to her primary care physician, who documented a pulse rate of 120 beats/min, blood pressure of 132/60 mm Hg, and goiter. Her family history is notable for a maternal great-grandmother and a maternal grandmother with Graves disease, both with history of thyroid storm. Her maternal great-grandmother died during thyroidectomy.

Laboratory test results 1 month ago:
 TSH = <0.008 mIU/L (0.5-5.0 mIU/L)
 Free T$_4$ = 8.3 ng/dL (0.7-1.8 ng/dL) (SI: 106.8 pmol/L [9.0-23.2 pmol/L])
 Total T$_3$ = 2279 ng/dL (60-181 ng/dL) (SI: 35.10 nmol/L [0.92-2.79 nmol/L])
 Thyroglobulin antibodies = 526 IU/mL (<40 IU/mL) (SI: 526 kIU/L [<40 kIU/L])
 TPO antibodies = 2896 IU/mL (<35 IU/mL) (SI: 2896 kIU/L [<35 kIU/L])
 Thyroid-stimulating immunoglobulin index = 6.1 (<1.3)

One month ago, thyroid ultrasonography showed a diffusely enlarged thyroid gland, with the right lobe measuring 2.0 × 2.2 × 6.6 cm and the left lobe measuring 2.1 × 2.4 × 6.5 cm, without thyroid nodules. She also saw an endocrinologist who prescribed atenolol, 25 mg daily, and methimazole, 7.5 mg in the morning, 5 mg in the afternoon, and 7.5 mg at night. Due to tachycardia that still persisted 3 days after treatment initiation, the atenolol dosage was increased to 50 mg daily. Two weeks later, the patient developed a rash on her lower back, abdomen, and legs. Her mother gave her diphenhydramine, which led to improvement, but the rash recurred and her parents were advised to stop methimazole and to consider radioactive iodine treatment or thyroidectomy.

She has been off methimazole for 6 days. At your office, her weight is 88 lb (40 kg), blood pressure is 118/60 mm Hg, and pulse rate is 86 beats/min. She has exophthalmos, eyelid retraction, and lid lag, without redness or periorbital swelling. She has decreased vision in the left eye, although the pupils are equally reactive to light. She has no diplopia or tenderness to eye movements. Her thyroid is diffusely enlarged, with thrill. She has fine tremors.

Laboratory test results:
 TSH = <0.01 mIU/L
 Free T$_4$ = 6.0 ng/dL (SI: 77.2 pmol/L)
 Total T$_3$ = 541 ng/dL (SI: 8.33 nmol/L)
 Complete blood cell count with differential, normal
 Liver enzymes, normal

In addition to referring her to an ophthalmologist, which of the following is the best management plan?
A. Continue atenolol and recommend radioactive iodine treatment within 1 to 2 weeks
B. Start steroids, continue atenolol, start potassium iodide drops, and repeat thyroid function studies in 4 weeks
C. Restart methimazole at 10 to 20 mg daily (pretreating with diphenhydramine) and repeat thyroid function studies in 2 weeks
D. Start potassium iodide drops and refer to a high-volume thyroid surgeon for thyroidectomy to be completed within 6 weeks
E. Start potassium iodide drops and refer for radioactive iodine treatment to be completed in 2 weeks

29 You are called to the neonatal intensive care unit to evaluate a male newborn with severe electrolyte abnormalities. The patient was born at 28 weeks' gestation with a birth weight of 2 lb 6.1 oz (1080 g). The pregnancy was complicated by preterm labor, and the mother was treated with magnesium sulfate, antibiotics, and betamethasone before delivery. At birth, the baby was intubated and started on intravenous fluids, and on the second day of life he began receiving total parenteral nutrition. On day 14 of life, he developed rapid-onset hypotonia, accompanied by hypotension and episodes of apnea and bradycardia.

Laboratory test results:
    Magnesium = 15.3 mEq/L (1.8-2.5 mEq/L) (SI: 6.3 mmol/L [0.7-1.0 mmol/L])
    Creatinine = 1.6 mg/dL (0.2-1.0 mg/dL) (SI: 141.4 µmol/L [17.7-88.4 µmol/L])
    Total calcium = 7.6 mg/dL (8.8-10.8 mg/dL) (SI: 1.9 mmol/L [2.2-2.7 mmol/L])

Electrocardiography shows sinus bradycardia with a prolonged QT-interval.

In addition to stopping any magnesium-containing fluids, which of the following is the best next step in this patient's management?
    A. Intravenous hydration with ½ normal saline
    B. Intravenous calcium gluconate
    C. Hemodialysis
    D. Loop diuretic
    E. Exchange transfusion

30 An 11-month-old boy presents to the emergency department at 3:00 PM with jerking of his right arm that has been happening on and off for the last 30 minutes. A screening point-of-care glucose measurement is 34 mg/dL (1.9 mmol/L). He had been well the day before, and ate a normal breakfast, midmorning snack, and lunch. The emergency department physician places an intravenous line, draws a critical sample, and gives him 2 mL/kg D10 followed by an infusion of D10 dextrose at a rate of 5 mL/kg per h. His seizure stops and his repeated point-of-care glucose value is 74 mg/dL (4.1 mmol/L). He is transferred to the regular inpatient care area.

He was born at term weighing 7 lb 8 oz (3420 g) and had no problems in the newborn period. One month ago, he started having twitching movements during the day (but not at night). The patient has always grown well. His immunizations are current. He was breastfed until 9 months of age. He started solids by spoon at 6 months. He is currently on whole milk with jars of baby food during the day and comfort breastfeeds at night. His family history is negative for seizures or hypoglycemia.

On physical examination, he is a typical-appearing child with no enlarged liver, no cleft lip or palate, and typical genitalia.

Laboratory test results:
    Glucose = 41 mg/dL (70-110 mg/dL) (SI: 2.3 mg/dL [3.9-6.1 mmol/L])
    Insulin = 14.0 µIU/mL (3.0-19.0 µIU/mL) (SI: 97.2 pmol/L [20.8-132.0 pmol/L])
    Cortisol = 18.0 µg/dL (5.5-18.9 µg/dL) (SI: 496.6 nmol/L [151.7-521.4 nmol/L])
    GH = 11.0 ng/mL (0.1-6.2 ng/mL) (SI: 11.0 µg/L [0.1-6.2 µg/L])
    Free fatty acids = 8.5 mg/dL (14.1-25.4 mg/dL) (SI: 0.3 mmol/L [SI: 0.5-0.9 mmol/L])
    β-Hydroxybutyrate = 4.2 mg/dL (2.1-29.1 mg/dL) (SI: 0.4 mmol/L [0.2-2.8 mmol/L])
    Lactate = 4.5 mg/dL (4.5-18.0 mg/dL) (SI: 0.5 mmol/L [0.5-2.0 mmol/L])
    Ammonia = 45 mmol/L (10-42 mmol/L)
    AST = 35 U/L (0-67 U/L) (SI: 0.58 µkat/L [0-1.12 µkat/L])
    ALT = 29 U/L (20-53 U/L) (SI: 0.48 µkat/L [0.33-0.89 µkat/L])

He is admitted to the inpatient endocrinology service. After electroencephalography and brain MRI (normal findings), he undergoes a fasting study. He starts fasting at 8:00 AM following a breakfast of pureed fruit, apple juice, and breastmilk:

Time	Glucose
Start	74 mg/dL (4.1 mmol/L)
10 hours	62 mg/dL (3.4 mmol/L)
12 hours	55 mg/dL (3.1 mmol/L)
14 hours	45 mg/dL (2.5 mmol/L)

Fourteen hours into the fast, samples are drawn and tested in the lab, which confirm hypoglycemia (glucose = 43 mg/dL [2.4 mmol/L]). He is given 1 mg of glucagon and his point-of-care glucose rises from 49 to 95 mg/dL (2.5 to 5.3 mmol/L). Over the next several days while awaiting the laboratory results (on a normal home diet without any treatment and fasting overnight as usual), he has 2 glucose values documented to be less than 50 mg/dL (<2.8 mmol/L) occurring at noon and before an evening meal.

Which of the following is the most likely diagnosis?
   A. Glycogen storage disease type 0 (glycogen synthase deficiency)
   B. Hyperinsulinism due to a pathogenic variant in the K_{ATP} channel genes (*ABCC8* or *KCNJ11*)
   C. Hereditary fructose intolerance (aldolase B deficiency)
   D. Hyperinsulinism due to a pathogenic variant in the *GLUD1* gene (glutamate dehydrogenase deficiency)
   E. Glycogen storage disease type 3 (debrancher enzyme deficiency)

31 You are evaluating a 9-year-old boy for a second opinion regarding short stature. He was growing along the 5th percentile until age 3 years. His growth velocity has since decelerated to 2.5 cm/y (average growth velocity 5.5 cm/y for 9-year-old boy). He has not been attending well-child visits with his primary care physician, but goes to the doctor for 1 to 2 sick visits per year. His weight has always been at the 1st percentile. His mother states that he is constantly hungry, and she often finds food in his room and hidden in drawers. She has also found him picking food from the garbage as well. He has been on a stimulant medication for attention deficit hyperactivity disorder for 3 years, and he performs poorly in school.

A pediatric endocrinologist at another center previously evaluated him with an arginine/clonidine GH stimulation test, and his peak level was 8 ng/mL (8 µg/L). GH therapy was initiated, and he has been on this regimen for the last 9 months.

After a social work investigation, he is removed from his mother's home and placed with a maternal grandmother. Over the next 6 months, his abnormal eating behavior and school performance improve.

Considering the most likely diagnosis, which of the following scenarios best describes the changes in growth velocity before and after removal from his mother's home?

Answer	Before GH (Mother's Home)	On GH (Mother's Home)	On GH (Grandmother's Home)
A.	2.5 cm/y	4.0 cm/y	5.0 cm/y
B.	2.5 cm/y	5.5 cm/y	6.5 cm/y
C.	2.5 cm/y	3.0 cm/y	5.5 cm/y
D.	2.5 cm/y	4.5 cm/y	4.5 cm/y
E.	2.5 cm/y	4.0 cm/y	7.0 cm/y

32 You are asked to evaluate a 16-year-old girl for lack of breast development. There is no family history of pubertal delay or infertility.

On physical examination, her height is 61 in (155 cm) and weight is 110 lb (50 kg). Examination findings are normal, including those from neurologic and complete cranial nerve exam. She has bilateral breast buds of less than 1 cm and Tanner stage 3 pubic hair.

Laboratory test results:
   LH = 0.4 mIU/mL (adult female >2.0 mIU/mL) (SI: 0.4 IU/L [>2.0 IU/L])
   FSH = 0.8 mIU/mL (adult female >1.8 mIU/mL) (SI: 0.8 IU/L [>1.8 IU/L])
   Estradiol = 11 pg/mL (adult female >18 pg/mL) (SI: 40.4 pmol/L [66.1 pmol/L])
   Prolactin = 11 ng/mL (3-24 ng/mL) (SI: 0.5 nmol/L [0.1-1.0 nmol/L])

A pathogenic variant in which of the following genes is the most likely cause of her pubertal delay?

- A. *KISS1* (KiSS-1 metastasis-suppressor)
- B. *FGFR1* (fibroblast growth factor receptor 1)
- C. *PROKR2* (prokineticin receptor 2)
- D. *ANOS1* (anosmin 1)
- E. *SOX10* (SRY-box 10)

33 You are asked to evaluate a 7-month-old girl for a second opinion. At birth she was noted to have mild clitoromegaly, a urogenital sinus, and bilateral inguinal hernias with palpable masses. Pelvic and inguinal ultrasonography revealed testicular-appearing structures in the upper portion of the inguinal canal without evidence of a uterus or ovaries. The karyotype was determined to be 46,XY.

Laboratory test results at age 6 weeks:

Testosterone = 20 ng/dL (60-400 ng/dL [male]; <10 ng/dL [female]) (SI: 0.69 nmol/L [2.1-13.9 nmol/L] [male]; <0.35 nmol/L [female])

Dihydrotestosterone = 11 ng/dL (12-85 ng/dL [male]; <3 ng/dL [female]) (SI: 0.38 nmol/L [0.42-2.9 nmol/L] [male]; [<0.10 nmol/L] [female])

LH = 9.0 mIU/mL (0.2-7 mIU/mL) (SI: 9.0 IU/L [0.2-7.0 IU/L])

FSH = 4.3 mIU/mL (0.16-4.1 mIU/mL) (SI: 4.3 IU/L [0.16-4.1 IU/L)

Genetic analysis of the androgen receptor gene identified no mutations, but the patient was presumed to have androgen insensitivity syndrome. At age 3 months, the patient underwent bilateral orchiectomy, bilateral inguinal hernia repair, and vaginoplasty and tolerated the procedure well. Histology of the gonads demonstrated prepubertal seminiferous tubules, spermatic cord with vas deferens, and epididymis. At 5 months of age, she developed respiratory distress and vomiting for which she was hospitalized.

Laboratory test results:

Sodium = 124 mEq/L (136-142 mEq/L) (SI: 124 mmol/L [136-142 mmol/L])

Potassium = 7.7 mEq/L (3.5-5.0 mEq/L) (SI: 7.7 mmol/L [3.5-5.0 mmol/L])

Despite aggressive intravenous hydration with 0.9% sodium chloride solution over a 3-day period, her sodium was slow to improve. The patient underwent a stimulation test with 250 mcg of ACTH, with the following results (*see table*). Treatment was subsequently initiated.

Analyte	Baseline	60 Minutes	Baseline Reference Ranges
17-Hydroxyprogesterone	22 ng/dL (0.67 nmol/L)	20 ng/dL (0.61 nmol/L)	<91 ng/dL (<2.76 nmol/L)
17-Hydroxypregnenolone	10 ng/dL (0.3 nmol/L)	22 ng/dL (0.67 nmol/L)	36-763 ng/dL (1.1-23.0 nmol/L)
Androstenedione	25 ng/dL (0.87 nmol/L)	33 ng/dL (1.15 nmol/L)	<10-37 ng/dL (<0.35-1.29 nmol/L)
DHEA	25 ng/dL (0.87 nmol/L)	22 ng/dL (0.67 nmol/L)	26-835 ng/dL (0.87-28.97 nmol/L)
DHEA-S	<10 µg/dL (<0.27 µmol/L)	<10 µg/dL (<0.27 µmol/L)	5-48 µg/dL (0.14-1.3 µmol/L)
Testosterone	<3.0 ng/dL (<0.1 nmol/L)	<3.0 ng/dL (<0.1 nmol/L)	<3-10 ng/dL (<0.1-0.35 nmol/L)
11-Deoxycortisol	54 ng/dL (1.87 nmol/L)	64 ng/dL (2.2 nmol/L)	<10-156 ng/dL (0.35-5.41 nmol/L)
Cortisol	10 µg/dL (275.9 nmol/L)	12 µg/dL (331.1 nmol/L)	>18 µg/dL (>496.6 nmol/L)
Aldosterone	Quantity not sufficient	...	...
Plasma renin activity	14,345 ng/dL per h	...	235-3700 ng/dL per h
ACTH	4781 pg/mL (1052 pmol/L)	...	6-48 pg/mL (1.3-10.6 pmol/L)

Values are presented in conventional units with SI units in parentheses.

Which of the following genes is most likely to have a pathogenic variant?
- A. *NR0B1* (X-linked adrenal hypoplasia congenita)
- B. *CYP17A1* (17α-hydroxylase/17,20-lyase deficiency)
- C. *HSD17B3* (17β-hydroxysteroid dehydrogenase type 3 deficiency)
- D. *STAR* (congenital lipoid adrenal hyperplasia)
- E. *MC2R* (ACTH resistance)

34 A 7-year-old boy presents for evaluation of short stature. He was born at 40 weeks estimated gestational age with a birth weight of 6 lb 4 oz (2834 kg) and a birth length of 19 in (48.3 cm) following an uncomplicated pregnancy. He has had normal developmental milestones and school performance.

On physical examination, his height is 42.5 in (108 cm) (–2.60 SDS) and weight is 44 lb (20 kg) (–1.13 SDS). Genital examination is prepubertal (Tanner stage 1 pubic hair and phallus, testicular volume of 2 mL bilaterally).

Radiographic evaluation of his left hand reveals a bone age of 10 years by the method of Greulich and Pyle.

His mother's height is 62 in (157.5 cm) (–0.65 SDS), and father's height is 62 in (157.5 cm) (–2.83 SDS). His father has osteoarthritis of the knees.

Which of the following is the most likely cause of this child's short stature?
- A. Pathogenic variant in the *COL1A1* gene
- B. Activating mutation in the *FGFR3* gene
- C. Pathogenic variant in the *ACAN* gene (aggrecan)
- D. Pathogenic variant in the *IDS* gene (iduronate 2-sulfatase)
- E. Methylation abnormality on chromosome 11

35 A 16-year-old girl comes for initial evaluation of a low TSH level. One year ago, Epstein-Barr virus was diagnosed and she has since had fatigue and decreased exercise performance. A recent TSH measurement was 0.01 mIU/L. She has no tremors, palpitations, tachycardia, heat intolerance, lose stools, weight loss, or increased appetite. Her parents have not noted changes in the appearance of her eyes. She has no problems swallowing or breathing and has no neck tenderness or fever.

On physical examination, her weight and BMI are at the 50th percentile. She is afebrile, pulse rate is 70 beats/min, and blood pressure is 112/63 mm Hg. Her thyroid is symmetric, nontender, mildly enlarged, firm, and without palpable nodules. The rest of her examination findings are unremarkable.

C-reactive protein measurement is normal.

Which of the following is characteristic of this patient's most likely condition?
- A. Thyroid tissue replaced by lymphocytes in a dense matrix of hyalinized connective tissue and inflammatory reaction in vascular structures
- B. Lymphoid follicular infiltration and epithelial cell destruction with or without fibrosis
- C. Polymorphonuclear infiltrate and necrosis
- D. Granulomas with giant cells and diffuse fibrosis
- E. A somatic gain-of-function mutation in the gene encoding the TSH receptor

36 You have been following the course of a 13-year-old boy who presented 1 year ago with the following fasting laboratory values:

Triglycerides = 619 mg/dL (<130 mg/dL) (SI: 7.00 mmol/L [<1.47 mmol/L])
LDL cholesterol = 139 mg/dL (30-140 mg/dL) (SI: 3.60 mmol/L [0.78-3.63 mmol/L])

He was started on a regimen of atorvastatin and dietary changes. The family has missed their last 2 appointments with you. When you see the patient in clinic today, the family reports that he has had marked generalized abdominal pain for the last 5 days, which started at the end of a family trip. During this time, he has lost 6.6 lb (3 kg), and yesterday he had 3 episodes of emesis.

On physical examination, his height is 61.2 in (155.5 cm) (50th percentile) and weight is 94.6 lb (43 kg) (42nd percentile), and BMI is 17.8 kg/m^2 (40th percentile). He has marked nonspecific abdominal pain. The rest of his exam findings are normal.

Which of the following is the best next step in this patient's evaluation?
- A. Endoscopic retrograde cholangiopancreatography to assess for cholecystitis
- B. Abdominal CT to assess for appendicitis
- C. Measurement of amylase and lipase to assess for pancreatitis
- D. C-reactive protein to assess for Crohn disease
- E. Measurement of transaminases to assess for hepatotoxicity

37 You are called by the floor team to consult on a child with hypocalcemia and hyperphosphatemia. The patient is a 5-year-old boy with quadriplegic cerebral palsy, nonverbal intellectual disability, and chronic constipation, who presented this afternoon for a scheduled bowel cleanout.

Laboratory test results (sample drawn at admission):
Calcium = 5.7 mg/dL (8.5-10.5 mg/dL) (SI: 1.4 mmol/L [2.1-2.6 mmol/L])
Phosphate = 29 mg/dL (3.41-6.19 mg/dL) (SI: 9.4 mmol/L [1.1-2.0 mmol/L])

His family states he had been in his usual state of health, although since this morning he has seemed sluggish and had 1 episode of emesis. On physical examination, you note a lethargic-appearing child with a pulse rate in the 120's. Review of his chart reveals documentation of normal calcium and phosphate levels 1 year ago, during an admission for pneumonia.

Which of the following is the most likely etiology for this patient's mineral abnormalities?
- A. Pseudohypoparathyroidism
- B. Renal failure
- C. Iatrogenic cause
- D. Vitamin D deficiency
- E. Malabsorption

38 A 16-year-old boy seeks evaluation for delayed puberty. He has a history of cleft lip, bilateral undescended testes, and bilateral inguinal hernias that have been repaired. He also has a history of third and fourth digit syndactyly of his right foot. He has a small amount of pubic hair and axillary hair that developed at age 13 years but has not progressed. He does not have adult body odor or penile or testicular growth. His voice has not deepened. He has had steady growth but no growth spurt. He does not have headaches. He has a normal sense of smell for strong scents such as coffee, but he is unable to identify weaker scents. Two of his teeth never formed. He takes no medications. There is no family history of delayed puberty or infertility. Midparental target height is 68.3 in (173.5 cm).

On physical examination, his blood pressure is 114/77 mm Hg and pulse rate is 128 beats/min. His height is 64.8 in (164.7 cm) (Z-score, –0.72), weight is 120.5 lb (54.8 kg) (Z-score, –1.20), and BMI is 20.2 kg/m^2. He has a normal arm span and upper-to-lower segment ratio. His genitals are Tanner stage 1, pubic hair is Tanner stage 2, and testicular volume is 2 mL bilaterally, but the testes are retractile and difficult to palpate. He has no axillary hair. There is syndactyly of the third and fourth digits on the right foot and no synkinesia.

Laboratory test results:
Free T$_4$ = 1.39 ng/dL (0.98-1.63 ng/dL) (SI: 17.9 pmol/L [12.6-21.0 pmol/L])
TSH = 1.07 mIU/L (0.51-4.3 mIU/L)
Prolactin = 7.7 ng/mL (2-10 ng/mL) (SI: 0.33 nmol/L [0.09-0.43 nmol/L])
LH = <0.1 mIU/mL (0.2-9.0 mIU/mL) (SI: <0.1 IU/L [0.2-9.0 IU/L])
FSH = 0.4 mIU/mL (2.6-11.0 mIU/mL) (SI: 0.4 IU/L [2.6-11.0 IU/L])
Testosterone = 8.9 ng/dL (31-733 ng/dL) (SI: 0.3 nmol/L [1.1-25.4 nmol/L])

Bone age is interpreted to be 13.5 years. Findings on renal ultrasonography are normal. MRI of the brain shows hypoplastic olfactory bulb/tracts bilaterally.

A pathogenic variant in which of the following genes is the most likely cause of this patient's delayed puberty?
  A. *ANOS1* (formerly *KAL1*) (anosmin 1)
  B. *FGFR1* (fibroblast growth factor receptor 1)
  C. *GNRH1* (gonadotropin releasing hormone 1)
  D. *CHD7* (chromodomain helicase DNA binding protein 7)
  E. *MKRN3* (makorin ring finger protein 3)

39 You are asked to evaluate a 4-month-old boy because of cushingoid features and poor growth. He was born prematurely at 26 weeks' gestation, and his medical course was complicated by a 3-month stay in the neonatal intensive care unit. He had a life-threatening event caused by nasal obstruction, and treatment with ciprofloxacin and dexamethasone drops was initiated. When the patient developed a rash 1 week after starting this treatment, the therapy was changed to dexamethasone ophthalmic solution administered intranasally. Four weeks after the change in therapy, the patient developed a progressively decreased energy level and facial swelling. He was also sleeping more, and his feeding frequency decreased.

On physical examination, the baby has large, ruddy cheeks with moon facies. He has no striae, edema, posterior cervical fat pad, or hypertrichosis. His blood pressure is 94/61 mm Hg.

His growth velocity markedly decreased after glucocorticoid therapy was initiated. Cortisol measurement (sample drawn at 6:30 AM) is less than 0.4 µg/dL (<11.0 nmol/L). Because of continued intermittent respiratory distress, treatment with dexamethasone drops is continued and slowly weaned over a 4-month period. Two months into the weaning process, the patient's growth improves significantly to 4 cm/month, and his energy level and feeding normalize. Two and a half months after treatment is discontinued, his cushingoid features resolve.

A 1-mcg ACTH-stimulation test is conducted:
  Baseline cortisol = 6.2 µg/dL (171.0 nmol/L)
  30-minute cortisol = 11.1 µg/dL (306.2 nmol/L)
  60-minute cortisol = 12.3 µg/dL (339.3 nmol/L)

Which of the following would you recommend as the best next step in this patient's management?
  A. Start hydrocortisone at a total daily dose of 8 mg/m², slowly wean, and repeat an ACTH-stimulation test at a later time
  B. Start hydrocortisone at a total daily dose of 10 to 15 mg/m², slowly wean, and repeat an ACTH-stimulation test at a later time
  C. Administer stress-dose glucocorticoid therapy during times of illness and other physiologic stress and repeat an ACTH-stimulation test at a later time
  D. Perform MRI of the pituitary gland
  E. Recommend no further follow-up

40 You are asked to evaluate a newborn in the neonatal intensive care unit born to a 38-year-old nulliparous woman with type 1 diabetes mellitus. The baby was born prematurely at 36 weeks' gestation, was small-for-gestational-age, and had hypoglycemia. The mother has had diabetes for 22 years, and her glycemic control has been poor (average hemoglobin A_{1c} level of 10% [86 mmol/mol] for the last 5 years), although she has not had any episodes of diabetic ketoacidosis. Before attempting pregnancy, she was treated with an ACE inhibitor for microalbuminuria. The ACE inhibitor was stopped before she became pregnant. She has a maternal grandmother with type 2 diabetes, but otherwise does not report any other affected family member.

Which of the following is the most likely cause of the newborn's small-for-gestational-age status?
  A. Maternal hyperglycemia during the pregnancy
  B. Excess production of IGF-2
  C. Dysfunctional insulin receptor regulation
  D. Placental insufficiency
  E. Fetal insulin hypersecretion in utero

41 A 14-year-old girl presents to your clinic for evaluation of bone health. She states that in childhood she was physically active and a competitive swimmer. However, at age 9 she began developing pain and weakness in her lower extremities, which led her to quit the swim team. At age 11, she stumbled on a curb and suffered a fracture of her left femur. One year later, she fractured her right femur after a small dog jumped into her lap.

Her growth chart is shown (*see image*).

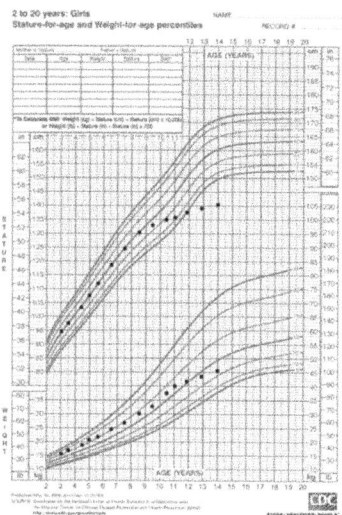

Laboratory test results (sample collected while fasting):

Phosphate =1.8 mg/dL (3.5-5.0 mg/dL) (SI: 0.6 mmol/L [1.1-1.6 mmol/L])

25-Hydroxyvitamin D = 29 ng/mL (20-80 ng/mL) (SI: 72.4 nmol/L [49.9-199.7 nmol/L])

PTH = 72.9 pg/mL (15-65 pg/mL) (SI: 72.9 ng/L [15-65 ng/L])

1,25-Dihydroxyvitamin D = 13.0 pg/mL (15.9-55.6 pg/mL) (SI: 33.8 pmol/L [41.3-144.6 pmol/L])

Serum creatinine = 0.6 mg/dL (0.3-1.0 mg/dL) (SI: 53.0 µmol/L [26.5-88.4 µmol/L])

Urinary phosphate = >200 mg/dL (7-148 mg/dL) (SI: >64.6 mmol/L [2.3-47.8 mmol/L])

Results from which of the following tests are most likely to lead to definitive therapy for this patient?

A. Calculation of tubular reabsorption of phosphate

B. Genetic testing for pathogenic variants in the *PHEX* gene

C. Measurement of serum FGF-23

D. Renal ultrasonography

E. Fluorodeoxyglucose PET/CT imaging

42 A 9-year-old boy presents for evaluation of short stature. He was born at 40 weeks estimated gestational age with a birth weight of 7 lb 8 oz (3401 g) to a 26-year-old mother (G1P0 to 1) following an uncomplicated pregnancy.

On physical examination, his height is 47.2 in (120 cm) (–2.25 SDS), and weight is 55 lb (25 kg) (–0.83 SDS). He has relative macrocephaly and a prominent forehead. Arm span is 44 in (112 cm).

His family history is unremarkable.

Genetic analysis documents a pathogenic variant in the *FGFR3* gene (fibroblast growth factor receptor 3).

Which of the following would be this child's most likely response to GH therapy?

A. Rapid advancement of bone age

B. Decreased NTproCNP levels

C. Worsening skeletal disproportion

D. Progressive improvement of height SDS

E. Increased risk of intracranial hypertension

43 A 4-year-old girl is referred to endocrinology after evaluation in the emergency department and subsequent follow-up by her primary care physician. Four months ago, she had an episode of gastroenteritis with vomiting and was unable to tolerate food or liquids on and off for 2 days. In the emergency department, she was found to be dehydrated and hypoglycemic with a plasma glucose concentration of 45 mg/dL (2.5 mmol/L). She was given intravenous saline to correct the dehydration, ondansetron to prevent vomiting, and juice to correct the hypoglycemia. After 4 hours in the emergency department and 90 minutes after eating a meal, her plasma glucose level was 180 mg/dL (10.0 mmol/L) and she was discharged home with a recommendation to follow-up with her primary care physician.

Her physician subsequently ordered a glucometer and, after properly demonstrating its use, asked the parents to monitor her glucose levels for 1 week and return for a follow-up appointment. After 3 days, the patient's mother called the primary care physician because her daughter was having "blood sugars all over the place." The physician asked her to continue monitoring and referred her to the endocrinology clinic.

On physical examination, she is a healthy appearing child with normal findings on physical examination. Her height is at the 40th percentile (target height 25th percentile), and weight is at the 50th percentile.

A review of her blood glucose profile shows a pattern of postmeal hyperglycemia in the range of 120 to 180 mg/dL (6.7-10.0 mmol/L) and fasting glucose in the range of 38 to 60 mg/dL (2.1-3.3 mmol/L). Her point-of-care glucose in clinic is 180 mg/dL (10.0 mmol/L), and urinalysis is normal except for the presence of glucose. A complete metabolic profile documents normal electrolytes and the following results:

Glucose = 192 mg/dL (70-120 mg/dL) (SI: 10.7 mmol/L [3.9-6.7 mmol/L])
Calcium = 9.2 mg/dL (8.4-10.2 mg/dL) (SI: 2.3 mmol/L [2.1-2.6 mmol/L])
Phosphate = 4.2 mg/dL (3.4-5.0 mg/dL) (SI: 1.4 mmol/L [1.1-1.6 mmol/L])
Alkaline phosphatase = 253 U/L (67-340 U/L) (SI: 2.4 μkat/L [1.1-5.7 μkat/L])
AST = 39 U/L (10-45 U/L) (SI: 0.65 μkat/L [0.17-0.75 μkat/L])
ALT = 42 U/L (22-60 U/L) (SI: 0.70 μkat/L [0.37-1.00 μkat/L])

Which of the following conditions is most likely to be present?
    A. Glycogen storage disease type 0 (glycogen synthase deficiency)
    B. GLUT2 deficiency (glucose transporter 2 deficiency; Fanconi Bickel syndrome)
    C. Fructose 1,6-bisphosphatase deficiency
    D. Glycogen storage disease IXa (phosphorylase kinase deficiency)
    E. Pathogenic variants in the insulin receptor gene

44 A 15-year-old girl with autoimmune hypothyroidism has routine surveillance laboratory tests performed to monitor levothyroxine therapy. Hypothyroidism was diagnosed 1 year ago, and she has been mostly adherent to the daily thyroid hormone regimen. Her TSH level has been between 2.0 and 3.0 mIU/L (mid-normal range).

Laboratory test results:

Measurement	Time Point #1
TSH (0.5-4.5 mIU/L)	0.02 mIU/L
Free T₄	>7.8 ng/dL (SI: 100.4 pmol/L)
Total T₃	>650 ng/dL (SI: 10.0 nmol/L)

You call the family immediately. The patient reports good adherence to her levothyroxine therapy and no change in the tablet's color or shape compared with the previous refill (current dosage, 88 mcg daily). She takes no other medications and reports that she is feeling fine. In response to your questions, you determine she has no signs or symptoms of hyperthyroidism, although she has intermittent anxiety.

You see the patient in clinic and confirm the absence of signs or symptoms of hyperthyroidism, but the patient has a goiter that is visible on neck inspection. There are no nodules or abnormal lymph nodes. You order a ^{123}I thyroid uptake and scan and the results show 10% uptake at 4 hours and 22% uniform uptake throughout the gland at 24 hours.

You repeat the laboratory tests with the addition of several more measurements:

Measurement	Time Point #1	Time Point #2
TSH (0.5-4.5 mIU/L)	0.02 mIU/L	0.03 mIU/L
Free T₄ (0.9-1.7 ng/dL [SI: 11.6-21.9 pmol/L])	>7.8 ng/dL (SI: 100.4 pmol/L)	>7.8 ng/dL (SI: 100.4 pmol/L)
Total T₃ (80-190 ng/dL [SI: 1.2-2.9 nmol/L])	>650 ng/dL (SI: 10.0 nmol/L)	>650 ng/dL (SI: 10.0 nmol/L)
Thyroid-stimulating immunoglobulin (<129%)	...	95%
Thyroglobulin (3-40 ng/mL [SI: 3-40 μg/L])	...	20 ng/mL (SI: 20 μg/L)
Thyroglobulin antibodies (<1.0 IU/mL [SI: <1.0 kIU/L])	...	<1.0 IU/mL (SI: <1.0 kIU/L)

Which of the following is the most likely explanation for the abnormal thyroid hormone levels?
- A. Autoimmune hyperthyroidism (Graves disease)
- B. Laboratory assay interference
- C. Autoimmune-associated Hashitoxicosis
- D. Silent thyroiditis
- E. Exogenous consumption of excess levothyroxine

45 A 15-year-old girl with congenital leptin deficiency has moved to your area and presents for a clinic visit. Leptin deficiency was diagnosed at age 5 years after evaluation of rapid-onset obesity. There was known consanguinity in the family. She was seen at a large referral center hospital, where she was prescribed a medication that resulted in a significant decrease in body weight (BMI decreased from the 99th percentile to the 80th percentile). Due to an unstable family situation, the girl has failed to receive treatment for the past 3 years, during which time she has rapidly gained weight.

Her parents report that although she underwent menarche at age 11, she has not had a menses since age 12. She has had progression of pubic hair development over the past 2 years, but no virilizing features. Her family has not noticed any polyuria or polydipsia.

On physical examination, her height is 63.8 in (162 cm) (50th percentile), weight is 202.4 lb (92 kg) (98th percentile), and BMI is 35 kg/m^2 (99th percentile). Breasts and pubic hair are Tanner stage 5.

The family is concerned about her lack of menstrual periods. Which of the following interventions best addresses the etiology of her secondary amenorrhea?
- A. Initiate an oral contraceptive pill
- B. Initiate metformin
- C. Initiate exenatide
- D. Initiate recombinant leptin
- E. Provide lifestyle counseling for improved physical activity and diet

46 A 9-year-old previously healthy boy is brought to the emergency department after falling at the playground. He had no loss of consciousness but he feels dizzy and nauseated. Findings on head CT are suspicious for a mass, so MRI is performed, which confirms the presence of a pituitary lesion. His parents report he has had recent polydipsia, polyuria, and nocturia, and has been keeping a water bottle near his bed at night. He feels hungry all the time and has had a 30-lb (13.6-kg) weight gain over the last year despite being an active child. He wears glasses but has not noticed any vision changes. His parents think he has grown slowly over the last year, and they report that his pediatrician had performed thyroid labs in the past that were slightly abnormal. His family history is noncontributory. His midparental height is 72 in (180 cm).

On physical examination, his blood pressure is 108/65 mm Hg and pulse rate is 92 beats/min. His height 51.2 in (130 cm) (Z-score, −0.66), weight is 99.5 lb (45.2 kg) (Z-score, +2.0), and BMI is 26.75 kg/m^2 (Z-score +2.33). He is overweight, with faint acanthosis nigricans noted on the back of the neck. His visual fields are normal to confrontation. He is prepubertal.

Laboratory test results:
Free T$_4$ = 0.7 ng/dL (0.8-1.5 ng/dL) (SI: 9.0 pmol/L [10.3-19.3 pmol/L])
TSH = 0.3 mIU/L (0.49-4.70 mIU/L)
IGF-1 = 59 ng/mL (123-257 ng/mL) (SI: 7.7 nmol/L [16.1-33.7 nmol/L])
Cortisol (8 AM) = 13 μg/dL (3-21 μg/dL) (SI: 358.6 nmol/L [82.8-579.3 nmol/L])
Prolactin = 26 ng/mL (2-10 ng/mL) (SI: 1.1 nmol/L [0.09-0.43 nmol/L])
Serum osmolality = 300 mOsm/kg (285-295 mOsm/kg) (SI: 300 mmol/kg [285-295 mmol/kg])
Urine osmolality = 185 mOsm/kg (50-1400 mOsm/kg) (SI: 185 mmol/kg [50-1400 mmol/kg])

MRI of the brain shows a 2.3 × 3.2 × 2.2-cm lobulated, mixed solid and cystic suprasellar mass with calcifications. The mass obscures the pituitary infundibulum, with mild extension into the superior pituitary gland not excluded. There is persistent mild mass effect on the ventral pons, midbrain, hypothalamus, and basilar artery.

Which of the following is the most likely diagnosis?
- A. Prolactinoma
- B. Adamantinomatous craniopharyngioma
- C. Germinoma
- D. Rathke cleft cyst
- E. Papillary craniopharyngioma

47 A healthy full-term newborn is found to have congenital hypothyroidism on routine newborn screening with a venipuncture confirmation sample showing the following results:

Measurement	Time Point #1
TSH (0.5-4.5 mIU/L)	316.0 mIU/L
Total T₄ (4.5-11.5 µg/dL [SI: 57.9-148.0 nmol/L])	4.3 µg/dL (SI: 55.3 nmol/L)

Levothyroxine, 50 mcg daily, is prescribed and the parents are instructed on the proper administration of the medication. One month later, thyroid function testing reveals a low TSH level, and the levothyroxine dosage is decreased to 37.5 mcg daily (*see table, 1 month later*). After another 2 months, thyroid function testing shows a suppressed TSH level, and the levothyroxine dosage is further reduced (*see table, 3 months later*).

Measurement	Time Point #1	1 Month Later	3 Months Later
TSH (0.5-4.5 mIU/L)	316.0 mIU/L	0.62 mIU/L	0.07 mIU/L
Total T₄ (4.5-11.5 µg/dL [SI: 57.9-148.0 nmol/L])	4.3 µg/dL (SI: 55.3 nmol/L)	10.9 µg/dL (SI: 140.3 nmol/L)	11.2 µg/dL (SI: 144.1 nmol/L)
Levothyroxine dosage	50 mcg daily	37.5 mcg daily	25 mcg daily

There is no family history of congenital hypothyroidism and no known maternal thyroid disease. Pregnancy and delivery were uncomplicated and both mother and baby were discharged just before 48 hours after delivery. The baby has been breastfed and has displayed normal growth and development. Physical examination findings are normal, with no goiter.

Which of the following is the most likely diagnosis to explain this patient's constellation of laboratory results?
- A. Thyroid agenesis
- B. Thyroxine-binding globulin deficiency
- C. Thyroid dyshormonogenesis
- D. Maternal TSH receptor–blocking antibodies
- E. Central hypothyroidism

48 You are called to the emergency department to evaluate a 5-week-old girl with a history of poor weight gain and vomiting for 2 days.

Laboratory test results:
  Serum sodium = 126 mEq/L (132-146 mEq/L) (SI: 126 mmol/L [132-146 mmol/L])
  Potassium = 7 mEq/L (3.5-5.1 mEq/L) (SI: 7 mmol/L [3.5-5.1 mmol/L])
  Chloride = 88 mEq/L (99-109 mEq/L) (SI: 88 mmol/L [99-109 mmol/L])
  Carbon dioxide = 16 mEq/L (20-31 mEq/L) (SI: 16 mmol/L [20-31 mmol/L])
  Serum urea nitrogen = 11 mg/dL (6-22 mg/dL) (SI: 11 mmol/L [3.9-7.9 mmol/L])
  Creatinine = 0.16 mg/dL (0.1-1.0 mg/dL) (SI: 14.1 µmol/L [8.8-88.4 µmol/L])

On physical examination, her blood pressure is 88/58 mm Hg and pulse rate is 170 beats/min. She is irritable and not easily consoled. Her skin appears normal without hyperpigmentation. She has typical female genitalia.

You begin intravenous fluids and hydrocortisone treatment.

An ACTH-stimulation test (125 mcg) is conducted after holding a hydrocortisone dose, and the results are as follows:

Measurements	Baseline	60 Minutes
Cortisol	17.0 µg/dL (SI: 469 nmol/L)	39 µg/dL (SI: 1076 nmol/L)
17-hydroxyprogesterone	98 ng/dL (13-106 ng/dL) (SI: 2.97 nmol/L [0.39-3.21 nmol/L])	138 ng/dL (SI: 4.18 nmol/L)
Androstenedione	27 ng/dL (<10-37 ng/dL) (SI: 0.94 nmol/L [<0.35-1.29 nmol/L])	40 ng/dL (SI: 1.40 nmol/L)
Testosterone	7 ng/dL (<10 ng/dL) (SI: 0.24 nmol/L [<0.35 nmol/L])	11 ng/dL (SI: 0.38 nmol/L)
Plasma renin activity	128 ng/mL per h (2.4-37.0 ng/mL per h)	...
Aldosterone	2.79 ng/dL (5-90 ng/dL) (SI: 77.4 pmol/L [138.7-2496.6 pmol/L])	...

Which of the following is the best long-term treatment for this patient?
A. Sodium chloride, sodium bicarbonate, and potassium-binding resin
B. 9α-fludrocortisone and sodium chloride
C. Hydrocortisone, 9α-fludrocortisone, and sodium chloride
D. Prednisolone, 9α-fludrocortisone, and sodium chloride
E. No treatment now as the electrolyte abnormalities are transient

49 A 16-year-old African American boy is brought to the emergency department by ambulance with a 24-hour history of vomiting and a 12-hour history of difficulty breathing. His older sister found him unresponsive; when she could not wake him, she called 911. She reports that he had been losing weight recently, which pleased his family because his primary care physician had said he was at risk for developing diabetes.

On physical examination, his height is 70 in (178 cm) (75th percentile) and weight is 226.5 lb (103 kg) (>97th percentile) (BMI = 32.5 kg/m^2). He has acanthosis nigricans on his neck, axillae, and abdomen. His respiratory rate is 25 breaths/min and deep, and pulse rate is 140 beats/min. He is assessed to be 10% to 15% dehydrated. The smell of ketones is detected on his breath.

Laboratory test results:
Glucose = 750 mg/dL (70-110 mg/dL) (SI: 41.6 mmol/L [3.8-6.1 mmol/L])
pH = 6.9 (7.35-7.45)
β-Hydroxybutyrate = 62.5 mg/dL (5.2-22.9 mg/dL [fasting]) (SI: 6.0 mmol/L [0.5 to 2.2 mmol/L])
Plasma sodium = 145 mg/dL (138-146 mg/dL) (SI: 145 mmol/L [138-146 mmol/L])
Serum osmolality = 336 mOsm/kg (275-295 mOsm/kg) (SI: 336 mmol/kg [275-295 mmol/kg])
Lactate = 36.0 mg/dL (4.5-18.0 mg/dL) (SI: 4.0 mmol/L [0.5-2.0 mmol/L])
Hemoglobin A$_{1c}$ = >14.0% (4.0%-5.6%) (>130 mmol/mol [20-38 mmol/mol])

The patient is admitted to the hospital and treated with intravenous insulin and intravenous fluids. He recovers well from diabetic ketoacidosis. Subsequent laboratory studies show that islet-cell antibodies, glutamic acid decarboxylase antibodies, and insulin autoantibodies are negative.

At the 6-week follow-up appointment, which of the following is the best surveillance plan?
A. Perform retinal exam, assess for microalbuminuria, order lipid panel, and assess for hypertension
B. Perform retinal exam, assess for microalbuminuria,, order thyroid function panel and celiac disease panel
C. Perform retinal exam, assess for microalbuminuria, order lipid panel, thyroid function panel, celiac disease panel, and assess for hypertension
D. Order thyroid function panel and celiac disease panel and plan for retinal exam and assessment for microalbuminuria in 3 years
E. Order lipid panel and assess for hypertension and plan for retinal exam and assessment for microalbuminuria in 3 years

50 You are asked to evaluate a 15-year-old boy who was recently diagnosed with Klinefelter syndrome by a developmental pediatrician. He has had normal growth, and puberty began at age 13 years. The family is concerned about the possibility of future fertility and wishes to pursue initial evaluation.

Other than semen analysis, you suggest that which of the following correlates best with the possibility of viable sperm production?
    A. Inhibin B level
    B. LH level
    C. Testicular volume
    D. Antimullerian hormone level
    E. FSH level

51 A 16-year-old boy presents for evaluation of hyperparathyroidism. The family states he was initially found to have an elevated PTH level as part of an evaluation for recurrent stress fractures. He is highly athletic, participating year-round on several elite soccer teams. After he developed his third stress fracture in 3 years, his primary care physician ordered the following laboratory tests:

Calcium = 9.9 mg/dL (8.2-10.6 mg/dL) (SI: 2.5 mmol/L [2.1-2.7 mmol/L])
Phosphate = 4.1 mg/dL (3.0-4.5 mg/dL) (SI: 1.3 mmol/L [10.0-1.5 mmol/L])
Alkaline phosphatase = 407 U/L (138-511 U/L) (SI: 6.8 μkat/L [2.3-8.5 μkat/L])
25-Hydroxyvitamin D = 19 ng/mL (20-80 ng/mL) (SI: 47.4 nmol/L [49.9-199.7 nmol/L])
1,25-Dihydroxyvitamin D = 27 pg/mL (13-87 pg/mL) (SI: 70.2 pmol/L [33.8-226.2 pmol/L])
PTH = 460 pg/mL (15-65 pg/mL) (SI: 460 ng/L [15-65 ng/L])
Random urine calcium-to-creatinine ratio = 0.04 (<0.2)

DXA scan is normal with a lumbar spine Z-score of 0.9 and total body less head Z-score of 0.2.

His medical and developmental history is otherwise unremarkable. The patient reports a good energy level and states that other than his stress fractures, he feels well. He reports a diet high in calcium and protein, consuming 4 servings of dairy and 3 protein shakes per day.

Which of the following is the most likely etiology for this patient's elevated PTH levels?
    A. Primary hyperparathyroidism
    B. Vitamin D deficiency
    C. PTH resistance
    D. Heterophile antibodies
    E. Excessive protein intake

52 A 9-and-5/12-year-old boy is referred by his primary care physician for evaluation of tall stature and concerns of early pubertal development (darkening pubic hair). Per his parents' report, he has always been tall. He was born by cesarean delivery at 34 weeks' gestation. Birth weight was 6 lb 11.2 oz (3039 g), and birth length was 20 in (50.8 cm). His father's height is 72 in (182.9 cm), and his mother's height is 67 in (170.2 cm). Midparental target height is 72 ± 4 in (183 ± 10 cm) with a range of 68 to 76 in (173-193 cm).

On physical examination, his height is 61.6 in (156.4 cm) (>97th percentile; SDS, +3.1), weight is 128.5 lb (58.4 kg) (>97th percentile; SDS, +2.6), and BMI is 23.87 kg/m^2 (>97th percentile; SDS, +1.99). His blood pressure is 91/53 mm Hg. No dysmorphism is noted. Pubic hair is Tanner stage 2. Testicular volume is 3 to 4 mL (right) and 2 to 3 mL (left). There is no gynecomastia.

Bone age assessment at age 9 and 2/12 years when his height was 60.6 in (154 cm) was interpreted to be 11 years. Predicted adult height according to the Bayley-Pinneau tables is 78.7 in (200 cm).

Laboratory test results:
  DHEA-S = 45 µg/dL (≤145 µg/dL) (SI: 1.2 µmol/L [≤3.9 µmol/L])
  17-Hydroxyprogesterone = 18 ng/dL (12-130 ng/dL) (SI: 0.54 nmol/L [0.36-3.94 nmol/L])
  Testosterone = 1 ng/dL (3-30 ng/dL) (SI: 0.03 nmol/L [0.10-1.04 nmol/L])
  LH = 0.04 mIU/mL (0.01-0.78 mIU/mL) (SI: 0.04 IU/L [0.01-0.78 IU/L])
  Prolactin = 2.6 ng/mL (≤6.1 ng/mL) (SI: 0.11 nmol/L [≤0.27 nmol/L])
  IGF-1 = 169 ng/mL (80-398 ng/mL) (SI: 22.1 nmol/L [10.5-52.1 nmol/L])
  Thyroid function, normal

At a follow-up visit 5 months later, his growth velocity is documented to be 5.63 cm/y. Pubic hair is Tanner stage 2, and testicular volume is 4 mL bilaterally.

Which of the following is the most likely diagnosis?
  A. Central precocious puberty
  B. Premature adrenarche
  C. Congenital adrenal hyperplasia
  D. Constitutional tall stature
  E. Gigantism

53 A 6-and-6/12-year-old girl began developing breast buds 6 months ago. Her parents have not noticed any body odor or pubic hair. Her height velocity over the last 6 months was 5 cm/y (10th percentile), and she has become heavier. Her midparental target height is at the 50th percentile.

On physical examination, her weight is at the 35th percentile, height is at the 10th percentile, and BMI is at the 75th percentile. Her pulse rate is 70 beats/min. She has early Tanner stage 3 breast buds extending beyond the areola. There is no axillary or pubic hair. No café-au-lait spots are observed. There is no hepatosplenomegaly.

Laboratory test results:
  LH = 0.02 mIU/mL (≤0.15 mIU/mL [Tanner stage 1]) (SI: 0.02 IU/L [≤0.15 IU/L])
  Ultrasensitive estradiol = 25 pg/mL (≤16 pg/mL [Tanner stage 1]) (SI: 91.8 pmol/L [≤58.8 pmol/L])

Her bone age is interpreted to be 5 years and 9 months at a chronologic age of 6 years and 6 months.

Which of the following tests would be diagnostic?
  A. Leuprolide-stimulation test
  B. Pelvic ultrasonography
  C. TSH measurement
  D. Repeated LH measurement
  E. Bone scan

54 A 15-year-old boy presents with asymptomatic hyperglycemia discovered on routine physical examination. His older sister and younger brother were diagnosed with type 1 diabetes mellitus at ages 8 and 5 years, respectively. His sister's most recent hemoglobin A_{1c} measurement is 9.1% (76 mmol/mol), which is attributed to lack of adherence to insulin therapy. His brother's most recent hemoglobin A_{1c} measurement is 6.2% (44 mmol/mol), but he has frequent hypoglycemia on insulin therapy.

Review of the family history (*see image*) reveals multiple affected members, some on insulin and some on oral hypoglycemic agents. The patient's father has had diabetes for more than 30 years. His condition is managed with insulin, and he reports a recent hemoglobin A_{1c} measurement of 6.9% (52 mmol/mol). Two of the patient's paternal aunts were diagnosed with diabetes in their late 20s and were initially treated with oral agents and later with insulin. His paternal grandfather experienced diabetes complications in his late 40s.

The patient has no polyuria, polydipsia, nocturia, or weight loss. Physical examination findings are normal. His BMI is at the 65th percentile. His fasting blood glucose measurement is 92 mg/dL (5.1 mmol/L) and his hemoglobin A_{1c} value is 7.4% (57 mmol/mol).

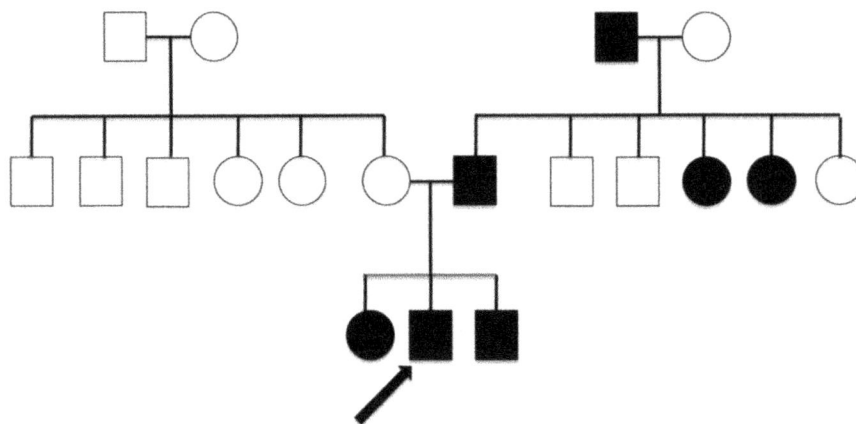

Figure. The index patient is marked with an arrow. Filled squares represent male family members with diabetes mellitus and filled circles represent female family members with diabetes mellitus.

Which of the following is the most likely etiology of diabetes in this family?

    A. Pathogenic variant in the *GCK* gene
    B. HLA class II DR-DQ genotype predisposing to type 1 diabetes
    C. Pathogenic variant in the *PDX* or *INS* genes
    D. Pathogenic variant in the transcription factor *HNF1A* or *HNF4A* genes
    E. Pathogenic variant in the *TCF7L2* gene

55   A 16-year-old girl presents to her pediatrician with concerns about leakage from her breasts and absent menstrual periods. She reports that she had menarche at age 13 years. Her periods were regular for several years; however, this year she has had only 3 periods and her last menstrual period was more than 3 months ago. The leakage from her breasts started in the past month. The discharge is milky in color and happens most often when she showers. She is sexually active with one partner and started taking an oral contraceptive pill 3 months ago. She reports excellent adherence. Her partner uses condoms. She has been having more headaches recently but attributes this to her seasonal allergies. She has had no vision changes. She has a history of depression for which she takes a serotonin reuptake inhibitor, and her psychiatrist recently changed her medication dosage.

On physical examination, her blood pressure is 120/79 mm Hg and pulse rate is 80 beats/min. Her height is 62 in (157.5 cm), weight is 107 lb (48.6 kg), and BMI is 19.6 kg/m^2. Her visual fields are normal to confrontation. She has easily expressible milky discharge from both breasts. The rest of her physical examination findings are normal.

Laboratory test results:
    Free T$_4$ = 1.39 ng/dL (0.98-1.63 ng/dL) (SI: 17.9 pmol/L [12.6-21.0 pmol/L])
    TSH = 1.07 mIU/L (0.5-5.0 mIU/L)
    Prolactin = 112 ng/mL (2-10 ng/mL) (SI: 0.33 nmol/L [0.09-0.43 nmol/L])
    Serum urea nitrogen = 9 mg/dL (8-23 mg/dL) (SI: 3.2 mmol/L [2.9-8.2 mmol/L])
    Serum creatinine = 0.63 mg/dL (0.6-1.1 mg/dL) (SI: 55.7 μmol/L [53.0-97.2 μmol/L])

Which of the following is the most likely cause of this patient's hyperprolactinemia?

    A. Estrogen-containing oral contraceptive pill
    B. Prolactinoma
    C. Antidepressant medication
    D. Craniopharyngioma
    E. Pregnancy

56 You are evaluating a 16-and-3/12-year-old girl for primary amenorrhea. She reports that breast development started 2 years ago and she has not had pubic or axillary hair development. Her review of systems is notable for occasional headaches and mild depression.

On physical examination, her blood pressure is 158/92 mm Hg and pulse rate is 82 beats/min. She has Tanner stage 2 breasts, Tanner stage 1 pubic hair, and no axillary hair development. She has normal female genitalia.

A laboratory evaluation is conducted; however, due to a laboratory incident, only some of the test results have been reported:

Sodium = 142 mEq/L (136-142 mEq/L) (SI: 142 mmol/L [136-142 mmol/L])
Potassium = 3.0 mEq/L (3.5-5.0 mEq/L) (SI: 3.0 mmol/L [3.5-5.0 mmol/L])
Plasma renin activity = 0.1 ng/mL per h (0.6-4.3 ng/mL per h)
Karyotype = 46,XX

Which of the following laboratory results do you expect to see in this patient?
 A. Elevated testosterone level
 B. Low LH and FSH
 C. Elevated deoxycorticosterone
 D. Normal ACTH level
 E. Low corticosterone

57 A 16-year-old girl presents for evaluation of primary amenorrhea and abnormal hormone levels. Breast development started at age 11 years and pubic and axillary hair growth started at age 13 to 14 years. She notes that her pubic hair has always been scant. She has never noticed facial hair. She reports that she has never been sexually active. She exercises on a regular basis, but she is not involved in competitive sports. She is a good student. Abdominal ultrasonography performed 5 years ago to rule out appendicitis revealed no abnormalities. She had no withdrawal bleeding after 10 days of oral progesterone.

On physical examination, she is at the 76th percentile for height and the 95th percentile for weight (BMI, 93rd percentile). Breasts are Tanner stage 5, and pubic hair is scant. Findings on external genital examination are normal.

Laboratory test results:
 β-hCG = 2.0 mIU/mL (0-5.0 mIU/mL) (SI: 2.0 IU/L [0-5.0 IU/L])
 FSH = 13.3 mIU/mL (1.7-21.5 mIU/mL) (SI: 13.3 IU/L [1.7-21.5 IU/L])
 LH = 38.5 mIU/mL (1.0-12.6 mIU/mL) (SI: 38.5 IU/L [1.0-12.6 IU/L])
 Estradiol = 34.5 pg/mL (12.5-211.0) (SI: 126.6 pmol/L [45.9-774.6 pmol/L])
 Total testosterone = 624 ng/dL (5-38 ng/dL) (SI: 21.7 nmol/L [0.2-1.3 nmol/L])
 TSH = 1.12 mIU/L (0.45-4.5 mIU/L)
 Free T$_4$ = 1.36 ng/dL (0.93-1.60 ng/dL) (SI: 17.5 pmol/L [11.9-20.6 pmol/L])
 Prolactin = 12.2 ng/mL (4.8-23.3 ng/mL) (SI: 0.5 nmol/L [0.2-1.0 nmol/L])

On pelvic ultrasonography, no uterus is identified. The radiologist reports that the left gonad measures 1.1 × 1.5 × 1.2 cm, and the right gonad measures 1.2 × 1.3 × 1.1 cm.

A laboratory test confirms the diagnosis.

Which of the following is the best next step in this patient's management?
 A. Laboratory testing for serum tumor markers
 B. Surgical referral for gonadectomy
 C. Counseling for the patient and her family regarding the condition and clinical monitoring
 D. MRI to assess for gonadoblastoma
 E. CT of the adrenal glands

58 A 16-year-old boy who is a childhood cancer survivor has been referred for evaluation of short stature. Medulloblastoma was diagnosed at age 6 years and his treatment consisted of surgery, radiation therapy (craniospinal irradiation of 36 Gy plus a posterior fossa boost of 18 Gy for a total dose of 54 Gy) and chemotherapy (carboplatin, vincristine, and cyclophosphamide). The pediatric oncology survivor clinic referred the patient to you after the family raised concerns about his height, which has not increased for at least 2 years. He has never seen an endocrinologist. He does well academically in high school and does not take any medications.

On physical examination, his height is 60 in (152.5 cm) (<1st percentile; –2.6 SD) and weight is 110 lb (50 kg) (10th percentile; –1.26 SD). His sitting height is at –3.0 SD. His midparental target height is 69.7 in (177 cm) (50th percentile). Vital signs are normal. Pubic hair is Tanner stage 5, and testicular volume is 8 mL bilaterally.

Preliminary workup by his oncologist includes normal complete blood cell count, basic metabolic panel, and erythrocyte sedimentation rate. His bone age is 14 years at a chronologic age of 16 years.

Which of the following is the best next step in this patient's management?
  A. Explain that his short stature is due to delayed puberty; recommend follow-up in 6 months to document growth velocity and pubertal progression
  B. Explain that his short stature is due to poor growth of the spine secondary to radiation; discharge him from clinic
  C. Screen for celiac disease; if negative, follow-up in 6 months to document growth velocity and pubertal progression
  D. Order screening lab tests including TSH, and IGF-1; if results are normal, recommend follow-up in 6 months
  E. Order screening lab tests including free T_4, TSH, IGF-1, LH, FSH, and testosterone and consider stimulation studies

59 A 12-year-old girl has a history of craniopharyngioma that was resected 12 months ago. Postoperatively, she had normal urine output and had no evidence of hypopituitarism. Your colleagues have been monitoring her clinical course for evidence of hormone abnormalities, with no signs of thyroid dysfunction and an IGF-1 level of 142 ng/mL (132-376 ng/mL) (SI: 18.6 nmol/L [17.3-49.3 nmol/L]). She has generally been in good health. However, lately her family has been worried that she is gaining excess weight.

On physical examination, she is obese (BMI, 28 kg/m^2; >97th percentile) and breast and pubic hair are Tanner stage 2. Her growth curve is shown (*see image*).

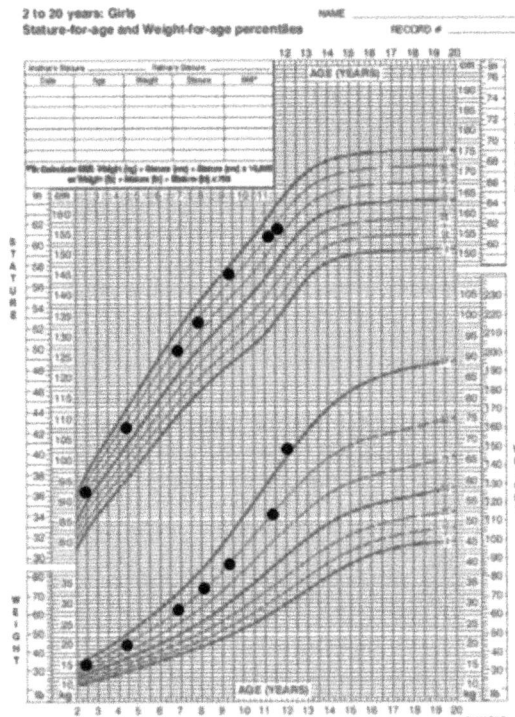

Her parents inquire what might be done to address her weight gain. Developing a management plan in response to which of the following diagnostic assessments is most likely to lead to a reduction in her accumulation of fat mass?

A. MRI to assess for damage to appetite-regulating nuclei of the hypothalamus
B. GH-stimulation test
C. 24-Hour urinary free cortisol measurement
D. Exploration in operating room for removal of possible recurrent craniopharyngioma
E. Assessment of high-caloric beverage consumption

60 You receive a phone consult regarding a 36-hour-old female baby born at 39 weeks' gestation to a 32-year-old woman (G5P4) with a history of Graves disease. Birth weight was 3175 g (6 lb 15.9 oz). The mother was treated with radioactive iodine about 1 year ago, and she has since been on levothyroxine treatment. Delivery was uncomplicated, and Apgar scores were 9 at both 1 minute and 5 minutes. The baby's TSH level from a sample obtained at 24 hours of life was 3.39 mIU/L. Her pediatrician tells you that the baby is asymptomatic and appears well on examination. She is feeding well and has normal vitals signs. The pediatrician calls for guidance before she discharges the baby from the nursery.

Which of the following is the best advice for this provider?

A. TSH is normal for age; the newborn may be discharged and TSH and free T_4 should be measured in 2 weeks as she may develop hyperthyroidism
B. TSH is normal for age; the newborn may be discharged and TSH and free T_4 levels should be measured in 4 weeks as she may develop hypothyroidism
C. TSH is normal for age; the newborn may be discharged and there is no need to repeat thyroid function studies unless she has symptoms or newborn screening is abnormal
D. TSH is low for age; the newborn should stay in the nursery for observation and be started on methimazole
E. TSH is low for age; the newborn may be discharged and TSH and free T_4 should be measured in 2 to 4 days, or sooner if symptomatic

61 A 10-and-7/12-year-old boy is referred for evaluation of poor growth and lack of weight gain. He has a history of vague gastrointestinal symptoms, including occasional abdominal pain since infancy. His father's height is 66 in (167.6 cm), and he had onset of puberty at age 15 years. His mother's height is 63 in (160 cm), and she had onset of puberty at age 13 years. Neither parent has any health issues. Midparental target height is 66.9 ± 4 in (170 ± 10 cm).

On physical examination, his height is 50 in (126.8 cm) (<3rd percentile; SDS, –2.23), weight is 56.1 lb (25.5 kg) (3rd percentile; SDS, –1.89), and BMI is 15.86 kg/m² (28th percentile; SDS, –0.59). Arm span is 50.7 in (128 cm), and the upper-to-lower segment ratio is normal for age and sex. He has no goiter. Findings on cardiopulmonary and abdominal examinations are unremarkable. Pubic hair and genitalia are Tanner stage 1. Testes are 2 to 3 mL bilaterally.

Bone age is interpreted to be 9 years and 6 months at a chronologic age of 10 years and 7 months. Predicted adult height according to the Bayley-Pinneau tables is 62.4 in (158.5 cm) (below the lower end of the midparental target height range).

Laboratory test results:
Hemoglobin = 9.6 g/dL (13.8-17.2 g/dL) (SI: 96 g/L [138-172 g/L])
Mean corpuscular volume = 60.6 μm³ (80-100 μm³) (SI: 60.6 fL [80-100 fL])
Platelet count = 150 × 10³/μL (150-450 × 10³/μL) (SI: 150 × 10⁹/L [150-450 × 10⁹/L])
Albumin = 3.4 g/dL (3.5-5.0 g/dL) (SI: 34 g/L [35-50 g/L])
Erythrocyte sedimentation rate = 80 mm/h (0-20 mm/h)
Total IgA, normal
tTG-IgA, negative
TSH = 6.3 mIU/L (0.7-5.7 mIU/L)
Free T_4 = 1.65 ng/dL (0.89-1.78 ng/dL) (SI: 21.2 pmol/L [11.5-22.9 pmol/L])
IGF-1 = 65 ng/mL (84-315 ng/mL) (SI: 8.5 nmol/L [11.0-41.3 nmol/L])

Which of the following causes of short stature most likely explains this patient's clinical picture?
   A. Hypothyroidism
   B. Ulcerative colitis
   C. Crohn disease
   D. GH deficiency
   E. Juvenile idiopathic arthritis

62 A 13-and-10/12-year-old boy presents with short stature (2nd percentile). His mother and maternal grandfather had constitutional growth delay. His midparental target height is 72.6 in (184.3 cm). He has a normal sense of smell, and he is a good student in school.

On physical examination, he has proportional short stature. His BMI is at the 23rd percentile. There is no goiter. He has Tanner stage 1 pubic hair, and testicular volume is 4 mL bilaterally (both testes descended).

His bone age is interpreted to be 12 years and 6 months at the chronologic age of 13 years and 10 months.

Laboratory test results:
   Celiac panel, normal
   Erythrocyte sedimentation rate, normal
   IGF-1= 209 ng/mL (168-576 ng/mL [Z-score −1.3]) (SI: 27.4 nmol/L [22.0-75.5 nmol/L])
   TSH = 1.07 mIU/L (0.5-5.0 mIU/L)
   Free T$_4$ = 0.98 ng/dL (0.71-1.85 ng/dL) (SI: 12.6 pmol/L [9.1-23.8 pmol/L])

Findings at follow-up visits are shown (*see table*).

Age	Testicular Volume	Testosterone	IGF-1	Free T$_4$	Peak GH Provocative Testing	Cortisol	Height Velocity
14 6/12 years	8 mL	16 ng/dL (SI: 0.56 nmol/L)	161 ng/mL (SI: 21.1 nmol/L) (reference range, 187-599 ng/mL [SI: 24.5-78.5 nmol/L])	...	...	...	4.2 cm/y
14 8/12 years	...	...	...	0.85 ng/dL (SI: 10.9 pmol/L)	26 ng/mL (SI: 26 µg/L) (reference range, ≥10 ng/mL [SI: ≥10 µg/L])	14.4 µg/dL (SI: 397.3 nmol/L)	...
15 6/12 years	12-15 mL	295 ng/dL (SI: 10.2 nmol/L)	295 ng/mL (SI: 38.6 nmol/L) (reference range, 201-609 ng/mL [SI: 26.3-79.8 nmol/L])	...	...	...	6.6 cm/y
15 10/12 years	20 mL	343 ng/dL (SI: 11.9 nmol/L)	...	0.76 ng/dL (SI: 9.8 pmol/L)	...	...	4.9 cm/y

At age 15 and 10/12 years, his height is at the 3rd percentile and additional test results are documented:
   TSH = 1.48 mIU/L (0.5-5.0 mIU/L)
   Free T$_4$ by equilibrium dialysis = 1.0 ng/dL (1.0-2.4 ng/dL) (SI: 12.9 pmol/L [12.9-30.9 pmol/L])
   Levothyroxine is initiated. Five months later, his testes are 25 to 30 mL bilaterally.

Which of the following is the best next step in making the diagnosis?
A. Head pituitary MRI with and without contrast
B. FSH and LH measurements
C. Total T_3 and reverse T_3 measurements
D. *IGSF1* genetic testing
E. Fragile X genetic testing

63 You are evaluating an 11-year-old girl for lipid abnormalities. She was adopted and her family medical history is not known. She has been healthy and had menarche 3 months ago.
On physical examination, her BMI is at the 80th percentile. Findings are otherwise normal.

Nonfasting lipid testing:
Total cholesterol = 310 mg/dL (<175 mg/dL) (SI: 8.0 mmol/L [<4.53 mmol/L])
Triglycerides = 80 mg/dL (30-140 mg/dL) (SI: 0.90 mmol/L [0.34-1.58 mmol/L])
HDL cholesterol = 48 mg/dL (30-70 mg/dL) (SI: 1.24 mmol/L [0.78-1.81 mmol/L])
LDL cholesterol = 246 mg/dL (<130 mg/dL) (SI: 6.37 mmol/L [<3.37 mmol/L])

Previous laboratory assessment revealed normal thyroid function.

Which of the following is the most appropriate next step in this patient's management?
A. Order another lipid panel in 6 months when fasting
B. Wait until age 12 years to start treatment with diet and medication
C. Initiate a low-cholesterol diet until age 18 years
D. Initiate a low-fat, low-cholesterol diet and start medication if cholesterol is still high after 3 months
E. Initiate a low-carbohydrate, low-cholesterol diet and high-potency statin medication now

64 You are considering the possibility of initiating bisphosphonate therapy in a 4-year-old girl who has a history of biliary atresia, resulting in cirrhosis and hepatic osteodystrophy. She has had 3 long bone fractures over the past year. She has gastrointestinal malabsorption and has been receiving phototherapy to maintain her 25-hydroxyvitamin D levels within the normal range. Her nutritional status and oral intake are poor, and her gastroenterologist has recommended placement of a gastrostomy tube. She has a history of asthma treated with daily inhaled corticosteroids. She underwent a cleft palate repair in infancy, and the family states there are plans to complete a palate expansion and alveolar bone graft over the next several years.

Which of the following risk factors makes you the most concerned about initiating bisphosphonate therapy in this patient?
A. Malabsorption—risk for hypocalcemia
B. Upcoming oral surgeries—risk for osteonecrosis of the jaw
C. Malnutrition—risk for unhealed osteomalacia
D. Asthma—risk for respiratory distress
E. Cirrhosis—risk for an acute phase reaction

65 A 17-year-old boy presents with peripheral vision loss that has been worsening over the past year. An ophthalmologist recommended a brain MRI, which showed a 4.5-cm, bi-lobed, heterogeneously enhancing cystic lesion extending from the sella to the suprasellar region with compression of the optic chiasm. The patient notes increased urinary frequency and thirst for a few weeks, dizziness upon standing up, and fatigue. He has no headaches or galactorrhea. He has not noticed any further changes of puberty for the past year, does not have erections, and is upset that his voice has not deepened. He has never shaved.
On physical examination, his blood pressure is 120/73 mm Hg and pulse rate is 82 beats/min. His height is 73 in (186 cm), weight is 186 lb (84.4 kg), and BMI is 24.4 kg/m². Ophthalmologic exam shows a bitemporal field cut on

confrontation visual fields. There is no expressible galactorrhea. Genitalia and pubic hair are Tanner stage 3, there is axillary hair present, and testicular volume is 6 mL bilaterally.

Laboratory test results (sample drawn at 8 AM):
    Cortisol = 1.9 μg/dL (8.0-19.0 μg/dL) (SI: 52.4 nmol/L [220.7-524.2 nmol/L])
    LH = 0.73 mIU/mL (0.2-9.2 mIU/mL) (SI: 0.73 IU/L [0.2-9.2 IU/L])
    FSH = 1.2 mIU/mL (2.0-9.2 mIU/mL) (SI: 1.2 IU/L [2.0-9.2 IU/L])
    Testosterone = <6 ng/dL (350-970 ng/dL) (SI: 0.2 nmol/L [12.1-33.7 nmol/L])
    TSH = 2.76 mIU/L (0.5-5.0 mIU/L)
    Free T$_4$ = 0.55 ng/dL (0.98-1.63 ng/dL) (SI: 7.1 pmol/L [12.6-21.0 pmol/L])
    Prolactin = >5000 ng/mL (2-10 ng/mL) (SI: 217.4 nmol/L [0.09-0.43 nmol/L])
    IGF-1 = 74 ng/mL (223-578 ng/mL) (SI: 9.7 nmol/L [29.2-75.7 nmol/L])
    GH = 0.06 ng/mL (0.06-4.30 ng/mL) (SI: 0.06 μg/L [0.06-4.30 μg/L])

He is started on replacement dosages of hydrocortisone, levothyroxine, and desmopressin for his hypopituitarism. Cabergoline is initiated with escalating doses and this resolves his visual field cut. His prolactin level decreases to 424 ng/mL, but it does not decrease further despite increases in the cabergoline dosage to 4.5 mg twice weekly. He continues to be very upset by his lack of further pubertal development. As his testosterone levels have remained below 6 ng/dL (<0.2 nmol/L), testosterone enanthate is started at a dosage of 100 mg intramuscularly monthly. After 2 months, his prolactin level rises to 875 ng/mL (38.0 nmol/L) without any vision changes or headaches.

Which of the following is the best next step in his treatment plan?
    A. Switch therapy to bromocriptine
    B. Increase the cabergoline dosage
    C. Add an aromatase inhibitor to his medication regimen
    D. Decrease the testosterone dosage
    E. Perform transsphenoidal tumor resection

66 A 12-year-old boy with Klinefelter syndrome presents to your clinic for management. Klinefelter syndrome was diagnosed prenatally when amniocentesis was performed due to an abnormal triple screen. His karyotype was documented to be 47,XXY. He has been followed up in the genetics clinic every 1 to 2 years and has had periodic endocrine visits. He reports that he has had underarm and pubic hair for about a year. He is treated with methylphenidate for attention-deficit/hyperactivity disorder.

Findings on physical examination are notable for Tanner stage 3 pubic hair and stage 3 development of the phallus with testicular volume less than 3 mL bilaterally. His height is at the 95th percentile and weight is at the 50th percentile for age (BMI, 10th percentile).

Laboratory test results:
    FSH = 1.3 mIU/mL (1.6-8.0 mIU/mL) (SI: 1.3 IU/L [1.6-8.0 IU/L])
    LH = 0.6 mIU/mL (0.2-5.0 mIU/mL) (SI: 0.6 IU/L [0.2-5.0 IU/L])
    Total testosterone = 67 ng/dL (21-719 ng/dL) (SI: 2.3 nmol/L [0.7-24.9 nmol/L])

At today's visit, his mother is mostly concerned about the timing of exogenous testosterone therapy and eventual sperm extraction for future fertility.

Which of the following should you advise in terms of treatment?
    A. Start testosterone treatment now to improve body composition
    B. Wait to start testosterone treatment until gonadotropin levels become elevated
    C. Refer now for sperm retrieval/extraction to optimize future fertility
    D. Defer sperm retrieval/extraction into adulthood
    E. Defer testosterone replacement until after attempts at sperm extraction

67 A 9-year-old prepubertal boy with type 1 diabetes mellitus is referred for poor growth. He has had diabetes since age 7 years, and his hemoglobin A_{1c} values have ranged from 7.0% to 8.0% (53 to 64 mmol/mol) while on insulin therapy. Review of systems is notable for chronic intermittent abdominal pain and constipation. Review of growth charts from the last 2 years shows that his height has crossed from the 25th to the 5th percentile, and his weight has decreased from the 10th to the 5th percentile. His growth velocity is 3 cm/y. Midparental target height is at the 75th percentile. His family history is positive for hypothyroidism in his mother and type 1 diabetes in a maternal uncle. His whole family has been on a gluten-free diet for the last 6 months since his older brother was diagnosed with celiac disease. However, there has been only minimal improvement in the patient's abdominal symptoms. Preliminary workup done by his pediatrician 1 month ago shows iron deficiency anemia, low serum total IgA, normal tissue transglutaminase IgA, and normal thyroid function. The patient's mother is worried that he might have celiac disease. She is reluctant to take him off the gluten-free diet.

Which of the following is the best next step to determine whether this patient has celiac disease?
- A. HLA genotyping
- B. Endoscopic biopsy
- C. Serologic testing with deamidated gliadin-derived peptide (anti-DGP) IgA antibodies
- D. Serologic testing with deamidated gliadin-derived peptide (anti-DGP) IgG antibodies
- E. Gluten challenge with 1 to 2 slices of wheat bread a day for 2 weeks and followed by repeated serologic testing

68 A 14-year-old obese girl is referred to you after her primary care physician documented a fasting blood glucose value of 100 mg/dL (5.6 mmol/L), a 2-hour postprandial glucose value of 209 mg/dL (11.6 mmol/L), and a hemoglobin A_{1c} value of 7.2% (55 mmol/mol). An antibody panel for type 1 diabetes is negative. The patient's family history is notable for type 2 diabetes mellitus in her mother and maternal grandmother. The patient underwent menarche at age 10 years, and she has had infrequent menstruation in recent years.

On physical examination, moderate acanthosis nigricans is noted on her neck. Her BMI is above the 97th percentile for age.

The patient unsuccessfully attempts lifestyle intervention for 6 months as guided by the weight management team. You then prescribe metformin extended-release, 500 mg daily to be taken with the evening meal. You instructed her parents to increase the dosage by 500 mg every 2 weeks until a daily dosage of 2000 mg is reached. The patient's mother calls you in 7 to 8 weeks, reporting that her daughter is experiencing severe abdominal pain and diarrhea after reaching the dosage of 2000 mg daily.

Which of the following should you recommend as the best next step in this patient's management?
- A. Discontinue metformin therapy
- B. Continue metformin therapy for another 2 weeks and reassure the patient that symptoms will improve
- C. Switch metformin extended-release to the immediate-release formulation (same dosage)
- D. Reduce the metformin dosage to the previously tolerated dosage
- E. Determine whether the patient has been exposed to any intravenous contrast or alcohol

69 A 9-and-2/12-year-old girl has multiple endocrine neoplasia type 2B due to the M918T mutation in the *RET* gene. Her condition was diagnosed at age 7 and 3/12 years, after her primary care physician noticed her prominent lips. Thyroidectomy with central neck dissection revealed multifocal medullary thyroid carcinoma with 4 positive nodes on the left side (T1bN1a). Calcitonin and carcinoembryonic antigen (CEA) levels are shown (*see table*).

Measurement	Preoperative	Postoperative	12 Months After Surgery	18 Months After Surgery
Calcitonin (reference range, <8 pg/mL [<2.3 pmol/L])	289 pg/mL (84.4 pmol/L)	16 pg/mL (4.7 pmol/L)	82 pg/mL (23.9 pmol/L)	190 pg/mL (55.5 pmol/L)
CEA (reference range, <2.5 ng/mL)	53.5 ng/mL	1.0 ng/mL	3.8 ng/mL	13 ng/mL

The doubling time is 134 days for calcitonin and 98 days for CEA. She now has 1 anterior upper cervical lymph node measuring 2 cm noted on ultrasonography at 12 and 18 months postoperatively.

Which of the following is the best next step?
  A. Perform ultrasonography 1 year after the last exam
  B. Perform CT of the neck and chest
  C. Continue to follow her calcitonin level
  D. Continue to follow her CEA level
  E. Measure urinary metanephrines

70 You are seeing a 10-year-old boy for a second opinion. He has a longstanding history of being at the low end of the normal growth curve, but he started experiencing excess weight gain 18 months ago after the family moved to your area from another state. His mother mentioned her concern for his lagging height to his primary care physician, who ordered multiple laboratory tests (morning blood draw):

IGF-1 = 171 ng/dL (123-275 ng/mL) (SI: 22.4 nmol/L [16.1-36.0 nmol/L])
Free T$_4$ = 1.4 ng/dL (0.8-2.2 ng/dL) (SI: 18.0 pmol/L [10.3-28.3 pmol/L])
TSH = 6.1 mIU/L (0.5-5.0 mIU/L)
Cortisol = 18 μg/dL (3-21 μg/dL) (SI: 496.6 nmol/L [87.8-579.3 nmol/L])

He was referred to a local pediatric endocrinologist who was concerned about his weight gain and performed a GH-stimulation test, the results of which are shown (*see table*).

	Time				
	0 min	15 min	30 min	45 min	60 min
GH	2 ng/mL (2 μg/L)	3 ng/mL (3 μg/L)	6 ng/mL (6 μg/L)	4 ng/mL (4 μg/L)	5 ng/mL (5 μg/L)

You review his growth curve (*see image*). His BMI is 24 kg/m^2 (>97th percentile). The rest of his examination findings are unremarkable.

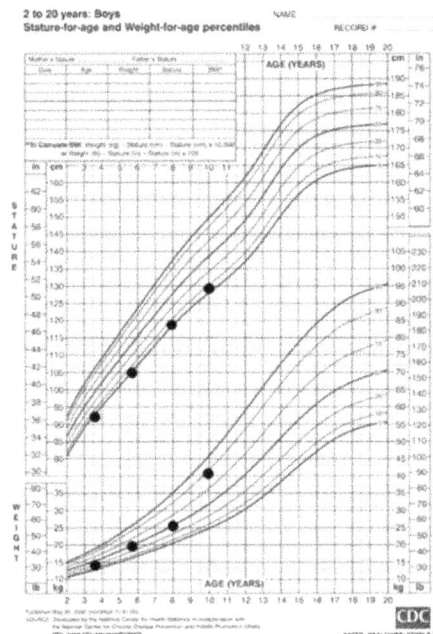

2 to 20 years: Boys
Stature-for-age and Weight-for-age percentiles

For which of the following should the patient be treated?
A. GH deficiency
B. Hypothyroidism
C. Obesity
D. Excess cortisol
E. Probable brain tumor

71 A 12-year-old girl seeks evaluation for thyroid nodules. She was initially seen by her primary care physician for lightheadedness and was noted to have goiter on examination. Primary hypothyroidism secondary to chronic lymphocytic thyroiditis was diagnosed and levothyroxine was initiated. Neck ultrasonography (*see images*) documents a solid right nodule (*thick arrow on right side*) measuring 1.8 × 1.04 × 1 cm with a halo (*thin arrow on right side*) and a less well-defined smaller nodule (*thick arrow on left side*) on the left lobe measuring 1.12 × 0.79 × 0.78 cm, with microcalcifications (*thin arrow on left side*).

Left Nodule   Right Nodule

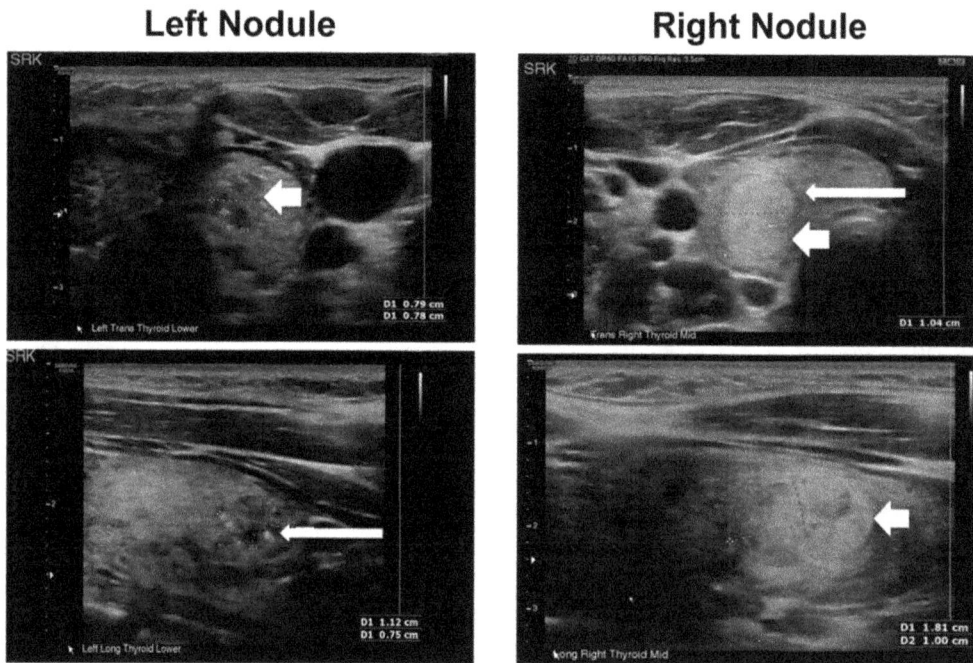

She undergoes ultrasonography-guided FNA. The right nodule is benign and the left nodule is indeterminate, with atypia of unclear significance. Counseling is provided and the patient undergoes total thyroidectomy. Pathology demonstrates a 0.9-cm papillary thyroid carcinoma, classic type, on the left lobe. Margins are negative and no lymphovascular invasion is identified. The nodule on the right lobe is determined to be a thyroid adenoma. She has background Hashimoto thyroiditis. Left level 6 (central neck) lymph node resection includes 13 lymph nodes, all of which are negative for thyroid carcinoma. Thyroid hormone replacement is started.

Which of the following is the best next step in this patient's management?
A. Arrange for ^{123}I whole-body scan following levothyroxine withdrawal after confirming that TSH is >30 mIU/L and treat with ^{131}I if she has radioactive iodine uptake
B. Arrange for treatment with 1.0 to 1.5 mCi/Kg ^{131}I following levothyroxine withdrawal after confirming that TSH is >30 mIU/L
C. Arrange for radioactive iodine ablation with 30 to 50 mCi ^{131}I to facilitate follow-up of thyroglobulin levels, as she most likely has thyroglobulin antibodies
D. Reassure the family, adjust levothyroxine to keep TSH between 0.5 and 1.0 mIU/L, and measure non-stimulated thyroglobulin and thyroglobulin antibodies in 3 to 6 months
E. Reassure the family that no further treatment is needed and adjust levothyroxine to maintain TSH in the normal range

72 You are called to the neonatal intensive care unit to evaluate a 1-day-old newborn with atypical genitalia. The baby was born at 39-and-5/7-weeks' gestation to a 22-year-old mother who did not receive prenatal care. She reports that her pregnancy was uneventful. Birth weight was 7 lb 2.6 oz (3250 g).

On physical examination, the baby appears well. Phallus length is 1.9 cm and width is 0.7 cm. The urethral opening is at the inferior aspect of the phallus. The labioscrotal folds are minimally rugated and no gonads or masses are palpable.

Ultrasonography demonstrates no mullerian structures, and gonads are visualized in the inguinal canals bilaterally.

Laboratory test results (sample drawn on day 3 of life):
Sodium = 138 mEq/L (136-144 mEq/L) (SI: 138 mmol/L [136-144 mmol/L])
Potassium = 5.0 mEq/L (3.2-5.2 mEq/L) (SI: 5.0 mmol/L [3.2-5.2 mmol/L])
Chloride = 109 mEq/L (101-111 mEq/L) (SI: 109 mmol/L [101-111 mmol/L])
Carbon dioxide = 24 mEq/L (22-32 mEq/L) (SI: 24 mmol/L [22-32 mmol/L])
17-hydroxyprogesterone = 228 ng/dL (<78 ng/dL) (SI: 6.9 nmol/L [<2.4 nmol/L])
17-hydroxypregnenolone = 5994 ng/dL (10-829 ng/dL) (SI: 180.4 nmol/L [0.3-25.0 nmol/L])
Testosterone = 30 ng/dL (75-400 ng/dL) (SI: 1.0 nmol/L [2.6-13.9 nmol/L])
Androstenedione = 28.7 ng/dL (<10-279 ng/dL) (SI: 1.0 nmol/L [0.3-9.7 nmol/L])
DHEA = 5813 ng/dL (41-1292 ng/dL) (SI: 201.7 nmol/L [1.4-44.8 nmol/L])
Cortisol = 3.1 μg/dL (SI: 85.5 nmol/L)
Karyotype analysis = 46,XY (*SRY* sequence is normal)

Which of the following genes most likely harbors a pathogenic variant?
   A. *CYP17A1* (17α-hydroxylase/17,20-lyase deficiency)
   B. *POR* (P450 oxidoreductase deficiency)
   C. *CYP11B1* (11β-hydroxylase deficiency)
   D. *NR0B1* (X-linked adrenal hypoplasia congenita)
   E. *HSD3B2* (3β-hydroxysteroid dehydrogenase deficiency)

73 You are called by a general pediatrician to consult on a 2-week-old male newborn. The baby was born at 38 weeks' gestation with a birth weight of 3460 g (7 lb 10 oz). The pregnancy was complicated by preeclampsia, and the baby was born via emergent cesarian delivery. Shortly after birth, he developed respiratory distress and temperature instability. He underwent a sepsis workup and treatment was initiated with broad-spectrum antibiotics. On day 2 of life, he developed hardened, edematous lesions on his lower limbs and back. All cultures returned negative, and the baby was discharged home on day 7 of life.

He now presents to his general pediatrician for routine follow-up. The family states that they have been feeding the baby 2 to 3 oz of 20 kcal/oz formula every 2 to 3 hours. He has been having 6 to 8 voids and 2 to 3 stools per day.

On physical examination, he appears well and has gained appropriate weight. Hardened nodules are apparent on his extremities and back, with no tenderness or overlying erythema.

Laboratory test results:
Calcium = 11 mg/dL (7.6-10.4 mg/dL) (SI: 2.8 mmol/L [1.9-2.6 mmol/L])
Phosphate = 4.3 mg/dL (4.2-8.0 mg/dL) (SI: 1.4 mmol/L [1.4-2.6 mmol/L])

Which of the following is the best next step in this baby's management?
   A. Change to low-calcium infant formula
   B. Prescribe oral prednisolone
   C. Increase formula feeds to 4 oz every 2 hours
   D. Admit to the hospital for intravenous fluids and furosemide
   E. Perform zoledronate infusion

74 You are evaluating a 17-year-old boy with type 1 diabetes mellitus. He transitioned to a hybrid closed-loop insulin delivery system with continuous glucose monitoring last year. He is efficiently using the system by wearing the continuous glucose monitor 97% of the time, allowing the pump to be in auto mode. The following data are downloaded:

Auto mode (per week)	98% (6 d 21 h)
Manual mode (per week)	2% (03 h)
Sensor wear (per week)	97% (6 d 20 h)
Average blood glucose (± SD)	150 mg/dL (±57 mg/dL)
Total daily dose (per day)	53 units
Bolus amount (per day)	27 units (51%)
Auto basal/basal amount (per day)	26 units (49%)

His pump download provides the following continuous glucose tracing (*see image*).

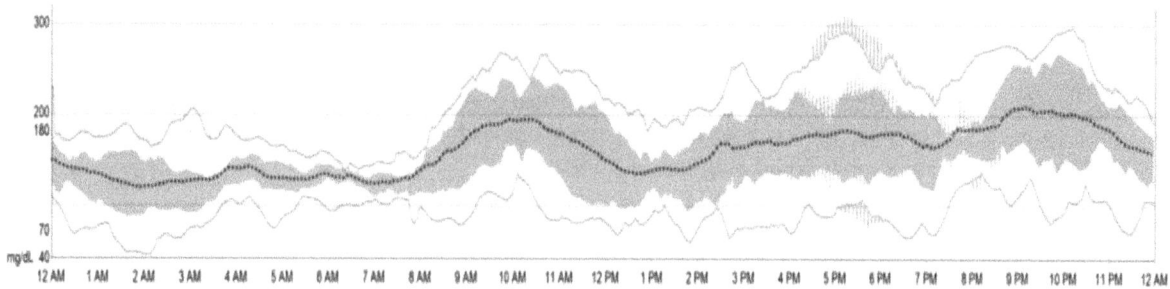

The insulin-to-carbohydrate ratio is 1:7 for 24 hours. The active insulin time is 2:00 hours, and the insulin sensitivity factor is 35 mg/dL (1.9 mmol/L). His manual basal rate is 0.9 units per hour.

During your discussion, he says that the hypoglycemia recordings overnight are probably due to pressure-induced sensor inaccuracies. He reports some hypoglycemia episodes during the day associated with exercise, and he is also bothered by hyperglycemia after meals.

Which of the following suggestions is the best next step in this patient's management?

  A. Set a temporary basal rate when he is physically active to avoid hypoglycemia while in auto mode
  B. Increase the manual basal rate to 1.1 units per hour to match the total daily auto basal in delivering adequate basal insulin if he is not in auto mode
  C. Decrease active insulin time to 1:45 hours to help avoid postprandial hyperglycemia late in the evening
  D. Lower his sensitivity to deliver more insulin bolus for correction of hyperglycemia in the evening when he is in auto mode
  E. Lower his insulin-to-carbohydrate ratio to 1:6 for breakfast and dinner intervals to deliver more insulin bolus to avoid postprandial hyperglycemia

75 A 12-year-old girl presents for evaluation of short stature. According to her parents, her height has always been at the lower end of the growth chart. Her pediatrician referred her for evaluation because her height was noted to be below the 3rd percentile at her recent well-child visit. She has no headaches, vision problems, abdominal pain, constipation, fatigue, or cold intolerance. She is in seventh grade and has an individualized education plan at school. Her parents are concerned that her height difference is causing social difficulties with her peers.

On physical examination, she has mild cubitus valgus, stage 3 pubic hair, and no breast development. Her height is 53.1 in (135 cm) (<3rd percentile) and weight is 110.2 lb (50.1 kg) (75th percentile). BMI is at the 97th percentile.

Bone age is interpreted to be 13 years at the chronologic age of 12 and 7/12 years.

Laboratory test results:

    IGF-1 = 128 ng/mL (105-499 ng/mL) (SI: 16.8 nmol/L [13.8-65.4 nmol/L])

    Estradiol = 4.0 pg/mL (7.0-60.0 pg/mL) (SI: 14.7 pmol/L [25.7-220.3 pmol/L])

    LH = 22.0 mIU/mL (0.5-41.7 mIU/mL) (SI: 22.0 IU/L [0.5-41.7 IU/L])

    FSH = 93.8 mIU/mL (1.6-17.0 mIU/mL) (SI: 93.8 IU/L [1.6-17.0 IU/L])

    TSH, normal

    Free T$_4$, normal

The underlying diagnosis is confirmed with additional testing.

Which of the following would be the most likely to help address her problems with school performance?
    A. Testing for intellectual disability
    B. Stimulant therapy
    C. Educational assessment for learning disability
    D. Evaluation for autistic spectrum disorder
    E. Estrogen replacement

76   A 10-year-old girl is referred by her pediatrician because of a goiter, weight loss of 3.3 lb (1.5 kg) over the past 2 weeks, and fatigue. She has been wearing dental braces for 6 months, and in the past 2 weeks she has had lower jaw pain. She has no abdominal pain and no nocturia.

Laboratory test results:

    TSH = <0.03 mIU/L (0.5-5.0 mIU/L)

    Free T$_4$ = 1.8 ng/dL (0.9-1.4 ng/dL) (SI: 23.2 pmol/L [11.6-18.0 pmol/L])

    Total T$_3$ = 245 ng/dL (105-207 ng/dL) (SI: 3.77 nmol/L [1.62-3.19 nmol/L])

    Thyroid-stimulating immunoglobulin antibodies, negative

    TPO antibodies = 30.0 IU/mL (<9.0 IU/mL) (SI: 30.0 kIU/L [<9.0 kIU/L])

    Thyroglobulin antibodies = 5.0 IU/mL (<1.0 IU/mL) (SI: 5.0 kIU/L [<1.0 kIU/L])

On physical examination, she is mildly tachycardic with a pulse rate of 112 beats/min. Blood pressure is normal. She has no proptosis, and findings on eye exam are normal. She has a small and mildly tender goiter. There is no bruit.

Which of the following is the best next step in this patient's management?
    A. Prescribe propranolol
    B. Measure erythrocyte sedimentation rate, perform thyroid iodine uptake scan, and prescribe propranolol
    C. Prescribe methimazole and propranolol
    D. Repeat thyroid-stimulating immunoglobulin antibody assessment
    E. Measure TSH-receptor antibodies

77   A 12-and-6/12-year-old boy is referred for evaluation of short stature. According to his parents, he has always grown below the 3rd percentile. They have not been too concerned because there is a history of short stature on both sides of the family. Over the last 2 years, his growth has slowed compared with that of his classmates. His father's height is 66 in (167.6 cm), puberty onset was at age 14 years, and he has no health issues. His mother's height is 63 in (160 cm), menarche was at age 15.5 years, and she has no health issues. Midparental target height is 67 ± 4 in (170 ± 10 cm).

    On physical examination, his height is 52.9 in (134.3 cm) (<3rd percentile; SDS, −2.46), weight is 59 lb (26.8 kg) (<3rd percentile; SDS, −2.88), and BMI is 14.9 kg/m^2 (3rd percentile; SDS, −1.92). No dysmorphic features are noted. Pubic hair and genitalia are Tanner stage 1. Testes are 2 to 3 mL bilaterally.

Bone age is interpreted to be 10 years and 6 months at a chronologic age of 12 years and 6 months. Predicted adult height according to the Bayley-Pinneau tables is 64.5 in (163.9 cm), in the lower half of the midparental height range.

Laboratory test results:
    Hemoglobin, normal
    Hematocrit, normal
    Mean corpuscular volume = 82 μm^3 (77-95 μm^3) (SI: 82 fL [77-95 fL])
    Glucose = 68 mg/dL (70-126 mg/dL) (SI: 3.8 mmol/L [3.9-7.0 mmol/L])
    TSH = 3.3 mIU/L (0.7-5.7 mIU/L)
    Free T_4 = 1.24 ng/dL (0.89-1.78 ng/dL) (SI: 16.0 pmol/L [11.5-22.9 pmol/L])
    IGF-1 = 55 ng/mL (100-330 ng/mL) (SI: 7.2 nmol/L [13.1-43.2 nmol/L]) (IGF-1 Z-score = –2.8 [Tanner stage 1 male])

Nutritional recommendations are provided to increase caloric intake along with the prescription of an appetite stimulant (cyproheptadine). At a follow-up visit 6 months later, his height is 53.3 in (135.5 cm) (<3rd percentile; SDS, –2.66), weight is 65.8 lb (29.9 kg) (<3rd percentile; SDS, –2.50), and BMI is 16.3 kg/m^2 (14th percentile; SDS, –1.09). Growth velocity is 2.4 cm/y. Pubic hair and genitalia are Tanner stage 1. Testes are 3 mL bilaterally.

His IGF-1 concentration is documented to be 62 ng/mL (105-350 ng/mL) (SI: 8.1 nmol/L [13.8-45.9 nmol/L]) (IGF-1 Z-score = –2.9 [Tanner stage 1 male]).

Which of the following is the most appropriate next step in this child's management?
A. Overnight blood sampling to measure spontaneous GH secretion every 20 minutes
B. Administration of 4 monthly testosterone injections
C. Arginine-insulin tolerance test preceded by administration of 50 mg of testosterone intramuscularly 1 week before the test
D. Random measurement of GH
E. MRI of the brain and pituitary gland with and without contrast

78 A male baby is born at 38 weeks' gestation after delivery is induced because of severe maternal preeclampsia. The prenatal course was complicated by concern for fetal hydrocephalus and polyhydramnios, both of which resolved before delivery. Following delivery, the baby is noted to have low blood glucose readings and poor temperature regulation.

On physical examination, his weight is 6 lb 5 oz (2870 g), length is 18 in (45.8 cm), head circumference is 13.4 in (34 cm), temperature is 98.8°F (37.1°C), pulse rate is 133 beats/min, blood pressure is 60/30 mm Hg, and respiratory rate is 54 breaths/min. The infant appears jittery, with mild hepatomegaly and hypotonia.

Laboratory test results:
    Glucose = 34 mg/dL (60-110 mg/dL) (SI: 1.9 mmol/L [3.3-6.1 mmol/L])
    Sodium = 121 mEq/L (136-142 mEq/L) (SI: 121 mmol/L [136-142 mmol/L])
    Potassium = 5.0 mEq/L (4.4-6.3 mEq/L) (SI: 5.0 mmol/L [4.4-6.3 mmol/L])
    Total bilirubin = 7.2 mg/dL (0.2-1.0 mg/dL) (SI: 123.1 µmol/L [3.4-17.1 µmol/L])
    Direct bilirubin = 3.1 mg/dL (<0.3 mg/dL) (SI: 53.0 µmol/L [<5.1 µmol/L])

Which of the following is the most likely diagnosis?
A. Congenital hyperinsulinemic hypoglycemia of infancy
B. Congenital adrenal hyperplasia
C. Glycogen storage disease type 1a
D. Stress-induced hypoglycemia
E. Congenital hypopituitarism

79 A 14-year-old girl diagnosed with acute lymphoblastic leukemia 10 years ago presents for a follow-up visit. She completed initial chemotherapy and relapsed 2 years later, receiving additional chemotherapy with idarubicin, vincristine, dexamethasone, PEG-asparaginase, and triple intrathecal chemotherapy. She then received conditioning with cyclophosphamide, 60 mg/kg, followed by fractionated total-body irradiation (13.2 Gy) and bone marrow transplant. She has remained in remission following bone marrow transplant; however, she has developed hypergonadotropic hypogonadism and central hypothyroidism. Her pituitary function is otherwise normal. She is taking hormone replacement for both complications of therapy.

At today's visit, she has no questions or concerns. She is asymptomatic.

On physical examination, she has normal vital signs. A small nodule is palpated under the right lobe of her thyroid, which does not move with deglutition. Neck ultrasonography is performed (*see images*) and reveals a subcentimeter right thyroid nodule with microcalcifications (*short arrows*) and a round lymph node on the right side of her neck, without hilum (*long arrow*).

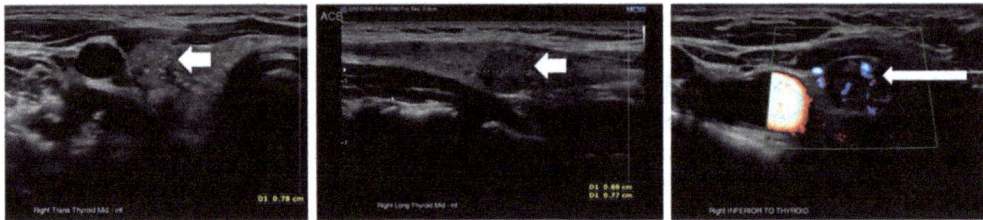

Which of the following is the best management recommendation for this patient?
A. Total thyroidectomy and central neck dissection
B. Complete neck ultrasonography and FNA of the thyroid nodule, the right inferior lymph node, and other suspicious lymph nodes (if found)
C. Complete blood cell count with differential, FNA of the thyroid nodule, and excision biopsy of the right lymph node to rule out lymphoma
D. Repeated neck ultrasonography in 4 to 6 months
E. Follow-up with palpation with additional evaluation if nodules enlarge or change over time

80 A 12-year-old boy is followed in pediatric endocrine clinic for idiopathic short stature and advanced bone age. His height is at less than the 1st percentile (–2.5 SD), and his weight is at –1.0 SD. He has no dysmorphic features and has proportional short stature. His midparental height is at the 50th percentile. He started noticing pubic hair at age 10 and 6/12 years. Pubic hair is currently Tanner stage 3, and his testes are 6 mL bilaterally. Bone age was interpreted to be 13 years at a chronologic age of 11 years. His predicted height from the bone age was at –2.8 SD. Results from the laboratory workup to evaluate for poor growth and short stature are normal.

An aromatase inhibitor (letrozole, 2.5 mg daily) was prescribed 6 months ago and he takes it regularly. He has noticed worsening acne since starting treatment. There has been no significant change to his predicted adult height or ratio of bone age to chronologic age.

Which of the following sets of laboratory test results would you be most likely to document in this patient?

Answer	LH	FSH	Testosterone
A.	<0.02 mIU/mL (<0.02 IU/L)	<0.02 mIU/mL (<0.02 IU/L)	115 ng/dL (4.0 nmol/L)
B.	<0.02 mIU/mL (<0.02 IU/L)	<0.02 mIU/mL (<0.02 IU/L)	628 ng/dL (21.8 nmol/L)
C.	6.1 mIU/mL (6.1 IU/L)	14.5 mIU/mL (14.5 IU/L)	628 ng/dL (21.8 nmol/L)
D.	<0.02 mIU/mL (<0.02 IU/L)	30 mIU/mL (30 IU/L)	628 ng/dL (21.8 nmol/L)
E.	42 mIU/mL (42 IU/L)	65 mIU/mL (65 IU/L)	115 ng/dL (4.0 nmol/L)

81 You are asked to evaluate a 1-month-old female infant with hyperthyroidism who presented to the emergency department with decreased oral intake, poor weight gain, and difficulty being consoled. Her heart rate was noted to be 200 beats/min. She does not take any medications. The pregnancy was unremarkable; however, the infant's mother has been on levothyroxine for several years, including during the pregnancy. She is unsure of the etiology of her thyroid condition.

Laboratory test results:
    TSH = 0.008 mIU/L (0.9-7.7 mIU/L)
    Free T_4 = 3.7 ng/dL (0.81-2.12 ng/dL) (SI: 47.6 pmol/L [10.4-27.3 pmol/L])
    Total T_4 and total T_3 are not measured.

On physical examination, the infant is crying and difficult to console. You note facial plethora and mild hypertrichosis (*see image*).

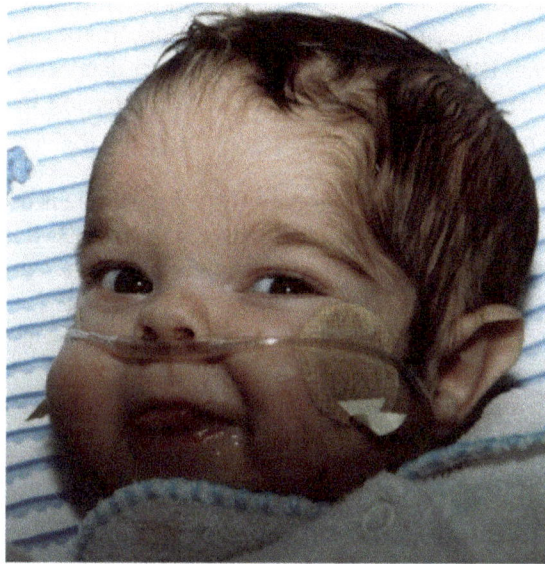

Which of the following is this child most likely to develop?
    A. Celiac disease
    B. Vitiligo
    C. Osteoporosis
    D. Precocious puberty
    E. GH deficiency

82 You are asked to evaluate a 16-year-old boy for small testes. He has a history of acute lymphocytic leukemia (pre-B cell) diagnosed at age 2 years that was treated with chemotherapy without complications. He had testicular and bone marrow relapse at age 7 years and underwent re-induction chemotherapy and radiation therapy, with a total radiation dose of 2400 cGy. He has had no disease recurrence since then. He has no family history of delayed puberty and has no other current medical concerns. Midparental target height is 71.5 in (181.6 cm).

On physical examination, his height is at the 24th percentile, weight is at the 26th percentile, and BMI is at the 32nd percentile. He has Tanner stage 3 pubic hair, and testicular volume is 3 mL bilaterally.

Laboratory test results:
    LH = 34 mIU/mL (0.2-5.0 mIU/mL) (SI: 34 IU/L [0.2-5.0 IU/L])
    FSH = 71 mIU/mL (1.5-12.9 mIU/mL) (SI: 71 IU/L [1.5-12.9 IU/L])
    Total testosterone = 83.3 ng/dL (350- 970 ng/dL) (SI: 2.9 nmol/L [12.1-33.7 nmol/L])
    β-hCG = 2.0 mIU/mL (0-3.0 mIU/mL) (SI: 2.0 IU/L [0-3.0 IU/L])
    Thyroid function, normal

He starts topical testosterone gel treatment, and repeated testing 3 months later documents the following laboratory test results:

LH = 7.0 mIU/mL (2.0-5.0 mIU/mL) (SI: 7.0 IU/L [2.0-5.0 IU/L])

FSH = 36.9 mIU/mL (1.5-12.9 mIU/mL) (SI: 36.9 IU/L [1.5-12.9 IU/L])

Total testosterone = 351.8 ng/dL (350-970 ng/dL) (SI: 12.2 nmol/L [12.1-33.7 nmol/L])

Which of the following is the best next step in this patient's management?
- A. Perform brain MRI
- B. Add an aromatase inhibitor
- C. Increase the testosterone dosage
- D. Switch to intramuscular testosterone
- E. Continue current management

83 An 8-year-old girl is brought to the endocrinology clinic for concerns of slow growth for the past 3 to 4 years. Her parents note that she has been growing significantly slower than her fraternal twin sister. Her overall energy has been low and her hair has become coarse and brittle. She is having frequent headaches. She has no polyuria or polydipsia. The primary care physician obtains an MRI of the brain, which shows a likely craniopharyngioma.

On physical examination, her blood pressure is 85/46 mm Hg and pulse rate is 65 beats/min. Her height is 44.5 in (113 cm) (0.1th percentile), weight is 44.7 lb (20.3 kg) (2.8th percentile), and BMI is 15.90 kg/m^2 (47th percentile). Her body surface area is 0.8 m^2. Her hair is coarse and brittle, and visual fields are grossly normal to confrontation. She is prepubertal.

The neurosurgeon is planning resection of the craniopharyngioma and is asking for perioperative management recommendations.

Laboratory test results:

TSH = 2.48 mIU/L (0.6-4.84 mIU/L)

Free T$_4$ = 0.5 ng/dL (0.97-1.67 ng/dL) (SI: 6.4 pmol/L [12.5-21.5 pmol/L])

IGF-1= 47.7 ng/mL (80-233 ng/mL) (SI: 6.2 nmol/L [10.5-30.5 nmol/L])

Cortisol (8 AM) = 4.0 µg/dL (2.3-15.0 µg/dL) (SI: 110.3 nmol/L [63.5-413.8 nmol/L])

First morning urine osmolality = 606 mOsm/kg (50-1400 mOsm/kg) (SI: 606 mmol/kg [50-1400 mmol/kg])

She is started on physiologic hydrocortisone replacement and then 2 days later is started on levothyroxine replacement. One week later, surgery is planned. The endocrinologist recommends stress-dose hydrocortisone, 50-100 mg/m^2 intravenously before surgery. Two hours after surgery, she develops markedly increased urine output of 4 mL/kg per h, and her sodium concentration is 150 mEq/L (150 mmol/L).

Which of the following is the most likely cause of her increased urine output?
- A. Central diabetes insipidus that was unmasked after replacement with hydrocortisone
- B. Hyperglycemia due to steroid administration
- C. Excess fluid administration in the operating room
- D. Dysfunction of the vasopressinergic neurons of the supraoptic and paraventricular nuclei
- E. The second stage of the triphasic response

84 A 9-day-old full-term male infant of a diabetic mother is noted to have a series of elevated blood glucose values in the newborn nursery:

Day 1 of life = 108-130 mg/dL (6.0-7.2 mmol/L)

Day 2 of life = 206 mg/dL (11.4 mmol/L)

Day 4 of life = 190 mg/dL (10.5 mmol/L)

Otherwise, he has reportedly been doing well. He breastfeeds for approximately 15 minutes every 2 to 3 hours and takes 1 to 2 supplemental 2-oz bottles daily. The patient was born to a 24-year-old woman. The pregnancy was complicated by gestational diabetes mellitus controlled with insulin. Findings from all prenatal laboratory tests were normal. His birth weight was 6 lb 4 oz (2835 g).

When interviewing his mother, you learn that there is an extensive family history of diabetes in the patient's maternal grandparents and uncles. The patient's mother has reportedly experienced hypoglycemia in her lifetime in addition to the gestational diabetes she had during this pregnancy.

Which of the following is the most common etiology of the neonatal diabetes present in this patient?

A. Autoimmune type 1 diabetes mellitus
B. Chromosome 6q24–related transient neonatal diabetes mellitus
C. Homozygous pathogenic variants in the *GCK* gene
D. Pathogenic variant in the *PDX1* gene
E. Pathogenic variant in the *KCNJ11* gene

85 A 17-year-old girl is pregnant for the first time. She is at 33 weeks' gestation and has had appropriate weight gain during her pregnancy, which has been uneventful to date. She does not drink milk and she has not been taking supplements or prenatal vitamins. In the past, she was followed by an endocrinologist for mild obesity and was previously documented to be euthyroid. She recently sought advice from a gynecologist about possibly taking supplements, and the gynecologist referred her to you. She recalls having a normal TSH measurement at her first-trimester check-up.

Which of the following is the best recommendation regarding the thyroid health of the mother and the fetus?

A. Start prenatal vitamins plus 100 mcg of iodine daily
B. Start prenatal vitamins plus iodine supplementation (total of 250 mcg of iodine daily)
C. Take a total of 150 mcg of iodine daily
D. Measure TSH and total T_3
E. Measure iodine in a spot urine specimen

86 A 13-and-5/12-year-old boy is referred by his primary care physician for evaluation of poor growth. His linear growth has slowed over the last year. His appetite is reportedly poor, although he likes a variety of foods. He has had poor focus in school, especially in the last 2 years, and he was prescribed methylphenidate, 30 mg orally daily, approximately 6 months before the current visit. His review of systems is otherwise negative.

He was born at 39 weeks' gestation with a birth weight of 7 lb 12 oz (3515 g) and birth length of 20 in (50.8 cm). He reached his developmental milestones normally. He is active in sports. His father's height is 67 in (170.2 cm), and his mother's height is 64 in (162.6 cm). His family history is noncontributory.

On physical examination, his height is 59.2 in (150.4 cm) (14th percentile; SDS, –1.08) and weight is 70.4 lb (32 kg) (<3rd percentile; SDS, –2.33). His growth charts are shown (*see images*). BMI is 14.15 kg/m^2 (<3rd percentile; SDS, –2.9). Vital signs are normal. He has no dysmorphic features. Pubic hair is Tanner stage 1 and genitalia are Tanner stage 2 to 3. Testicular volume is 6 mL bilaterally.

Bone age is interpreted to be 13 years at a chronologic age of 13 years and 5 months. Predicted adult height according to the Bayley-Pinneau tables is 67.6 in (171.6 cm). This falls within the target height range calculated based on reported parental heights. Target height is 68.1 ± 3.9 in (173 ± 10 cm).

Laboratory test results:
IGF-1 = 172 ng/mL (152-540 ng/mL) (SI: 22.5 nmol/L [19.9-70.7 nmol/L]) (Z-score, –1.4)
IGFBP-3 = 4.8 mg/L (3.1-9.5)
Testosterone = 125 ng/dL (100-320 ng/dL) (SI: 4.3 nmol/L [3.5-11.1 nmol/L])

Thyroid function, complete blood cell count, and a comprehensive chemistry panel are normal. Screening for celiac disease is negative.

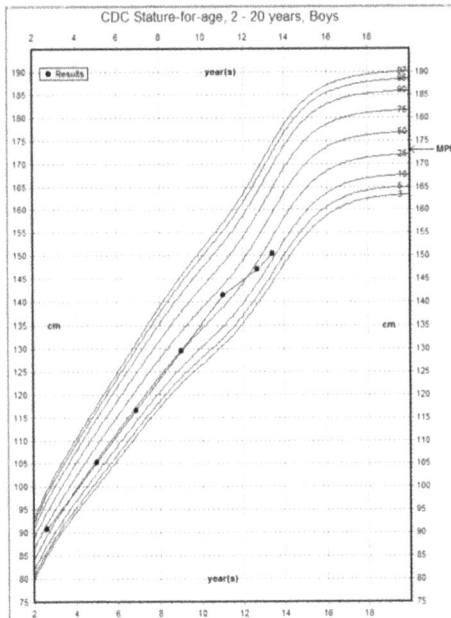

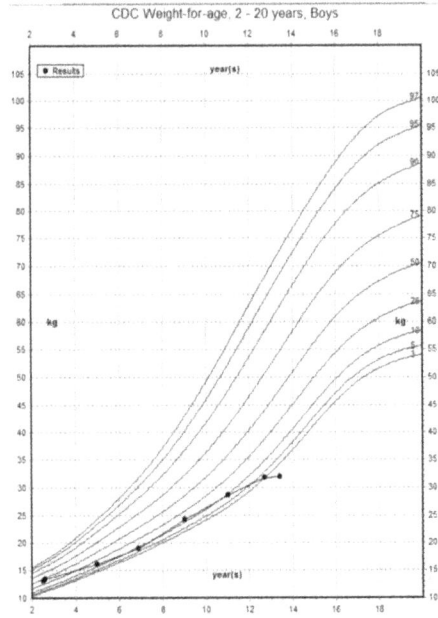

Which of the following is the most appropriate intervention to help improve this patient's growth?
- A. Start a series of testosterone injections every month for 4 months
- B. Start a gluten-free diet
- C. Start recombinant human GH
- D. Start an aromatase inhibitor
- E. Discuss with the patient's psychiatrist the possible use of nonstimulant medications

87 A 12-year-old boy presents to the clinic for evaluation of a thyroid mass. Neck ultrasonography identified a 3.5 × 2.6 × 3-cm nodule in his left thyroid lobe that was predominantly solid with internal vascular flow. A smaller 2.2 × 1.9 × 2-cm isoechoic nodule was observed in the lower pole of the same lobe. He underwent FNA of both nodules. The lower nodule had benign cytology. The larger nodule was reported as follicular lesion of unclear significance.

Which of the following is the best recommendation for this patient?
- A. Recommend left lobectomy
- B. Recommend total thyroidectomy
- C. Reassure the family that the patient most likely has thyroid adenomas
- D. Repeat neck ultrasonography in 6 months
- E. Repeat ultrasound-guided FNA and perform molecular genetic testing

88 You are evaluating a child with almond-shaped eyes, small hands, and a triangular mouth. Her BMI is at the 99th percentile. Genetic testing reveals maternal uniparental disomy of chromosome 15.

Which of the following is most likely associated with her weight gain?
- A. A molecularly based insensitivity to leptin
- B. Underdevelopment of the central melanocortin system
- C. Resistance to a pituitary hormone
- D. Overproduction of cortisol
- E. Overproduction of a gut-derived hormone

89 You are called to the pediatric intensive care unit to evaluate a 7-year-old boy who was admitted with left-sided hemiparesis after suffering a basal ganglion hemorrhage. He has an elevated blood pressure of 185/128 mm Hg. The parents report that he has been complaining of headaches and blurry vision. The patient's father has untreated mild hypertension.

Laboratory test results:
   Sodium = 139 mEq/L (136-144 mEq/L) (SI: 139 mmol/L [136-144 mmol/L])
   Potassium = 2.0 mEq/L (3.2-5.2 mEq/L) (SI: 2.0 mmol/L [3.2-5.2 mmol/L])
   Bicarbonate = 33 mEq/L (22-32 mEq/L) (SI: 33 mmol/L [22-32 mmol/L])
   Serum urea nitrogen = 14 mg/dL (8-20 mg/dL) (SI: 5.0 mmol/L [2.9-7.1 mmol/L])
   Creatinine = 0.7 mg/dL (0.2-1.0 mg/dL) (SI: 61.9 µmol/L [17.7-88.4 µmol/L])

On physical examination, he is a frail-appearing boy whose height and weight are at the 1st percentile for age. His skin findings are normal. He has no axillary odor or hair. He has Tanner stage 1 pubic hair and 2-mL testes bilaterally.

Additional laboratory test results:
   Aldosterone = 2.2 ng/dL (4-48 ng/dL) (SI: 61 pmol/L [111-1332 pmol/L])
   Plasma renin activity = 0.1 ng/mL per h (0.3-3.0 ng/mL per h)
   Cortisol = 15 µg/dL (5-21 µg/dL) (SI: 414 nmol/L [138-579 nmol/L])
   17-Hydroxyprogesterone = 25 ng/dL (<83 ng/dL) (SI: 0.78 nmol/L [<2.5 nmol/L])
   17-Hydroxypregnenolone = 45 ng/dL (10-186 ng/dL) (SI: 1.35 nmol/L [0.30-5.60 nmol/L])
   Androstenedione = 18 ng/dL (<10-17 ng/dL) (SI: 0.63 nmol/L [<0.35-0.59 nmol/L])
   Testosterone = 5 ng/dL (<2.5-10.0 ng/dL) (SI: 0.17 nmol/L [<0.09-0.35 nmol/L])
   Deoxycorticosterone = 5 ng/dL (2-19 ng/dL) (SI: 0.15 nmol/L [0.06-0.57 nmol/L])

Which of the following genes is most likely to harbor a pathogenic variant?
   A. *HSD11B2* (11β-hydroxysteroid dehydrogenase type 2 causing apparent mineralocorticoid excess)
   B. *CYP11B1* (11β-hydroxylase deficiency)
   C. *CYP17A1* (17α-hydroxylase/17,20-lyase deficiency)
   D. Chimeric *CYP11B2/CYP11B1* gene (glucocorticoid remediable aldosteronism)
   E. *PRKAR1A* (Carney complex)

90 You are seeing a 4-month-old female infant for transfer of care. She was born at 39 weeks' gestation with a birth weight of 7 lb 8 oz (3401 g). Newborn screening (sample collected at 24 hours of life) documented a TSH value greater than 500 mIU/L. Confirmatory serum testing reported a TSH value of 382 mIU/L (0.5-5.0 mIU/L) and a free T$_4$ value of 0.32 ng/dL (0.8-1.8 ng/dL) (SI: 4.1 pmol/L [10.30-23.17 pmol/L]). Her knee bone age was delayed, and additional diagnostic evaluation confirmed athyreosis. Levothyroxine, 50 mcg daily (15 mcg/kg per day), was initiated.
   The following measurements were obtained over the next several months:

Measurement	Age			
	2 Weeks	1 Month	2 Months	3 Months
TSH	4.7 mIU/L	14.6 mIU/L	0 mIU/L	0.2 mIU/L
Free T$_4$	2.3 ng/dL (29.6 pmol/L)	1.9 ng/dL (24.5 pmol/L)	3.1 ng/dL (39.9 pmol/L)	1.8 ng/dL (23.2 pmol/L)
Treatment	Levothyroxine, 50 mcg daily	Levothyroxine increased to 62.5 mcg daily	Levothyroxine decreased to 50 mcg daily	Levothyroxine, 50 mcg daily

Her parents state that they are still administering levothyroxine, 50 mcg daily, with good adherence. They report that no changes were made in treatment at a visit 1 month ago with their previous physician, and they indicate that she has been doing well, gaining weight, and meeting all her developmental milestones.

On physical examination, her vital signs are normal. Weight and length are at the 50th percentile.

Laboratory tests obtained today document a TSH value of 2.1 mIU/L and a free T_4 value of 1.6 ng/dL (21.0 pmol/L).

Her parents are concerned about the length of time she has been hyperthyroid and ask about possible adverse effects of treatment.

You counsel the parents that their child is at most risk to have which of the following?
   A. Craniosynostosis
   B. Attention deficit/hyperactivity disorder
   C. Decreased bone density
   D. Intelligence quotient <90
   E. Accelerated skeletal maturation

91 You are called by an orthopedic surgeon to consult on a 13-year-old boy with McCune-Albright syndrome. The patient has been followed in your clinic for several years for management of polyostotic fibrous dysplasia, hyperthyroidism, and FGF-23–mediated hypophosphatemia. You saw him 2 months ago, at which point you decreased his methimazole dosage and continued his current dosages of phosphorus and calcitriol.

The patient presented to orthopedic surgery clinic for a postoperative evaluation 1 week after undergoing elective bilateral femoral rod placement. At that time, he reported nausea, vomiting, and fatigue.

You recommend laboratory evaluation, which documents the following results:
   Calcium = 11.9 mg/dL (7.6-10.4 mg/dL) (SI: 3.0 mmol/L [1.9-2.6 mmol/L])
   Phosphate = 3.3 mg/dL (4.0-5.5 mg/dL) (SI: 1.1 mmol/L [1.3-7.8 mmol/L])
   PTH = 9 pg/mL (16-87 pg/mL) (SI: 9 ng/L [16-87 ng/L])
   TSH = 0.13 mIU/L (0.45-4.50 mIU/L)
   Total T_3 = 210 ng/dL (80-180 ng/dL) (SI: 3.2 nmol/L [1.2-2.8 nmol/L])

Which of the following actions would have been most appropriate to prevent the development of hypercalcemia?
   A. Optimizing hyperthyroidism management before surgery
   B. Discontinuing calcitriol and phosphate before surgery
   C. Encouraging ambulation within 24 hours after surgery
   D. Postponing elective surgery until completion of skeletal growth
   E. Prescribing bisphosphonate treatment before surgery to decrease activity of fibrous dysplasia lesions

92 A 5-year-old boy presents to your clinic for evaluation of obesity. The growth curve (*see image*) from his primary care physician reveals that he had a normal birth weight and began gaining excess weight at approximately 1 year of age. His current BMI is at the 99th percentile.

His mother, who is also obese, reports that he has been in early intervention services because of developmental delay. She says that he has been healthy overall, although she has noticed that he has recently been stumbling and tripping more. Also, she intended to bring him to an ophthalmologist because he has been insisting on getting closer to objects that he is viewing.

On physical examination, he has mild ataxia and a stretched penis length of 3 cm (normal 4-7 cm) with Tanner stage 1 pubic hair and 1-mL testes bilaterally.

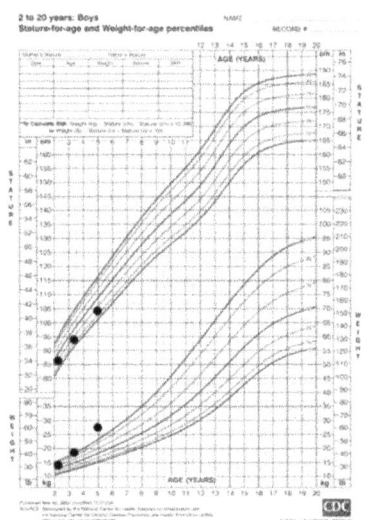

For which of the following conditions are you most likely to order genetic testing?
A. Prader-Willi syndrome
B. Neurofibromatosis type 2
C. Angelman syndrome
D. Bardet-Biedl syndrome
E. Carpenter syndrome

93 An 11-month-old infant born at 41 weeks' gestation via emergent cesarean delivery because of fetal distress has been admitted to the hospital for evaluation of continued poor growth, recent weight loss, and developmental delay.

Since birth, he has had difficulty feeding and gaining weight. His mother previously met with a lactation consultant to improve her breast milk supply and feeding technique. Formula was also used to supplement breastfeeding. He takes no medications. Between 2 and 7 months of age, his feeding improved, and he was gaining weight well. However, between 8 and 10 months of age, he had 2 episodes of respiratory illness, his appetite decreased significantly, and he lost 2.2 lb (1 kg) in 1 month. He has been delayed in achieving developmental milestones.

Laboratory test results:

Sodium = 134 mEq/L (136-142 mEq/L) (SI: 134 mmol/L [136-142 mmol/L])
Potassium = 4.4 mEq/L (4.1-5.3 mEq/L) (SI: 4.4 mmol/L [4.1-5.3 mmol/L]
Chloride = 100 mEq/L (96-106 mEq/L) (SI: 100 mmol/L [96-106 mmol/L])
Bicarbonate = 24 mEq/L (21-28 mEq/L) (SI: 24 mmol/L [21-28 mmol/L])
Serum urea nitrogen = 33 mg/dL (8-23 mg/dL) (SI: 11.8 mmol/L [2.9-8.2 mmol/L])
Creatinine = 0.72 mg/dL (0.7-1.3 mg/dL) (SI: 63.6 μmol/L [61.9-114.9 μmol/L])
Glucose = 84 mg/dL (70-99 mg/dL) (SI: 4.7 mmol/L [3.9-5.5 mmol/L])
Calcium = 14.9 mg/dL (8.2-10.2 mg/dL) (SI: 3.7 mmol/L [2.1-2.6 mmol/L])
Magnesium = 2.3 mg/dL (1.5-2.3 mg/dL) (SI: 0.9 mmol/L [0.6-0.9 mmol/L])
Phosphate = 4.1 mg/dL (4.0-6.5 mg/dL) (SI: 1.3 mmol/L [1.3-2.1 mmol/L])
25-Hydroxyvitamin D = 30 ng/mL (30-80 ng/mL [optimal]) (SI: 74.9 nmol/L [62.4-199.7 nmol/L])
1,25-Dihydroxyvitamin D = 20 pg/mL (16-65 pg/mL) (SI: 52.0 pmol/L [41.6-169.0 pmol/L])
PTH = 7 pg/mL (10-65 pg/mL) (SI: 7 ng/L [10-65 ng/L])
Liver function, normal
Thyroid function, normal

Which of the following is the best next step to diagnose this patient's condition?
A. Fluorescent in situ hybridization probe for the *ELN* gene (elastin)
B. Fluorescent in situ hybridization probe for chromosome 15q11.2-q13 deletion
C. Fluorescent in situ hybridization probe for 22q11.2 deletion
D. DNA methylation analysis of the *H19/IGF2* region of chromosome 11p15
E. Sweat chloride test for cystic fibrosis

94 A 10-year-old boy is referred for rapid weight gain of 30 lb (13.6 kg) over the past 6 months, especially noted in his face. His mother also reports that he has grown more slowly than he has in the past. His cheeks are often flushed and he has stretch marks on his upper arms and legs. His mood changes very rapidly, and he often loses his temper. He takes no medications.

On physical examination, his blood pressure is 116/77 mm Hg (blood pressure percentiles are 93% systolic and 93% diastolic based on 2000 NHANES data) and pulse rate is 109 beats/min. His height is 53 in (134.8 cm) (20th percentile; Z-score, –0.86), weight is 141.1 lb (64 kg) (99th percentile; Z-score, 2.50), and BMI is 35.22 kg/m^2. He is an obese boy with moon facies, his cheeks are flushed, and there are faint striae in the axillae and on the thighs. Pubic hair is Tanner stage 2, and testes are prepubertal. His midparental height is at the 50th percentile.

Laboratory test results:

Hemoglobin = 15.4 g/dL (11.5-15.5 g/dL) (SI: 154 g/L [115-155 g/L])

Hemoglobin A_{1c} = 5.4% (4.0%-5.6%) (36 mmol/mol [20-38 mmol/mol])

TSH = 2.3 mIU/L (0.5-5.0 mIU/L)

Urinary free cortisol = 235 µg/24 h (4-50 µg/24 h) (SI: 648.6 nmol/d [11-138 nmol/d])

A low-dose dexamethasone suppression test is performed followed by a high-dose dexamethasone suppression test.

Measurement	Baseline (8 AM)	Low-Dose Dexamethasone	High-Dose Dexamethasone
ACTH	42 pg/mL (9.2 pmol/L)	36 pg/mL (7.9 pmol/L)	30 pg/mL (6.6 pmol/L)
Cortisol	27 µg/dL (744.9 nmol/L)	13 µg/dL (358.6 nmol/L)	16 µg/dL (441.4 nmol/L)

This patient's disorder is characterized by the primary overproduction of a hormone that acts via which type of receptor?

A. G-protein–coupled membrane receptor

B. Transforming growth factor β receptor

C. Tyrosine kinase receptor

D. Cytokine receptor

E. Nuclear receptor

95 The family of a 4-year-old boy with salt-wasting congenital adrenal hyperplasia seeks a second opinion. His parents are concerned because he just had his first bone age assessment (interpreted to be 8 years). He takes liquid hydrocortisone, 2 mg/mL, at a dosage of 3.5 mg in the morning, 2 mg in the afternoon, and 6 mg at bedtime (16.4 mg/m^2; his body surface area is 0.7 m^2). He also takes 9α-fludrocortisone, 0.1 mg tablet in the morning. The patient's adrenal control has fluctuated quite a bit, and his 17-hydroxyprogesterone level has ranged from 50 ng/dL (1.5 nmol/L) to 7800 ng/dL (236.3 nmol/L) over the past 2 years, although most measurements have been elevated. His goal 17-hydroxyprogesterone range is between 200 and 1000 ng/dL (6.1-30.3 nmol/L). He has had frequent dosage adjustments of hydrocortisone. His parents have recently started to note that he has axillary odor, but he has no acne, pubic hair, or axillary hair. His growth rate over the last year has been 9.1 cm/y. His parents report that he is occasionally tired and has been hospitalized 4 times with vomiting that required intravenous hydrocortisone treatment and intravenous hydration.

Which of the following is the most likely reason for this patient's advanced bone age?

A. Suboptimal prescribed hydrocortisone dosage

B. Use of liquid hydrocortisone

C. Nonadherence to treatment regimen

D. Need for a higher hydrocortisone dose in the morning

E. Suboptimal prescribed fludrocortisone dosage

96 A 12-and-11/12-year-old boy is referred for evaluation of short stature, low body weight, and absence of pubertal development. Six months ago, his family came to the United States as part of a refugee program that provides protection to victims of domestic violence. He was a full-term baby born by vaginal delivery. His birth weight was 6 lb 4.5 oz (2850 g), and birth length was 18.9 in (48 cm). His mother breastfed him for 1 month before transitioning him to cow's milk. He reportedly had appropriate weight gain for the first 6 months of life, after which his weight gain slowed significantly. At age 6 months, he had a 2-month admission in a rural hospital for pneumonia and prolonged respiratory illness. He has never been diagnosed with a chronic illness. He started walking at age 2 years, but his other developmental milestones were met at appropriate ages. Frequent antibiotic therapy in infancy was associated with dental issues and early loss of primary teeth. Before coming to the United

States, the patient lived in a very stressful environment, as he was a victim of domestic violence by an abusive parent.

His mother's height is 56 in (143 cm) and weight is 110 lb (50 kg). She has no known medical issues. His father's height is reportedly 67 in (170 cm), and his weight is unknown. His health status is unknown. The patient has 2 half-siblings (different father).

On physical examination, the patient's height is 52.2 in (132.7 cm) (<3rd percentile; SDS, –3.00), weight is 59 lb (26.8 kg) (<3rd percentile; SDS, –3.24), and BMI is 15.22 kg/m² (4th percentile; SDS, –1.79). His blood pressure is 92/55 mm Hg, and pulse rate is 65 beats/min. He has no dysmorphic facial features. He has dark skin but no birth marks. Findings on cardiopulmonary and abdominal examinations are normal. He has no limb length discrepancy. There is no shortening of metacarpals. Pubic hair and genitalia are Tanner stage 1. Testicular volume is 1 to 2 mL bilaterally. He has no axillary hair. On oral examination, he has 6 teeth in each quadrant.

Bone age is interpreted to be 11 years and 0 months at a chronologic age of 12 years and 11 months. Predicted adult height according to the Bayley-Pinneau tables is 63.5 in (161.2 cm), which falls within the target height range based on parental heights. Target height is 64.6 ± 3.9 in (164 cm ± 10 cm).

Laboratory test results:
TSH = 1.34 mIU/L (0.70-5.70 mIU/L)
Free T$_4$ = 1.31 ng/dL (0.89-1.78 ng/dL) (SI: 16.9 pmol/L [11.5-22.9 pmol/L])
IGFBP-3 = 5.10 mg/L (1.73-5.11 mg/L)
IGF-1 (by LC-MS/MS) = 101 ng/mL (105-350 ng/mL) (SI: 13.2 nmol/L [13.8-45.9 nmol/L]) (IGF-1 Z-score, –1.8)
Hemoglobin = 10.1 g/dL (13.5-17.5 g/dL) (SI: 101 g/L [135-175 g/L])
Hematocrit = 31% (37.0%-49.0%) (SI: 0.31 [0.37-0.49])
Mean corpuscular volume = 62.5 μm³ (78.0-98.0 μm³) (SI: 62.5 fL [78.0-98.0 fL])
Erythrocyte sedimentation rate (automated) = 25 mm/h (0-20 mm/h)
C-reactive protein = <2.9 mg/L (0.8-7.6 mg/L) (SI: 27.6 nmol/L [7.6-72.4 nmol/L])
IgA = 165 mg/dL (40-218 mg/dL)
Tissue transglutaminase antibody IgA = <0.5 U/mL (<15.0 U/mL)
Albumin = 3.6 g/dL (3.8-5.4 g/dL) (SI: 36 g/L [38-54 g/L])

Which of the following sets of diagnoses most likely explains this patient's short stature?
A. Familial short stature, celiac disease, pseudohypoparathyroidism
B. Crohn disease, psychosocial dwarfism, Russell-Silver syndrome
C. GH deficiency, malnutrition, Crohn disease
D. Familial short stature, iron deficiency, psychosocial dwarfism
E. Celiac disease, constitutional delay, hypothyroidism

97 A 15-year-old girl with a 3-year history of type 1 diabetes mellitus and no other notable medical history presents with mild diffuse abdominal pain, increased thirst, increased urine output, and elevated blood glucose levels, confirming that she is in diabetic ketoacidosis (DKA).

She had her first episode of DKA 10 months ago, and she regularly sees a pediatric endocrinologist. Her diabetes management regimen includes multiple daily injections of basal and bolus insulin. She admits to occasionally missing insulin doses. After the first DKA episode, her parents increased supervision of daily diabetes management. However, she has recently been more independent because of summer break. Her hemoglobin A$_{1c}$ levels are as follows:

Measurement	Before 1st Episode of DKA	At the Time of 1st Episode of DKA	Interval Visits	At the Time of 2nd Episode of DKA
Hemoglobin A$_{1c}$	8.4% (68 mmol/mol)	10.7% (93 mmol/mol)	7.8% (62 mmol/mol) 8.1% (65 mmol/mol) 8.3% (67 mmol/mol)	10.8% (95 mmol/mol)

The patient lives with her parents and 17-year-old sister. Her paternal grandmother, who is a retired nurse, provides after-school care. The patient receives special education support for language and learning difficulties. It is difficult to engage the patient's mother in problem-solving barriers to care. She is defensive when discussing the diabetes education needs of the family in the presence of her mother-in-law. The grandmother initiates discussion about caregiver-child communication. She states that it is often difficult to talk to the patient about diabetes tasks and blood glucose values. She describes the patient as responding to questions with anger and frustration. The patient agrees, noting that she often feels blamed for out-of-range glucose values and therefore falsifies information when asked.

Which of the following should be the first step in clinical management to avoid a third episode of DKA?
   A. Mental health referral
   B. Admission to long-term inpatient care facility
   C. Responsible adult supervision of all diabetes-related tasks
   D. Initiation of insulin pump therapy
   E. Referral to state child protection agency for medical neglect

98 A 14-year-old girl is referred for evaluation of severe acanthosis nigricans involving the neck, axillae, and groin. She is also concerned about increasing and excessive body hair. The darkening and thickening of the skin on the back of her neck has become so severe that she has been teased about it and has stopped playing soccer because she does not want to put her hair in a ponytail.

She was born at 40 weeks' gestation with a birth weight of 5 lb 2 oz (2330 g). The pregnancy was complicated by type 2 diabetes mellitus in her mother (treated with metformin). The patient's pubic hair development started at age 6 years, breast development started at age 9 years, and she underwent menarche at age 11 years. Menses were initially regular and then became irregular and infrequent. She reports being less physically active, having a depressed mood, and gaining weight.

On physical examination, her height is at the 40th percentile, weight is at the 98th percentile, and BMI is at the 98th percentile. She has a significant amount of hair on her face, abdomen, arms, and legs with some hair on her chest and back (Ferriman-Gallwey score of 15). She does not have acne but does have very dark, thickened skin covering the neck, groin, and axillae. Breast development and pubic hair are Tanner stage 5, and she has normal female external genitalia.

Laboratory test results:
   Testosterone = 106 ng/dL (8-60 ng/dL) (SI: 3.7 nmol/L [0.3-2.1 nmol/L])
   LH = 3.3 mIU/mL (0.5-18.0 mIU/mL) (SI: 3.3 IU/L) [0.5-18.0 IU/L])
   FSH = 4.3 mIU/mL (1.0-12.0 mIU/mL) (SI: 4.3 IU/L [1.0-12.0 IU/L])
   Estradiol = 39 pg/mL (10-300 pg/mL) (SI: 143 pmol/L [37-1101 pmol/L])
   DHEA-S = 334.8 µg/dL (67.8-328.7 µg/dL) (SI: 9.1 µmol/L [1.8-8.9 µmol/L])
   Androstenedione = 291 ng/dL (28-288 ng/dL) (SI: 10.2 nmol/L [0.98-10.1 nmol/L])
   17-Hydroxyprogesterone = 46 ng/dL (20-265 ng/dL) (SI: 1.4 nmol/L [0.6-8.0 nmol/L])
   Hemoglobin A_{1c} = 5.5% (5.0%-5.6%) (37 mmol/mol [31-38 mmol/mol])
   Glucose (fasting) = 85 mg/dL (70-99 mg/dL) (SI: 4.7 mmol/L [3.9-5.5 mmol/L])
   Insulin (fasting) = 179.3 µIU/mL (1.4-14.0 µIU/mL) (SI: 1245 pmol/L [9.7-97.0 pmol/L])
   Free T_4 = 1.17 ng/dL (0.8-1.8 ng/dL) (SI: 15.1 pmol/L [10.3-23.2 pmol/L])
   TSH = 2.92 mIU/L (0.5-5.0 mIU/mL)
   Total cholesterol = 170 mg/dL (<200 mg/dL) (SI: 4.40 mmol/L [<5.18 mmol/L])
   LDL cholesterol = 107 mg/dL (<100 mg/dL) (SI: 2.77 mmol/L [<2.59 mmol/L])
   HDL cholesterol = 27 mg/dL (>60 mg/dL) (SI: 0.70 mmol/L [>1.55 mmol/L])
   Triglycerides = 179 mg/dL (<150 mg/dL) (SI: 2.02 mmol/L [<1.70 mmol/L])

Which of the following is the most likely underlying diagnosis?
   A. Type A insulin resistance syndrome
   B. Type B insulin resistance syndrome
   C. Lawrence syndrome
   D. Polycystic ovary syndrome
   E. Alstrom syndrome

99 A 16-year-old boy presents for follow-up of poor growth and short stature. When reviewing his medical record, you note that he was seen by your colleague for an initial consultation at age 15 years. At that time, his height was 58.3 in (148 cm) (<3rd percentile; –2.6 SD) and weight was 88 lb (40 kg) (<3rd percentile; –2.1 SD). His father's height is 67.7 in (172 cm) (30th percentile, –0.5 SD), and his mother's height is 63 in (160 cm) (33rd percentile, –0.4 SD). He was born at term; birth weight was 7 lb 0.9 oz (3200 g) and birth length was 18.5 in (47 cm). Results of initial laboratory workup at age 15 years were normal except for a low IGF-1 level of 40 ng/mL (5.2 nmol/L) and an IGFBP-3 level less than 0.5 mg/L. He passed the GH-stimulation test with a peak GH level of 11 ng/mL (11 µg/L). His bone age was interpreted to be 12 and 6/12 years at a chronologic age of 15 years.

GH therapy was started 6 months ago for the indication of idiopathic short stature. His growth velocity before GH therapy was 6 cm/y, and since starting GH therapy, it has decreased to 5 cm/y. His current height is 59.7 in (152 cm) (<3rd percentile; –2.7 SD) and weight is 96.8 lb (44 kg) (<3rd percentile; –2.2 SD). His pubic hair and genitalia are Tanner stage 2 on examination today. His IGF-1 level continues to be low at 60 ng/mL (7.9 nmol/L) (reference range, 201-648 [SI: 26.3-88.9 nmol/L] for Tanner stage 2 males) despite GH therapy for 6 months.

Which of the following is this patient's most likely diagnosis?
  A. Constitutional delay of growth and puberty
  B. Complete GH insensitivity due to a pathologic variant in the GH receptor gene (*GHR*)
  C. IGF-1 deficiency due to a pathogenic variant in the IGF-1 gene (*IGF1*)
  D. IGF-1 instability due to a pathogenic variant in the acid-labile subunit gene (*IGFALS*)
  E. IGF-1 resistance due to a pathogenic variant in the IGF-1 receptor gene (*IGF1R*)

100 A 13-month-old boy is admitted to the hospital for seizure activity. He was born the full-term product of an uncomplicated pregnancy. He was formula-fed until last month and is now drinking one 8-oz bottle of milk per day. He began crawling at age 11 months and is not yet pulling to stand.

Laboratory test results:
  Calcium = 7.0 mg/dL (9.0-10.8 mg/dL) (SI: 1.8 mmol/L [2.3-2.7 mmol/L])
  Phosphate = 1.9 mg/dL (4.0-5.5 mg/dL) (SI: 0.6 mmol/L [1.3-1.8 mmol/L])
  Alkaline phosphatase = 1387 U/L (70-250 U/L) (SI: 23.2 µkat/L [1.2-4.8 µkat/L])
  25-Hydroxyvitamin D = 25 ng/mL (20-80 ng/mL) (SI: 62.4 nmol/L [49.9-199.7 nmol/L])
  PTH = 683 pg/mL (16-87 pg/mL) (SI: 683 ng/L [16-87 ng/L])
  1,25-Dihydroxyvitamin D = 84 pg/mL (24-86 pg/mL) (SI: 218.4 pmol/L [62.4-223.6 pmol/L])

Which of the following is the most likely diagnosis?
  A. Pseudohypoparathyroidism
  B. Hereditary vitamin D–resistant rickets
  C. Dietary calcium deficiency
  D. FGF-23–mediated hypophosphatemia
  E. 1α-Hydroxylase deficiency

PEDIATRIC ENDOCRINE SELF-ASSESSMENT PROGRAM 2019-2020

Part II

1 **ANSWER: A) Aluminum toxicity**

Patients receiving long-term parenteral nutrition are at high risk for fractures due to metabolic bone disease. The etiology of bone disease in these patients is multifactorial and incompletely understood. Early reports of fractures and bone pain in patients receiving long-term parenteral nutrition are now thought to be primarily related to aluminum toxicity (Answer A), resulting from exposure to casein hydrolysates that contained high concentrations of aluminum in early parenteral nutrition solutions. In aluminum toxicity, exposure to high serum levels leads to incorporation of aluminum into the skeleton, resulting in impaired mineralization and osteomalacia. Newer formulations of parenteral nutrition have substantially reduced aluminum exposure by replacing casein hydrolysates with crystalline amino acids, which contain very little aluminum. However, aluminum exposure remains an ongoing problem in parenteral nutrition due to contamination of component products, including calcium gluconate and phosphate salts. Byproducts from the manufacturing process are another source of contamination, during which aluminum leaches from autoclaved glass vials. Since 2000, the US FDA has required manufacturers to label the aluminum content of parenteral nutrition solutions and has recommended limiting daily exposure to 4 to 5 mcg/kg. However, several studies have shown this recommendation is not feasible in neonates and children when using currently available parenteral nutrition solutions, most of which exceed these limits between 3- and 12-fold. Patients with suspected aluminum toxicity should be screened with serum aluminum levels.

Selenium is a trace element that has an essential role in immune function and various enzymatic processes. Patients receiving long-term parenteral nutrition require preparations that include selenium. Selenium deficiency (Answer B) may increase risk for cardiovascular disease and other conditions involving oxidative stress; however, it is not associated with metabolic bone disease.

Administration of adequate calcium and phosphorus in parenteral nutrition is essential to promote bone mineralization. Calcium and phosphorus should be administered in a 1:1 molar ratio to optimize mineral use. Premature infants have relatively high requirements for both calcium and phosphorus in comparison to children and adolescents. Administration of adequate mineral content to this population may be limited by the solubility of calcium and phosphorus in parenteral nutrition solutions, which frequently contributes to metabolic bone disease of prematurity. Given the relatively lower calcium and phosphorus requirements for children and adolescents, delivery of these nutrients in parenteral nutrition solutions is less likely to be impaired (thus, Answer C is incorrect).

Parenteral nutrition may be associated with metabolic acidosis (not alkalosis [Answer D]) through multiple mechanisms, including increased acid load, metabolism of amino acids, and disruption of carbohydrate and lipid metabolism. Metabolic acidosis promotes osteoclast activity and increases bone resorption, placing patients at increased risk for metabolic bone disease. Patients receiving long-term parenteral nutrition should be monitored for the development of metabolic acidosis, and may require adjustment of parenteral nutrition solution with the addition of acetate or other basic components.

Protein content of parenteral nutrition should be individualized on the basis of age, body weight, and illness severity. Acute stress factors such as trauma, surgery, sepsis, and burns increase protein requirements. While protein content should be evaluated in this patient to ensure it is sufficient to meet her nutritional needs, protein deficiency (Answer E) is a less common contributor to metabolic bone disease in stable patients receiving long-term parenteral nutrition.

Educational Objective

Diagnose aluminum toxicity that may occur with parenteral nutrition in neonates, and explain how osteopenia can occur with parenteral nutrition.

Reference(s)

Poole RL, Pieroni KP, Gaskari S, Dixon TK, Park K, Kerner JA Jr. Aluminum in pediatric parenteral nutrition products: measured versus labeled content. *J Pediatr Pharmacol Ther.* 2011;16(2):92-97. PMID: 22477831

Hamilton C, Seidner DL. Metabolic bone disease in the patient on long term parenteral nutrition. *Pract Gastroenterol.* 2008;58:18-32.

2 **ANSWER: D) Amiodarone-induced decreased conversion of T_4 to T_3**

Amiodarone is a potent antiarrhythmic medication used to treat life-threatening cardiac disease. Within the cardiac myocyte, amiodarone's actions are believed to be primarily related to its functioning as a potassium channel blocker. The endocrine adverse effects of amiodarone are mostly targeted at the thyroid secondary to the high iodine content of the medication (iodine comprises approximately 37%). The most commonly reported adverse effects of amiodarone are hypothyroidism and thyrotoxicosis, with the incidence of these disorders related to the iodine status of the population; amiodarone-induced thyrotoxicosis is more common than amiodarone-induced hypothyroidism in iodine-replete communities. In adults, amiodarone-induced hypothyroidism typically occurs 3 to 6 months after initiation of amiodarone when there is a failure to escape the Wolff-Chaikoff effect—iodine-induced decreased expression of the sodium-iodine symporter and thyroid peroxidase. Amiodarone-induced thyrotoxicosis is also associated with chronic use and it may be secondary to iodine-induced excessive thyroid hormone production (type I amiodarone-induced thyrotoxicosis) or destructive thyroiditis (type II amiodarone-induced thyrotoxicosis).

In addition to the direct effect of amiodarone on thyroid hormone synthesis and the thyroid gland itself, amiodarone may be associated with acute effects on thyroid hormone metabolism and transport within the first weeks after initiation of medication. Amiodarone strongly inhibits T_3 and T_4 entry into cells and decreases binding of T_3 to its nuclear receptor. In addition, amiodarone inhibits 5′-monodeiodination of T_4, resulting in decreased intrapituitary T_3 concentrations (type II deiodination; D2), as well as decreased peripheral conversion of T_4 to T_3 in the liver (type I deiodination; D1). The structures and interrelationships between the principal iodothyronines activated or inactivated by the selenodeiodinases are shown (*see figure*).

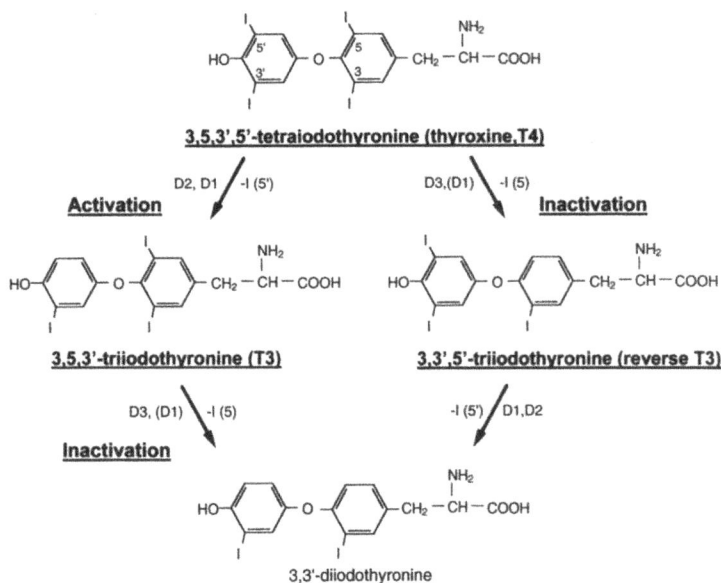

Reprinted from Bianco AC, Salvatore D, Gereben B, Berry MJ, Larsen PR. Biochemistry, cellular and molecular biology, and physiological roles of iodothyronine selenodeiodinases. *Endo Rev.* 2002;23(1):38-39.

The sum of these effects is reflected in the patient's laboratory values at time point #1 and 1 week later where the increase in TSH was secondary to reduced concentration of T_3 in the pituitary and the relative increase in serum T_4 was due to decreased peripheral conversion of T_4 to T_3 (inhibition of D1) (thus, Answer D is correct). The elevated reverse T_3 is caused by an amiodarone-induced decrease in renal clearance of reverse T_3, not from increased D3 activity, and the increase in reverse T_3 has no impact on TSH secretion (thus, Answers B and E are incorrect). These changes in thyroid hormone metabolism and transport are transient and most commonly resolve without treatment. The potential negative impact of reduced T_3 levels and reduced binding of T_3 to its nuclear receptor in the CNS of a developing child is not known.

Amiodarone-induced hypothyroidism (Answer A) typically occurs 3 to 6 months after initiation of treatment and is associated with low T_4 and elevated TSH. All patients who are acutely ill may have nonthyroidal illness (Answer C); however, the most common changes in thyroid values are an increase in reverse T_3 but with a low T_3 level associated with nonelevation in TSH. Free T_4 and total T_4 may be high, normal, or low.

Educational Objective
Describe the effect of amiodarone on thyroid hormone metabolism and transport.

Reference(s)

Loh K. Amiodarone-induced thyroid disorders: a clinical review. *Postgrad Med J.* 2000;76(893):133-140. PMID: 10684321

Martino E, Bartalena L, Bogazzi F, Braverman LE. The effects of amiodarone on the thyroid. *Endocr Rev.* 2001;22(2):240-254. PMID: 11294826

Bianco AC, Salvatore D, Gereben B, Berry MJ, Larsen PR. Biochemistry, cellular and molecular biology, and physiological roles of iodothyronine selenodeiodinases. *Endo Rev.* 2002;23(1):38-39. PMID: 11844744

3 ANSWER: D) GH-binding protein measurement

The pertinent findings in this case are marked small stature with preservation of weight and head circumference, a history of a relatively normal birth size, mild neonatal hypoglycemia, very low IGF-1 and IGFBP-3 levels, and an elevated GH level. These findings are consistent with GH insensitivity syndrome, also known as Laron dwarfism.

GH is a peptide hormone that is synthesized and secreted by the pituitary gland in response to stimulation from GHRH produced by the hypothalamus. GHRH stimulates GH, and somatostatin inhibits GH. GHRH and somatostatin act in conjunction to maintain adequate levels of GH in the blood. About half of circulating GH is bound to GH-binding protein, which protects it from metabolic clearance and provides a mechanism for transport to target tissues. GH binds to protein receptors on cell surfaces, primarily the liver hepatocytes. The GH receptor is composed of 3 domains: the extracellular domain, to which the GH molecule binds, the transmembrane domain that anchors the receptor in the cell membrane, and the intracellular domain that interacts with proteins of the intracellular signaling pathway. The extracellular domain of the membrane-bound GH receptor is also believed to be the source of GH-binding protein, resulting from proteolytic cleavage of the extracellular domain of the receptor. GH insensitivity syndrome was first reported in 1966 in a boy with marked short stature and the appearance of classic GH deficiency, with increased adiposity, frontal bossing, midfacial hypoplasia, and hypoglycemia. Subsequently, more than 50 genetic defects (variable exon deletions, missense mutations, splice mutations) of the GH receptor causing GH insensitivity syndrome have been described. In patients with GH receptor defects leading to GH insensitivity syndrome, GH-binding protein levels are typically low. Thus, measuring GH-binding protein (Answer D) is the best test to do now.

Achondroplasia is caused by autosomal dominant pathogenic variants in the gene encoding the fibroblast growth factor receptor 3 (*FGFR3*) and is the most common form of dwarfism in humans. A skeletal survey (Answer A) would reveal limb shortening with proximal segments affected disproportionately. Children with achondroplasia have short stature, frontal bossing, and midfacial hypoplasia. However, GH, IGF-1, and IGFBP-3 levels are normal. Thus, a skeletal survey is unnecessary in this case.

Endogenous Cushing syndrome or Cushing disease is a rare cause of linear growth failure in children and occurs even more rarely in infancy. The hallmark of this disorder in children is growth retardation or growth arrest with preservation of weight or weight gain. Urinary free cortisol levels (Answer B) are elevated in Cushing syndrome. GH levels can be low, but IGF-1 and IGFBP-3 levels are typically normal in Cushing syndrome.

This infant has many features of classic congenital GH deficiency. MRI may show a small anterior pituitary gland and an ectopic posterior pituitary gland in congenital GH deficiency. Although IGF-1 and IGFBP-3 levels would be low in this setting, the GH level would not be elevated as in this case. Thus, MRI of the pituitary and hypothalamus (Answer C) is incorrect.

The short stature seen in Turner syndrome is due to haploinsufficiency of the *SHOX* gene located in the pseudoautosomal region of the X chromosome. The growth failure in Turner syndrome does not usually present at such an early age, and hypoglycemia is not a feature of this disorder. The GH-IGF-1 axis is normal in Turner syndrome, so karyotype analysis (Answer E) is incorrect.

Educational Objective
Explain the relationship between plasma GH-binding protein concentrations and GH insensitivity syndrome.

Reference(s)
Savage MO, Attie KM, David A, Metherell LA, Clark AJ, Camacho-Hübner C. Endocrine assessment, molecular characterization and treatment of growth hormone insensitivity disorders. *Nat Clin Pract Endocrinol Metab.* 2006;2(7):395-407. PMID: 16932322

4 ANSWER: B) Relative excess insulin and exercise

This 16-year-old boy with longstanding type 1 diabetes mellitus had a severe nocturnal hypoglycemia event. He has a history of frequent mild-to-moderate asymptomatic hypoglycemia and very tightly controlled hemoglobin A_{1c}.

Hypoglycemia in diabetes is defined as mild (54 mg/dL > glucose <70 mg/dL [3.0 mmol/L > glucose < 3.9 mmol/L]), moderate (<54 mg/dL [<3.0 mmol/L]), and severe (<54 mg/dL [<3.0 mmol/L] *with* altered mental and or physical status). It typically results from the interplay of relative or absolute insulin excess and compromised physiologic and behavioral defenses against a falling plasma glucose. Thus, although all of the listed options could contribute to the occurrence of hypoglycemia, relative excess insulin and exercise (Answer B) is the most likely cause because he administered extra insulin, exercised, was in a hot tub (which increases insulin absorption), and was asleep (thus, eliminating the behavioral defense).

Loss of glucagon secretion due to loss of intra-islet insulin secretion (Answer C), the 4 to 6 episodes of moderate hypoglycemia the week before (Answer D), and hypoglycemia-associated autonomic failure (Answer E) are associated with a higher risk of developing severe hypoglycemia. Simply increasing the insulin glargine dosage (Answer A) a few days ago is unlikely to be the cause.

Normal physiologic steps in the prevention of hypoglycemia are incremental decreases in insulin secretion that occur when the glucose is falling to less than 80 mg/dL (<4.4 mmol/L), but this is lost in patients with diabetes taking insulin or insulin secretogogues. Next, there is an incremental increase in glucagon secretion, which is in part mediated by intra-islet insulin secretion, and this is also lost in patients with diabetes who have insulin deficiency (both type 1 diabetes and type 2 diabetes in the insulin-dependent stage). The next defense is the elevation of epinephrine, which stimulates glycogen release and generates symptoms (neurogenic) such as sweating, pallor, and hunger. These symptoms trigger the behavioral response of eating. This epinephrine response becomes attenuated with recent antecedent hypoglycemia, prior exercise, and sleep. The attenuated sympathetic neural response increases the risk of hypoglycemia by 25-fold and leads to hypoglycemia-associated autonomic failure, which itself further increases the risk of severe hypoglycemia 6-fold. In patients with diabetes, this causes a vicious cycle of frequent mild hypoglycemia leading to factors associated with severe hypoglycemia; in this 16-year-old boy's case, it culminated in a hypoglycemic seizure due to insulin excess and the inability to sense it and react to it.

If scrupulous attention is paid to preventing even mild hypoglycemia for 2 to 3 weeks, hypoglycemic awareness may return. However, there are reports that in patients with longstanding diabetes or in those with diabetic autonomic neuropathy, even post islet-cell transplant hypoglycemia-associated autonomic failure may not reverse. Finally, adrenal secretion of catecholamines can also be blunted and nonreversible.

Educational Objective
Identify factors that contribute to hypoglycemia in patients with diabetes mellitus and review how frequent hypoglycemia can cause permanent harm.

Reference(s)

Cryer PE, Axelrod L, Grossman AB, et al; Endocrine Society. Evaluation and management of adult hypoglycemic disorders: an Endocrine Society Clinical Practice Guideline. *J Clin Endocrinol Metab*. 2009;94(3):709-728. PMID: 19088155

Cryer PE. Mechanisms of hypoglycemia-associated autonomic failure in diabetes. *N Engl J Med*. 2013;369(4):362-372. PMID: 23883381

5 **ANSWER: B) She may develop neurologic manifestations but likely no adrenal manifestations**
The boy in this vignette has X-linked adrenoleukodystrophy (ALD), a peroxisomal disorder that can affect the adrenal cortex, nervous system, and testicular function. There are multiple phenotypes. The childhood cerebral form of ALD is a progressive condition that initially presents with behavioral changes such as attention deficit and hyperactivity followed by decline in school performance, dementia, unsteady gait, hemiparesis or quadriparesis, and seizures. Adrenal insufficiency is present in most, but not all patients. Symptoms typically onset around 4 to 8 years of age. This patient has neurologic findings, with white matter changes typical of the disorder, as well as adrenal insufficiency. He is quite young, hence he has the childhood cerebral form. Other forms include:

- Adolescent ALD, which presents similarly to the childhood form, just later in life and with slower progression
- Adrenomyeloneuropathy, which presents in adulthood with progressive spastic paraparesis, sphincter dysfunction, sexual dysfunction, and depression, with most patients also having adrenal insufficiency
- Adult cerebral ALD, which presents with dementia, behavioral disturbances, and focal neurologic deficits without preceding adrenomyeloneuropathy
- Adrenal insufficiency only

ALD is caused by pathogenic variants in the *ABCD1* gene, which encodes the ALD protein, an ATP-binding cassette protein transporter that is responsible for the transport of very long-chain fatty acids (VLCFAs) across the peroxisome membrane. When the ALD protein is defective, VLCFAs cannot be transported properly, which leads to their accumulation. This in turn causes cell membrane disruption and induction of oxidative stress and apoptosis, leading to cerebral ALD and adrenomyeloneuropathy. VLCFA accumulation directly in the adrenal cortex (mostly in the zona reticularis and zona fasciculata) and Leydig cells leads to adrenal and testicular dysfunction.

Because the disorder is inherited in an X-linked manner, when the mother is a mutation carrier, a male fetus has a 50% chance of inheriting the mutation and being affected with the disorder. The phenotype is variable, however, with no clear genotype-phenotype correlation, and it has been reported to vary within the same family with the same mutation. Likewise, when the mother is a mutation carrier, a female fetus has a 50% chance of inheriting the mutation. Most females carrying an *ABCD1* pathogenic variant go on to develop neurologic manifestations that resemble those observed in adrenomyeloneuropathy, yet the onset of symptoms occurs later in life and with manifestations that are less severe than in males (Answer B). About 65% of women develop neurologic manifestations by age 60 years. The parents cannot be told with complete certainty that the baby will remain asymptomatic (Answer A). Adrenal manifestations (Answers C and D) are exceedingly rare, affecting less than 1% of carrier women. Affected female patients have not been reported to develop adrenal tumors (Answer E).

Educational Objective
Counsel patients regarding the mode of inheritance of X-linked adrenoleukodystrophy and the clinical presentation in males and females.

Reference(s)
Burtman E, Regelmann MO. Endocrine dysfunction in X-linked adrenoleukodystrophy. *Endocrinol Metab Clin North Am.* 2016;45(2):295-309. PMID: 27241966

Kemp S, Huffnagel IC, Linthorst GE, Wanders RJ, Engelen M. Adrenoleukodystrophy - neuroendocrine pathogenesis and redefinition of natural history. *Nat Rev Endocrinol.* 2016;12(10):606-615. PMID: 27312864

6 **ANSWER: B) Maternal uniparental disomy of chromosome 15**

A methylation defect in the imprinted region on chromosome 15q11 is the most common cause of Prader-Willi syndrome. However, maternal uniparental disomy of chromosome 15 (Answer B), when 2 copies of the maternally expressed genes are present, is another etiology. A number of maternally expressed genes are silenced due to imprinting. Maternal uniparental disomy of chromosome 15 is more common in women of advanced maternal age. Children with Prader-Willi syndrome have small, almond-shaped eyes, small hands and feet, and hypogonadism leading to small genitals. Affected persons tend to have failure to thrive early in life followed by excessive weight gain expected to occur by age 8 years.

The caloric intake, metabolism, and food response vary by nutritional phase in children with Prader-Willi syndrome. In phase 1a, they have failure to thrive with poor caloric intake. In phase 1b, they begin to eat and gain weight normally. In phase 2a, they begin to gain weight despite no change in caloric intake. In phase 2b, they begin to gain weight due to an increase in caloric intake and are focused on food, but are still able to be sated. In phase 3, they are hyperphagic and are unable to be sated. In phase 4, their appetite is insatiable and they can become aggressive related to food access. The clinical characteristics of this child are consistent with a diagnosis of Prader-Willi syndrome.

Genetic abnormalities causing Russell-Silver syndrome include a methylation defect on chromosome 11p15.5 in 65% of cases (Answer C) and maternal uniparental disomy of chromosome 7 in 10% (Answer E). Children with Russell-Silver syndrome have short stature related to early failure to thrive, but do not later develop severe obesity. Affected individuals also have an increased frequency of relative macrocephaly with frontal bossing, a triangular-shaped face, limb asymmetry, and dental crowding. These features are not seen in the described child. Beckwith-Wiedemann syndrome is characterized by postnatal overgrowth, exomphalos, macroglossia, linear ear creases, and hemihypertrophy and is caused by mutation or deletion of imprinted genes in the chromosome region 11p15.5, particularly the *CDKN1C* gene. This child does not have features of Beckwith-Wiedemann syndrome (thus, Answer E is incorrect for this reason as well).

Proprotein convertase is an enzyme involved in the processing of numerous peptide hormones during the secretory process. Substrates of proprotein convertase include proinsulin, pro-opiomelanocortin, proglucagon, progastrin, and pro-oxytocin leading to lower levels of insulin, melanocyte-stimulating hormone, oxytocin, glucagon, gastrin, and ACTH. Proprotein convertase deficiency results in the inability to cleave these substrates, leading to hypocortisolism, red hair, and obesity. These clinical manifestations are due to lack of cleavage of pro-opiomelanocortin into functional melanocyte-stimulating hormone and ACTH. Proprotein convertase has numerous substrates that are known to be involved in energy homeostasis, including pro-opiomelanocortin, Agouti-related peptide, cholecystokinin, and glucagonlike peptide 1. However, the disrupted pro-opiomelanocortin processing in the hypothalamus most likely has a role in the development of obesity due to reduced melanocortin signaling in the hypothalamus. Children with proprotein convertase deficiency do not have failure to thrive (thus, Answer D is incorrect). In this vignette, the red hair is a red herring.

Children with homozygous mutations in the *MC4R* gene (melanocortin 4 receptor) (Answer A) have severe obesity from an early age. They do not have failure to thrive.

Educational Objective
Diagnose Prader-Willi syndrome on the basis of clinical characteristics and history and describe the underlying genetic etiology.

Reference(s)

Netchine I, Rossignol S, Dufourg MN, et al. 11p15 imprinting center region 1 loss of methylation is a common and specific cause of typical Russell-Silver syndrome: clinical scoring system and epigenetic-phenotypic correlations [published correction appears in *J Clin Endocrinol Metab*. 2007;92(11):4305]. *J Clin Endocrinol Metab*. 2007;92(8):3148-3154. PMID: 17504900

Miller JL. Approach to the child with Prader-Willi syndrome. *J Clin Endocrinol Metab*. 2012;97(11):3837-3844. PMID: 23129592

Farooqi IS, Volders K, Stanhope R, et al. Hyperphagia and early-onset obesity due to a novel homozygous missense mutation in prohormone convertase 1/3. *J Clin Endocrinol Metab*. 2007;92(9):3369-3373. PMID: 17595246

Mason K, Page L, Balikcioglu PG. Screening for hormonal, monogenic, and syndromic disorders in obese infants and children. *Pediatr Ann*. 2014;43(9):e218-e224. PMID: 25198446

Farooqi IS. Monogenic human obesity. *Front Horm Res*. 2008;36:1-11. PMID: 18230891

7 ANSWER: A) Three-day dietary history

While excessive weight gain is usually the result of exogenous forces of excessive food intake in the setting of low physical activity, it can be a warning sign of underlying endocrine causes such as severe hypothyroidism or Cushing syndrome. These causes of obesity share common features, but also have characteristics that help distinguish among underlying etiologies. This adolescent girl has findings that can be seen in patients with either Cushing syndrome or exogenous obesity. Because the treatment of endogenous Cushing syndrome is removal of the causative tumor (with the potential for significant complications), it is important to be cautious in making this diagnosis.

While a dorsocervical fat pad (sometimes called a "buffalo hump") is seen in patients with Cushing syndrome, it also occurs in the setting of marked obesity. Rapid weight gain can be associated with stretching of skin leading to pink-colored striae, which is in contrast to purple, tortuous striae typically associated with Cushing syndrome.

During periods of childhood marked by linear growth, a lack of linear growth is a critical feature distinguishing Cushing syndrome from exogenous obesity. Cortisol has a suppressive effect on linear growth due to suppression of osteoblastogenesis and stimulation of apoptosis of osteoblasts. However, this patient appears to have had early puberty, with menarche by age 10 years and a likely physiologic cessation of puberty at age 12 years. She continued gaining weight over this time frame, which supports the idea that the weight gain was not linked to growth suppression during her period of linear growth. Her lack of growth now would be expected from her timing of puberty and would not be supportive of a diagnosis of Cushing syndrome.

Diagnostic studies to evaluate for Cushing syndrome include:

- Measurement of 24-hour urinary free cortisol
- Measurement of midnight salivary free cortisol
- Low-dose dexamethasone suppression test (Answer B)
- Adrenal CT (Answer D)
- Pituitary MRI (Answer E)

In this patient's case, the 24-hour urinary free cortisol excretion was in the upper normal range, in contrast to findings in individuals with Cushing syndrome who typically have levels approximately 2-fold above the upper normal limit. If she had had an abnormal urinary free cortisol measurement, proceeding with one of the other laboratory tests listed above (Answers B, C, D, and E) would have been indicated.

"Pseudo-Cushing syndrome" is sometimes used to describe elevated cortisol associated with other underlying diseases such as depression. This should be included in the differential diagnosis of a patient with a clinical presentation suggestive of Cushing syndrome, even in the presence of abnormal laboratory testing. When this is suspected, one can perform a dexamethasone corticotropin-releasing hormone test (Answer C) in which corticotropin-releasing hormone is administered to assess for appropriate increases in ACTH and cortisol. This would not be necessary for the current patient, given that her 24-hour urinary cortisol excretion is in the normal range.

This patient most likely has exogenous obesity. While this is difficult to treat in any setting, beginning with an assessment of food intake (Answer A) is a reasonable start.

Educational Objective
Distinguish Cushing syndrome from exogenous obesity.

Reference(s)

Mushtaq T, Ahmed SF. The impact of corticosteroids on growth and bone health. *Arch Dis Child.* 2002;87(2):93-96. PMID: 12138051

Findling JW, Raff H. Diagnosis of endocrine disease: differentiation of pathologic/neoplastic hypercortisolism (Cushing's syndrome) from physiologic/non-neoplastic hypercortisolism (formerly known as pseudo-Cushing's syndrome). *Eur J Endocrinol.* 2017;176(5):R205-R216. PMID: 28179447

8 **ANSWER: E) Below midparental target height because of the duration of hypothyroidism before treatment**
This patient has had longstanding hypothyroidism as evidenced by her delayed bone age 1 year after diagnosis. Although her bone age is delayed and she has not yet entered puberty, children with severe, longstanding hypothyroidism have only partial catch-up growth (thus, Answers A, B, and C are incorrect). Final adult height will most likely be compromised, and this has been associated with longer duration of hypothyroidism before treatment (Answer E).

Although children with hypothyroidism may have rapid progressing puberty, this can also occur in children who are not hypothyroid and it does not occur in all hypothyroid children. The deficit in adult height observed in children with longstanding hypothyroidism also affects those who do not have rapidly progressing puberty (thus, Answer D is incorrect).

The loss of final adult height seems to be associated with the height deficit that occurs before diagnosis, and it is related to bone maturation that exceeds the rate of skeletal growth. This has been noted to occur within the first 18 months of treatment. Faster bone maturation is observed regardless of whether patients start puberty, and the mechanism is not well understood. Some hypotheses have been postulated, including overtreatment and rapid replacement with thyroid hormone, a direct effect of hypothyroidism reducing the potential for catch-up growth, and sex steroids during puberty exerting a limiting effect on final height.

Although no evidence-based data are available, most pediatric endocrinologists start replacement at a small dosage and gradually increase the dosage until thyroid function is normalized. This approach is applied because of the theoretical benefit of minimizing rapid maturation of growth plates. In addition, this approach has been associated with a decreased risk for pseudotumor cerebri (idiopathic intracranial hypertension) when initiating thyroid hormone replacement in severely hypothyroid patients.

Attempts have been made to improve final adult height in pediatric patients with severe, longstanding hypothyroidism by initiating GnRH analogues at the onset of puberty, as well as growth-promoting agents; however, the benefit of these approaches is still debated.

Educational Objective
Predict the effect that longstanding acquired hypothyroidism may have on final height.

Reference(s)

Rivkees SA, Bode HH, Crawford JD. Long-term growth in juvenile acquired hypothyroidism: the failure to achieve normal adult stature. *N Engl J Med.* 1988; 318(10):599-602. PMID: 3344006

Quintos JB, Salas M. Use of growth hormone and gonadotropin releasing hormone agonist in addition to L-thyroxine to attain normal adult height in two patients with severe Hashimoto's thyroiditis. *J Pediatr Endocrinol Metab.* 2005;18(5):515-521. PMID: 15921183

Nebesio TD, Wise MD, Perkins SM, Eugster EA. Does clinical management impact height potential in children with severe acquired hypothyroidism? *J Pediatr Endocrinol Metab.* 2011;24(11-12):893-896. PMID: 22308838

9 ANSWER: B) Placental insufficiency

Intrauterine growth retardation or small-for-gestational-age is a condition with multiple potential etiologies:

- Maternal factors such as inadequate nutrition, chronic maternal diseases, birth order, multiple births, and parental genetic factors
- Placental pathology, mainly placental vascular damage that may lead to placental insufficiency (often found in maternal diseases such as preeclampsia and thrombophilia)
- Intrauterine infections
- Specific fetal syndromes, including chromosomal aberrations
- Nonclassified causes such as adolescent pregnancy; maternal cigarette smoking, substance abuse, and alcohol use; prolonged living at high altitudes; and severe malnutrition

Placental insufficiency (Answer B) causes a reduction in fetal insulin concentrations and subsequent hyperglycemia. Several studies have shown a reduction in β-cell volume in patients with intrauterine growth retardation. The mechanism of the reduced insulin secretion continues to be studied. Animal studies evaluating elevated fetal catecholamines (due to low oxygen concentrations from placental insufficiency) suggest an association. The hypothesis purports that sustained high catecholamine concentrations produce developmental adaptations in pancreatic β cells that impair fetal insulin secretion. Elevated catecholamines can be the explanation for maintenance of a normal fetal basal metabolic rate despite low fetal insulin and glucose concentrations while suppressing fetal growth.

Insulin resistance (Answer D) and its association with type 2 diabetes in children and adults with a history of intrauterine growth retardation has been a topic of intense investigation. However, the usual cause of hyperglycemia in neonates with intrauterine growth retardation is primarily insulin insufficiency rather than resistance. Research investigating insulin resistance in muscles suggests that it can contribute to hyperglycemia in the cachectic neonate, but it does not appear to be the primary cause.

Although hyperthyroidism (Answer C) is a cause of intrauterine growth retardation, it would be unlikely in a newborn with a normal heart rate.

Cortisol excess (Answer E) in newborns is extremely rare. Cushing syndrome in infants is usually due to adrenocortical tumors. Older affected patients have linear growth failure and obesity and are unlikely to present at birth.

Hypopituitarism (Answer A) generally does not present with intrauterine growth retardation, but usually presents with hypoglycemia due to insufficient cortisol and GH.

Educational Objective

Describe the hormonal mechanisms that contribute to growth restriction in small-for-gestational-age newborns.

Reference(s)

Gatford KL, Simmons RA. Prenatal programming of insulin secretion in intrauterine growth restriction. *Clin Obstet Gynecol.* 2013;56(3):520-528. PMID: 23820120

Terauchi Y, Kubota N, Tamemoto H, et al. Insulin effect during embryogenesis determines fetal growth: a possible molecular link between birth weight and susceptibility to type 2 diabetes. *Diabetes.* 2000;49(1):82-86. PMID: 10615953

10

ANSWER: B) *NKX2-1* **(formerly** *TITF1***) (NK2 homeobox 1)**

Disclaimer: the goal of the following explanation is to remind the reader of genetic causes of clinical associations between congenital hypothyroidism with pathogenic variants that may affect development of other organs and be inherited, most commonly, in an autosomal dominant pattern.

Epithelial thyroid follicular cells simultaneously express 4 transcription factors that are critical for thyroid gland formation, migration, expression of thyroid-specific proteins (sodium iodide symporter, thyroglobulin, TSH receptor, DUOX1, and DUOXA2, and thyroperoxidase). Several of these transcription factors are also expressed during development of non-thyroid organs resulting in a combination of development malformations and/or dysfunction in patients with an inherited or de novo mutation (*see table*).

Gene	Chromosomal Localization	OMIM #	Phenotype
NKX2-1	14q13	610978	Choreoathetosis and congenital hypothyroidism with or without pulmonary dysfunction (brain-lung-thyroid syndrome): benign hereditary chorea and ataxia, infant respiratory distress syndrome, and thyroid dysgenesis or agenesis
PAX8	2q12-14	218700	Thyroid hypoplasia or ectopia, urogenital tract abnormalities
FOXE1	9q22	241850	Thyroid dysgenesis or agenesis, cleft palate, choanal atresia, spiky hair (autosomal recessive)
NKX2-5	5q34	600584	Ectopic thyroid, heart disease
TSHR	14q31	275200	Thyroid hypoplasia (autosomal recessive or autosomal dominant)
SLC26A4	7q31	601843	Thyroid agenesis, goiter secondary dyshormonogenesis, sensorineural hearing loss/enlarged vestibular aquaduct

NKX2-1 (Answer B) is expressed in the brain (basal ganglia), lung, and thyroid with pathogenic variants either associated with single-organ disease (neurologic phenotype is the most common single-organ disease) or with the complete triad known as brain-lung-thyroid syndrome (OMIM #610978). The neurologic sequelae include hypotonia, motor delay, and benign hereditary chorea, with up to 20% of patients having structural CNS malformations, including agenesis of the corpus callosum and holoprosencephaly. The lung disease may include fatal infant respiratory distress syndrome, pulmonary fibrosis, or a less severe phenotype associated with recurrent respiratory infections. Thyroid dysfunction correlates with the degree of thyroid gland dysgenesis; patients with near or complete agenesis present with profound congenital hypothyroidism, and patients with mild gland hypoplasia may have only mild elevations in TSH with normal T_4 levels (compensated hypothyroidism). Thus, for patients who do not present with congenital hypothyroidism, thyroid ultrasonography can be performed to assess the size and location of the thyroid followed by annual thyroid function testing surveillance. Mild dysmorphisms, such as micrognathia and hypertelorism, may also be present.

Brain-lung-thyroid syndrome is typically inherited in an autosomal dominant manner. De novo mutations are common, constituting up to 60% of cases. Clinically, up to 50% of affected patients develop the complete triad of the syndrome, 30% are affected with the neurologic and thyroid phenotype, 40% have only pulmonary disease, and 10% have the isolated neurologic phenotype. There is a weak association between pathogenic variants in *NKX2-1* and thyroid cancer. Current opinion suggests that physical examination is adequate for surveillance with follow-up thyroid ultrasonography if any concerns are found on physical exam.

The remaining pathogenic variants associated with multiorgan disease are shown in the table. With the exception of *FOXE1*, these syndromes are inherited in an autosomal dominant manner.

Educational Objective

Describe the molecular etiology of thyroid dysgenesis syndromes and how the clinical phenotype predicts the underlying pathogenic variant.

Reference(s)

Shetty VB, Kiraly-Borri C, Lamont P, Bikker H, Choong CS. NKX2-1 mutations in brain-lung-thyroid syndrome: a case series of four patients. *J Pediatr Endocr Metab*. 2014;27(3-4):373-378. PMID: 24129101

Kharbanda M, Hermanns P, Jones J, Pohlenz J, Horrocks I, Donaldson M. A further case of brain-lung-thyroid syndrome with deletion proximal to NKX2-1. *Eur J Med Genet*. 2017;60(5):257-260. PMID: 28286255

Fernandez LP, Lopez-Martinez A, Santisteban P. Thyroid transcription factors in development, differentiation and disease. *Nat Rev Endocrinol*. 2015;11(1):29-42. PMID: 25350068

11

ANSWER: D) Antimullerian hormone

With advances in modern assisted reproductive techniques, specifically the advent of fertility preservation, there is increasing likelihood that some young women diagnosed with Turner syndrome will have the potential of future fertility. As per the most recent guidelines, cardiac clearance should be obtained for women contemplating pregnancy. Early identification of potential fertility will be a mainstay of fertility preservation. Biochemical and radiographic indicators appear to be the best early markers of future fertility, and an algorithm has been developed for evaluation of such patients.

In addition to sex steroids, the gonads produce a series of nonsteroidal peptides that are important mediators of sexual development, gonadotropin regulation, and germ-cell maturation. Members of the transforming growth factor β superfamily—activin, inhibin, and mullerian inhibitory substance (also known as antimullerian hormone)—are glycoprotein hormones that have been characterized in both normal and aberrant states. As assays for these substances have been developed and standardized, they are routinely being used in clinical practice.

Antimullerian hormone (Answer D) currently appears to be the best marker of ovarian reserve because it decreases over time as ovarian reserve is depleted. Hence, along with antral follicle count on ultrasonography, antimullerian hormone is used as a basis for reproductive endocrinologists to initiate discussions about maintaining future fertility and possible early intervention geared towards fertility preservation. Antimullerian hormone has been detected at a higher rate in girls and young women with a 45,X/46,XX karyotype than in those with a classic 45,X karyotype. This hormone has been noted to decrease over time, from childhood through adolescence, and ultimately may be a trigger for intervention in late childhood. Current data suggest that an antimullerian hormone value greater than 2 ng/mL in a prepubertal girl speaks to the presence of ovarian reserve.

The inhibin B level (Answer A) reflects the number of activated small follicles in the early follicular phase, as well as the presence of a dominant follicle, and it inversely correlates with FSH levels, as it inhibits FSH production. While it correlates with current ovarian function, it is less reflective than antimullerian hormone of future reserve.

Although FSH (Answer B) is usually elevated and estradiol (Answer C) is usually low in girls and women with ovarian failure, neither is sufficiently sensitive nor specific to predict fertility potential in many cases.

Follistatin (Answer E) is an activin-binding protein important in ovarian folliculogenesis, but it does not have clinical utility in prediction of fertility.

Educational Objective

Explain the role of measuring gonadal peptides in predicting future fertility in girls with ovarian failure.

Reference(s)

McNeilly AS. Diagnostic applications for inhibin and activins. *Mol Cell Endocrinol.* 2012;359(1-2):121-125. PMID: 21741437

Oktay K, Bedoschi G, Berkowitz K, et al. Fertility preservation in women with Turner syndrome: a comprehensive review and practical guidelines. *J Pediatr Adolesc Gynecol.* 2016;29(5):409-416. PMID: 26485320

Gravholt CH, Andersen NH, Conway CS, et al. Clinical practice guidelines for the care of girls and women with Turner syndrome: proceedings from the 2016 Cincinnati International Turner Syndrome Meeting. *Eur J Endocrinol.* 2017;177(3):G1-G70. PMID: 28705803

12

ANSWER: D) Increased calcium requirements due to rapid skeletal mineralization

Hypocalcemia is a common complication of parathyroid surgery, and it may arise from several etiologies. In this adolescent with longstanding hyperparathyroidism and resultant bone disease, hypocalcemia is most likely the result of extensive skeletal remineralization (Answer D), otherwise known as "hungry bone syndrome." Patients with hungry bone syndrome typically require vigorous calcium supplementation to support remineralization, which may persist for weeks or months. This patient has several factors placing her at risk for hungry bone syndrome, including very elevated preoperative alkaline phosphatase, calcium, and PTH levels, a large parathyroid adenoma (>5 cm), and osteitis fibrosa cystica. Also known as "brown tumors," these focal areas of increased osteoclast activity are classically associated with hyperparathyroidism. In addition to hungry bone syndrome, suppression of nonadenomatous parathyroid tissue through longstanding hyperparathyroidism may potentially cause or contribute to hypocalcemia in this patient.

Damage or removal of the parathyroid glands during surgery may result in either transient or permanent hypoparathyroidism. This patient's hyperparathyroidism was due to an ectopic gland in the mediastinum; therefore, damage to the normally located parathyroid glands (Answer A) is unlikely.

Calcitonin lowers blood calcium levels by suppressing osteoclast activity and is a relatively weak agent with a therapeutic window limited to 48 hours. While preoperative administration of calcitonin in this patient was appropriate, the effects (Answer B) are unlikely to persist into the postoperative period.

Isotonic saline is an important initial step in the management of hypercalcemia because it promotes urinary calcium excretion and corrects volume depletion from hypercalcemia-induced salt wasting. In adolescents with severe hypercalcemia who have normal cardiac and renal function, normal saline infusion rates between 2 and 3 times maintenance are typically effective and well tolerated (thus, Answer E is incorrect).

Vitamin D deficiency (Answer C) impairs absorption of dietary calcium; however, given this patient's mild decrease in 25-hydroxyvitamin D, this is unlikely to be a significant contributor to her hypocalcemia.

Educational Objective

Identify the biochemical profile consistent with hungry bone syndrome after parathyroidectomy for severe hyperparathyroidism.

Reference(s)

Witteveen JE, van Thiel S, Romijn JA, Hamdy NA. Hungry bone syndrome: still a challenge in the post-operative management of primary hyperparathyroidism: a systematic review of the literature. *Eur J Endocrinol.* 2013;168(3):R45-R53. PMID: 23152439

Marcocci C, Cetani F. Primary hyperparathyroidism [published correction appears in *N Engl J Med.* 2012;366(22):2138]. *N Engl J Med.* 2011;365(25):2389-2397. PMID: 22187986

13 **ANSWER: A) Most affected: IGF-1; moderately affected: IGFBP-3; least affected: IGF-2**

IGF-1, IGF-2, and IGFBP-3 are excellent markers of GH levels. Serum IGF-1 is the most GH-dependent and is usually used as a screening tool for GH levels. IGFBP-3 is next most likely factor to be affected by GH deficiency, followed by IGF-2 (thus, Answer A is correct and Answers B, C, D, and E are incorrect). IGF-1 levels are, however, age-dependent, and in younger children they may not reflect GH status as well as IGFBP-3, which is age-independent. IGF-2 is age-independent and adult levels are often reached by 1 year of age.

IGF-1's primary role is to mediate the effects of GH. Primarily produced in the liver, IGF-1 is known to stimulate growth in many cells of the body, especially skeletal muscle, bone, and liver, and to contribute to overall body growth. When produced in the periphery by connective tissues such as bone, muscle, and cartilage, IGF-1 can have both autocrine and paracrine effects on that tissue or surrounding tissue.

IGFBP-3 is the most abundant plasma IGFBP, and it carries IGF proteins in the bloodstream to target areas in a complex with acid-labile subunit. Other hormones besides GH, such as testosterone, estrogen, and T_4, also regulate IGFBP-3 synthesis. IGFBP-3 levels are reduced in the presence of deficiencies in sex steroids and T_4. It is produced in multiple tissues, in addition to hepatocytes, and its gene is located on chromosome 7.

In early life, the primary role of IGF-2 is to promote growth in gestation, and it is involved in the development of fetal pancreatic β cells. It works through the IGF-1 receptor preferentially and is carried by IGF-binding proteins. The *IGF2* gene is located on chromosome 11 and is expressed through imprinting, with the paternal allele being active. IGF-2 is the most abundant IGF in adults and its role in oncogenesis has been studied extensively. IGF-2 binds to IGFBP-6, which appears to act as a suppressor of its effects.

In a consensus statement on the diagnosis and treatment of children with idiopathic short stature, IGF-1 measurement is recommended in the initial screening, but IGFBP-3 measurement is not recommended except in children younger than 3 years. IGF-2 is not recommended for evaluation of growth and is currently used in research settings, mostly in adults and in cancer research.

Educational Objective

Explain the effects of growth hormone deficiency on IGF-1, IGF-2, and specific binding proteins.

Reference(s)

Cohen P, Rogol AD, Deal CL, et al; 2007 ISS Consensus Workshop participants. Consensus statement on the diagnosis and treatment of children with idiopathic short stature: a summary of the Growth Hormone Research Society, the Lawson Wilkins Pediatric Endocrine Society, and the European Society for Paediatric Endocrinology Workshop. *J Clin Endocrinol Metab.* 2008;93(11):4210-4217. PMID: 18782877

Bajpai A, Menon PS. Insulin like growth factors axis and growth disorders. *Indian J Pediatr.* 2006;73(1):67-71. PMID: 16444065

Butler AA, Le Roith D. Control of growth by the somatropic axis: growth hormone and the insulin-like growth factors have related and independent roles. *Annu Rev Physiol.* 2001;63:141-164. PMID: 11181952

14 ANSWER: C) *AQP2* (aquaporin 2)

The pertinent findings in this case are a history of marked polyuria and polydipsia (with a clear preference for water starting at about 6 months of age), slow weight gain, hypernatremia, dilute urine in the setting of increased serum osmolality, and an absent posterior pituitary bright spot, consistent with a diagnosis of diabetes insipidus. Diabetes insipidus may be caused by inadequate production of arginine vasopressin (AVP) by the posterior pituitary gland (neurohypophyseal diabetes insipidus or central diabetes insipidus), signaling defects of vasopressin in the kidneys (nephrogenic diabetes insipidus), or increased AVP degradation by placental vasopressinase during pregnancy (gestational diabetes insipidus). Rarely it may be due to suppression of AVP production after excessive amounts of fluid intake, as seen in primary polydipsia. Diabetes insipidus can be acquired or familial. Acquired forms are most often central and are due to hypothalamic or pituitary injury by tumors or infiltrating disease (eg, craniopharyngioma, Langerhans cell histiocytosis), trauma, or post surgically. Acquired nephrogenic diabetes insipidus can be due to use of a variety of medications such as lithium. Children with nephrogenic diabetes insipidus tend to present early in life.

Prepro-AVP, which consists of a signal peptide, the AVP moiety, neurophysin II (NPII), and a co-peptin, is produced by the magnocellular neurons of the supraoptic and paraventricular nuclei of the hypothalamus. These neurons project from the hypothalamus through the diaphragma sellae and form the posterior pituitary gland. Prepro-AVP undergoes proteolytic cleavage into AVP, its carrier protein NPII, and co-peptin. All 3 peptides are stored in neurosecretory granules in the posterior pituitary. AVP secretion is regulated by plasma and interstitial osmotic pressure sensed by osmoreceptors in the hypothalamus, as well as by circulating blood volume, sensed by carotid, aortic, and atrial baroreceptors. After AVP is released into the circulation, it binds to its receptor, AVPR2, on the basolateral or interstitial side of the renal collecting duct. AVPR2 is a G-protein–coupled receptor. Binding of AVP to the receptor results in activation of adenylyl cyclase, an increase in cAMP release, and activation of protein kinase. The protein kinase phosphorylates AQP2, which stimulates the translocation of subapical AQP2-containing vesicles to the apical (luminal) membrane. Water is then able to enter the apical side of the collecting duct and leave the cell to the interstitium on the basolateral side via AQP3 and AQP4 channels (*see image*).

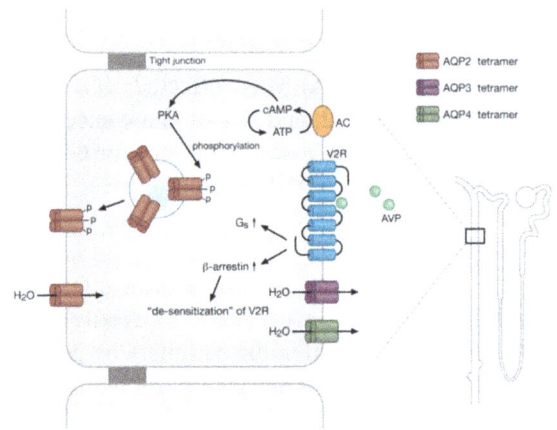

Reprinted from Moeller HB, Rittig S, Fenton RA. Nephrogenic diabetes insipidus: essential insights into the molecular background and potential therapies for treatment. *Endocr Rev.* 2013;34(2):278-301.

A serum osmolality greater than 300 mOsm/kg with a urine osmolality less than 300 mOsm/kg establishes the diagnosis of diabetes insipidus. However, often a water deprivation test is needed to diagnose diabetes insipidus. During this test, if the serum osmolality is greater than 300 mOsm/kg and the urine osmolality is less than 600 mOsm/kg, the patient has diabetes insipidus. DDAVP or vasopressin administration increases the urine concentration in neurohypophyseal diabetes insipidus, but has little to no effect in nephrogenic diabetes insipidus.

This child has nephrogenic diabetes insipidus as she had no response to vasopressin. Although absence of a posterior pituitary bright spot is usually seen in central diabetes insipidus, it can also be absent in nephrogenic diabetes insipidus presumably due to depletion of AVP stores in the vasopressinergic neurons. Homozygous or compound loss-of-function mutations in *AQP2* lead to autosomal recessive diabetes insipidus in approximately 10% of patients with nephrogenic diabetes insipidus and rarely an autosomal dominant form. The lack of response to vasopressin, the young age at presentation, and the lack of a family history of diabetes insipidus make autosomal recessive nephrogenic diabetes insipidus due to a pathogenic variant in *AQP2* (Answer C) the most likely diagnosis.

The most common form of nephrogenic diabetes insipidus is X-linked due to pathogenic variants in *AVPR2* (Answer B). This accounts for 90% of patients with familial nephrogenic diabetes insipidus. The lack of family history and the fact that girls with this form of diabetes insipidus are less likely to have such a severe phenotype make this form of nephrogenic diabetes insipidus much less likely. Familial neurohypophyseal diabetes insipidus is most frequently caused by pathogenic variants in the *AVP* gene (Answer A). Most are inherited in an autosomal dominant fashion. The AVP mutants are expressed but retained in the endoplasmic reticulum where they accumulate and are thought to lead to cell death of the vasopressinergic neurons. Familial neurohypophyseal diabetes insipidus typically presents between 1 and 6 years of age due to the gradual, progressive destruction of vasopressinergic neurons. Pathogenic variants in the *WFS1* gene (Answer D) cause Wolfram syndrome, a rare autosomal recessive disorder of central diabetes insipidus, diabetes mellitus, optic atrophy, and deafness (DIDMOAD). This child did not respond to vasopressin administration, so she therefore does not have neurohypophyseal diabetes insipidus. *HESX1* pathogenic variants (Answer E) are a rare cause of septo-optic dysplasia. This child has nephrogenic diabetes insipidus and no evidence of septo-optic dysplasia on MRI.

Educational Objective
Describe the site and mechanism of action of arginine vasopressin, V1 and V2 receptors, and aquaporin II.

Reference(s)

Schernthaner-Reiter MH, Stratakis CA, Luger A. Genetics of diabetes insipidus. *Endocrinol Metab Clin North Am.* 2017;46(2):305-334. PMID: 28476225

Moeller HB, Rittig S, Fenton RA. Nephrogenic diabetes insipidus: essential insights into the molecular background and potential therapies for treatment. *Endocr Rev.* 2013;34(2):278-301. PMID: 23360744

15 ANSWER: C) Thyroid hormone replacement

This patient has pituitary hyperplasia. The initial diagnosis was a suprasellar mass, possibly a macroadenoma; however, additional evaluation revealed severe primary hypothyroidism. Pituitary hyperplasia is reported in 25% to 81% of patients with primary hypothyroidism, usually in those who have a TSH concentration greater than 50 mIU/L. There is a positive correlation between the size of the pituitary gland and TSH levels. This patient also had hyperprolactinemia. This is a rare presentation of a common disease. Making the correct diagnosis of pituitary hyperplasia is critical because of the potential for prolonged, extremely elevated thyrotropin-releasing hormone levels. This patient developed thyrotroph and lactotroph hyperplasia in response to thyrotropin-releasing hormone stimulation, causing increased TSH and prolactin secretion. Pituitary hyperplasia secondary to hypothyroidism can present as severe hypothyroidism (usually short stature), amenorrhea/galactorrhea, or neurologic/vision problems.

Although imaging studies and the very high TSH level may lead to the diagnosis of a TSH-secreting adenoma, this kind of tumor is rare and the patient's low free T_4 level is not consistent with this diagnosis. Also, although his prolactin level is high, his TSH level is comparatively much higher and prolactinomas do not secrete TSH. Therefore, transsphenoidal resection (Answers A and E) and use of a dopamine agonist (cabergoline) (Answers B and D) are incorrect management choices.

The hyperprolactinemia in primary hypothyroidism is caused by elevated thyrotropin-releasing hormone that stimulates prolactin secretion, in addition to TSH. Also, it has been shown that T_3 decreases prolactin mRNA and that thyroid hormones are important for the clearance of prolactin from the circulation. Pituitary stalk compression and less dopamine inhibitory action may also be contributing factors to the elevated prolactin levels seen in patients with severe hypothyroidism.

Management requires thyroid hormone replacement (Answer C). Treatment with levothyroxine normalizes the size of the pituitary gland and prolactin levels. It is recommended to start at a low dosage and gradually increase the dosage to normalize thyroid function. This approach has been advocated in order to prevent increased intracranial hypertension (pseudotumor cerebri), pituitary apoplexy, empty sella syndrome due to rapid shrinkage of the pituitary gland, potentially faster maturation of the growth plates, and shorter final adult height.

This patient also has testicular enlargement, as has been described in some patients with very high TSH levels (Van Wyk-Grumbach syndrome). This is thought to be secondary to the weak intrinsic FSH activity of TSH, leading to cross-stimulation of the FSH receptor.

Educational Objective
Recommend appropriate management for a patient with pituitary hyperplasia associated with longstanding hypothyroidism.

Reference(s)

Anasti JN, Flack MR, Froehlich J, Nelson LM, Nisula BC. A potential novel mechanism for precocious puberty in juvenile hypothyroidism. *J Clin Endocrinol Metab*. 1995;80(1):276-279. PMID: 7829625

Joshi AS, Woolf PD. Pituitary hyperplasia secondary to primary hypothyroidism: a case report and review of the literature. *Pituitary*. 2005;8(2):99-103. PMID: 16195776

Larson NS, Pinsker JE. Primary hypothyroidism with growth failure and pituitary pseudotumor in a 13-year-old female: a case report. *J Med Case Rep*. 2013;7:149. PMID: 23725039

Neves CP, Massolt ET, Peeters RP, Neggers SJ, de Herder WW. Pituitary hyperplasia: an uncommon presentation of a common disease. *Endocrinol Diabetes Metab Case Rep*. 2015;2015:150056. PMID: 26279852

16 ANSWER: D) Congenital hyperinsulinism due to a pathogenic variant in the glucokinase gene (*GCK*)

This vignette represents a very tricky but classic presentation of a rare form of hyperinsulinism, which is the finding of hypoglycemia with ketosis in combination with hypoglycemia and the classic features of hyperinsulinism (ie, hypoglycemia despite increased glucose intake, short-duration hypoketotic fasting, and glycemic response to glucagon). It also reminds us that a critical sample drawn during hypoglycemia but while on intravenous dextrose should be interpreted similarly to one drawn in the fasted state.

This child had vomiting, diarrhea, very poor food intake, and dehydration with prolonged fasting. On presentation to the emergency department, he was found to have hypoglycemia with ketones. This is a normal response to a prolonged fast in a child of this age. However, when his hypoglycemia was treated with intravenous glucose, he continued to have glucose levels in the range of 50 to 60 mg/dL (2.8-3.3 mmol/L) and required a high glucose infusion rate of 10 mg/kg per min to raise his glucose above 60 mg/dL (>3.3 mmol/L). This indicates increased glucose use, which happens in the setting of hyperinsulinism. A subsequent critical sample obtained while on a glucose infusion rate of 7 mg/kg per min showed a classic hyperinsulinism pattern of low free fatty acids and ketones with measurable insulin and a positive glucagon stimulation test. Thus, idiopathic ketotic hypoglycemia (Answer B) is incorrect.

Congenital hyperinsulinism due to pathogenic variants in the glucokinase gene (*GCK*) (Answer D) can be diagnosed clinically by patterns of glucose dysregulation. Glucokinase acts as the glucose sensor of the β cell, and inactivating mutations that cause decreased activity of glucokinase cause a form of monogenic diabetes that is unresponsive to medications and does not need treatment. Conversely, activating mutations lower the threshold for glucose-stimulated insulin release. Thus, if glucose drops low enough, as occurred in the patient in this vignette, the normal process of switching off insulin secretion occurs (at a glucose level of approximately 50 to 60 mg/dL compared with when it normally does at 80 mg/dL) and normal fasting adaptation occurs. The evidence in this vignette supporting an etiology of a pathogenic variant in the *GCK* gene is as follows: the patient became ketotic when his glucose was low enough and the fasting was long enough, and at a glucose concentration of 50 mg/dL while on intravenous fluids, he was still secreting insulin and had suppressed free fatty acids and β-hydroxybutyrate production with a subsequent positive glucagon stimulation test. The insulin prevented glycogenolysis in the liver, which was overcome by glucagon.

Glycogen storage disease type 0 due to deficiency of glycogen synthetase (Answer C) is incorrect. Patients with glycogen storage disease type 0 are unable to make glycogen, so they will have postmeal hyperglycemia and lactic acidemia and fasting ketotic hypoglycemia with no glycemic response to glucagon. In addition, routine administration of glucose at 4 to 6 mg/kg per min prevents hypoglycemia.

The protein challenge showed a low glucose level at the start and no significant drop, and a random ammonia measurement was normal, making congenital hyperinsulinism due to glutamate dehydrogenase deficiency (Answer A) incorrect. In glutamate dehydrogenase hyperinsulinism, leucine inappropriately causes glutamate to be converted to α-ketoglutarate, which enters the Krebs cycle and generates ATP, which in-turn causes the K_{ATP} channels to close and stimulates insulin secretion, thus mimicking the effect of glucose-stimulated insulin release. Patients with this condition have protein sensitivity; following a 1 g per kg dose of protein, the plasma glucose typically drops by 50% and to less than 50 mg/dL (<2.8 mmol/L).

Congenital hyperinsulinism due to pathogenic variants in the K_{ATP} channel genes (*ABCC8* and *KCNJ11*) (Answer E) is more likely to present in the newborn period, to be more severe, and—no matter how long the fasting duration—the free fatty acids and β-hydroxybutyrate will always be low at the time of hypoglycemia.

Educational Objective
Clinically differentiate among different forms of hyperinsulinism.

Reference(s)
Glaser B, Kesavan P, Heyman M, et al. Familial hyperinsulinism caused by an activating glucokinase mutation. *N Engl J Med*. 1998;338(4):226-230. PMID: 9435328

Mohamed Z, Ayra VB, Hussein k. Hyperinsulinaemic hypoglycaemia: genetic mechanisms, diagnosis and management. *J Clin Res Pediatr Endocrinol*. 2012; 4(4):189-192. PMID: 23032149

17   ANSWER: E) Assessment for Y-chromosome–specific markers

Approximately 10% of girls with Turner syndrome have Y-chromosomal sequences. The risk of gonadoblastoma developing in these girls has previously been estimated at rates up to 30%; however, more recent review of the literature has revised the rate down to approximately 10% to 15%. The presence of pericentromeric Y-specific genes in the gonadoblastoma Y-specific locus of the Y chromosome (including *TSPY1*, testis-specific protein Y-linked 1) is associated with increased risk. While there is most likely more than 1 gene that confers risk, *TSPY1* is the gene that has been identified to date. Hence, assaying, via real-time PCR, for multiple Y-specific pericentromeric markers (Answer E) in the gonadoblastoma Y-specific locus is the current recommendation for evaluating the need for possible prophylactic gonadectomy. If markers are present, gonadectomy is recommended.

While the *SRY* gene (Answer A) may be present in some patients with mosaic Turner syndrome, the gene does not map in the region of the gonadoblastoma Y-specific locus, so it is not specific enough to rule out increased risk for gonadoblastoma. Although virilization, elevated testosterone (Answer C), and tumor markers (Answer B) (including α-fetoprotein and hCG) are ultimately harbingers of tumor presence, they would most likely appear later, once the tumor has already developed. Imaging (Answer D) is neither sensitive nor specific enough to surveil for possible tumor development.

Educational Objective
Explain the role of Y-chromosome–specific genes in the development of gonadoblastoma in Turner syndrome.

Reference(s)
Silveri M, Grossi A, Bassani F, Orazi C, Camassei FD, Zaccara A. Ullrich-Turner syndrome and tumor risk: is there another chance to early gonadectomy in positive TSPY and SRY patients? *Eur J Pediatr Surg*. 2016;26(3):273-276. PMID: 25978024

Kwon A, Hyun SE, Jung MK, et al. Risk of gonadoblastoma development in patients with Turner syndrome with cryptic Y chromosome material. *Horm Cancer*. 2017;8(3):166-173. PMID: 28349385

Gravholt CH, Andersen NH, Conway CS, et al. Clinical practice guidelines for the care of girls and women with Turner syndrome: proceedings from the 2016 Cincinnati International Turner Syndrome Meeting. *Eur J Endocrinol*. 2017;177(3):G1-G70. PMID: 28705803

18   ANSWER: A) DNMT3A overgrowth syndrome; pathogenic variant in the *DNMT3A* gene (DNA methyltransferase 3 alpha)

The child in this vignette has a syndrome characterized by prenatal and postnatal overgrowth. The differential diagnosis includes Sotos syndrome, Marfan syndrome, Weaver syndrome, homocystinuria, DNMT3A overgrowth syndrome, Klinefelter syndrome, and Beckwith-Wiedemann syndrome. DNMT3A overgrowth syndrome (also known as Tatton-Brown-Rahman syndrome) (Answer A) is characterized by prepubertal tall stature and a characteristic facial appearance (round face, heavy horizontal eyebrows, and narrow palpebral fissures). Scoliosis, umbilical hernia, epilepsy, intellectual disability, and atrial septal heart defects are associated features. This condition is caused by pathogenic variants in the gene encoding DNA methyltransferase 3 alpha (*DNMT3A*). *DNMT3A* is important in DNA methylation during embryogenesis and sex-dependent methylation of imprinted genes. This is the most likely diagnosis in this patient.

DNMT3A overgrowth syndrome is similar to other syndromes associated with overgrowth and intellectual disability such as Sotos and Weaver syndromes. Sotos syndrome is characterized by prepubertal tall stature, a high, broad forehead, prominent chin, and macrocephaly. This condition is caused by pathogenic variants in the histone methyltransferase gene *NSD1* (nuclear receptor-binding SET domain-containing protein 1). Weaver syndrome is characterized by tall stature, a high, broad forehead, prominent chin, large, fleshy ears, hypertelorism, and almond-shaped eyes. It is caused by pathogenic variants in the histone methyltransferase gene *EZH2* (enhancer of zeste 2 polycomb repressive complex 2 subunit). Proportional tall stature and developmental delay are present in Tatton-Brown-Rahman syndrome, Sotos syndrome, and Weaver syndrome and these features are caused by altered epigenetic regulation leading to activation of the PI3K/mTor pathway.

Marfan syndrome, caused by pathogenic variants in the *FBN1* gene (Answer B), is characterized by disproportionate tall stature (high upper-to-lower segment and arm span-to-height ratios) with pectus excavatum, upward dislocation of the lens, hyperflexibility, arachnodactyly, heart and aortic disease, and normal intelligence. Individuals with Marfan syndrome tend to have dolichocephaly and micrognathia.

Klinefelter syndrome (Answer C) is characterized by hypergonadotropic hypogonadism, small testes, gynecomastia, disproportionate tall stature (low upper-to-lower segment ratio and high arm span-to-height ratio), and learning disabilities.

Beckwith-Wiedemann syndrome (Answer D) is caused by mutation or deletion of imprinted genes in the chromosomal region 11p15.5, particularly *CDKN1C*. Affected individuals have exomphalos, macroglossia, linear ear creases, and hemihypertrophy.

Homocystinuria is caused by pathogenic variants in the *CBS* gene (Answer E) and is characterized by disproportionate tall stature, arachnodactyly, pectus excavatum, downward dislocation of the lens, and cognitive delay.

Educational Objective
Construct a differential diagnosis for overgrowth and tall stature.

Reference(s)

Tatton-Brown K, Seal S, Ruark E, et al. Mutations in the DNA methyltransferase gene DNMT3A cause an overgrowth syndrome with intellectual disability [published correction appears in *Nat Genet.* 2014;46(6):657]. *Nat Genet.* 2014;46(4):385-388. PMID: 2461470

Tatton-Brown K, Loveday G, Yost S, et al. Mutations in epigenetic regulation genes are a major cause of overgrowth with intellectual disability. *Am J Hum Genet.* 2017;100(5):725-736. PMID: 28475857

Albuquerque EV, Scalco RC, Jorge AA. Management of endocrine disease: diagnostic and therapeutic approach of tall stature. *Eur J Endocrinol.* 2017;176(6): R339-R353. PMID: 28274950

Neylon OM, Werther GA, Sabin MA. Overgrowth syndromes. *Curr Opin Pediatr.* 2012;24(4):505-511. PMID: 22705997

19 ANSWER: B) TSH measurement

Musculoskeletal symptoms occur in 30% to 80% of persons with hypothyroidism. Muscle weakness, myalgias, muscle stiffness, cramps, and exercise intolerance are common symptoms of hypothyroidism. Isolated elevation of serum creatine kinase and other muscle enzymes may also occur in hypothyroid patients, and hypothyroidism must be considered in the differential diagnosis of patients with persistently elevated creatine kinase and/or lactic dehydrogenase levels, especially because it is treatable with thyroid hormone replacement. More rarely, hypothyroidism presents as muscle enlargement (muscle pseudohypertrophy) or atrophy. Kocher described muscle hypertrophy in this setting in 1892. This syndrome was also studied by Debre and Semelaigne in 1935. Kocher-Debre-Semelaigne syndrome usually occurs in the pediatric population in patients with longstanding, moderate or severe hypothyroidism. It is characterized by increased muscle mass, usually in the calf muscles, with concomitant diminished strength. Hoffman syndrome is the adult form of hypertrophic myopathy.

In 1970, Golding described 9 patients with musculoskeletal symptoms, illustrating that generalized pain to muscles or joints is the most common complaint; however, pain may be severe and different parts may be affected at different times. Muscle cramps and paresthesias are also common symptoms.

Hypertrophy can be more severe on one side and is not always symmetric. Compartment syndrome has also been described. However, the symmetric "Herculean" appearance of patients has been the classic description of hypertrophic myopathy.

The diagnosis of hypothyroid myopathy is made in patients in whom the symptoms of muscle involvement dominate the clinical picture. T_3 is an important regulator of muscular fiber function, and it regulates numerous genes involved in the citric acid cycle and ATP synthesis. It also acts on the transcription of genes involved in muscle function, including MyoD, which is important in regulating muscle regeneration and proliferation, as well as muscle tight junctions. T_3 is also involved in muscle plasticity by influencing the expression of myosin heavy chain. Skeletal muscle fibers are classified into type 1 (slow contraction fibers) and type 2 (fast contraction fibers) depending on the expression of myosin heavy chain. Hypothyroidism causes loss and atrophy of type 2 fibers and hypertrophy of type 1 fibers.

Thyroid hormones also regulate proteins involved in the synapsis of neuromuscular transmission. In addition, T_3 regulates the metabolism of the connective tissue, including glycosaminoglycans important to form proteoglycans, which are involved in cell migration and adhesion. It is also thought that some of the changes seen in the muscles of hypothyroid patients may be secondary to denervation and myofiber necrosis. Apoptosis has not been demonstrated in hypothyroid myopathy.

Myoedema is one of the classic—and usually overlooked—signs of hypothyroid myopathy. It can be elicited either by percussion or by applying a light pressure stimulus with the thumb and index fingers, which produces a visible and palpable, nontender, hard nodule. The nodule does not spread and reaches maximal size after 1 to 2 seconds, subsiding after 5 to 10 seconds. This is due to a localized release of calcium ions and delayed uptake by the sarcoplasmic reticulum.

Thyroid dysfunction symptoms are nonspecific, so the diagnosis depends on measurement of TSH and thyroid hormone levels (Answer B). When she presented to her primary care physician, this patient had a TSH level of 150 mIU/L and a free T_4 level of 0.2 ng/dL (2.6 pmol/L). She acknowledged lack of adherence to her thyroid hormone treatment regimen. Levothyroxine was reinitiated, and her parents were instructed to supervise daily intake. Her symptoms resolved 2 weeks later, with improvement in thyroid function studies, thus confirming the diagnosis.

Although this patient could have an autoimmune myopathy or a neurologic condition, her history should raise suspicion for hypothyroid myopathy. Therefore, electromyography (Answer A) and creatine kinase measurement (Answer C) are not the best answers. Although electromyography could demonstrate changes consistent with myopathy in this patient, electrographic abnormalities are seen in only about 50% of cases. Furthermore, electromyography does not differentiate among the different types of myopathies. Documenting an elevated serum creatine kinase level may be helpful, but it is not diagnostic or specific and the concentration does not correlate with disease severity. Although autoimmune myositis is a possibility, myositis-specific autoantibody assessment (Answer D) is not the best step in this patient's evaluation but could be considered after ruling out hypothyroidism or if her symptoms do not improve with thyroid hormone replacement. MRI of the limb (Answer E) would show left muscle edema and swelling, but it would not provide information regarding the etiology of the findings or help to determine the best treatment.

Educational Objective
Describe the association between hypothyroidism and myopathy.

Reference(s)

Golding DN. Hypothyroidism presenting with musculoskeletal symptoms. *Ann Rheum Dis.* 1970;29(1):10-14. PMID: 5309049

Khaleeli AA, Griffith DG, Edwards RH. The clinical presentation of hypothyroid myopathy and its relationship to abnormalities in structure and function of skeletal muscle. *Clin Endocrinol (Oxf).* 1983;19(3):365-376. PMID: 6627693

Mastaglia FL, Ojeda VJ, Sarnat HB, Kakulas BA. Myopathies associated with hypothyroidism: a review based upon 13 cases. *Aust N Z J Med.* 1988;18(6): 799-806. PMID: 3071995

Sindoni A, Rodolico C, Pappalardo MA, Portaro S, Benvenga S. Hypothyroid myopathy: a peculiar clinical presentation of thyroid failure. Review of the literature. *Rev Endocr Metab Disord.* 2016;17(4):499-519. PMID: 27154040

Vignesh G, Balachandran K, Kamalanathan S, Hamide A. Myoedema: a clinical pointer to hypothyroid myopathy. *Indian J Endocrinol Metab.* 2013;17(2):352. PMID: 23776921

20 ANSWER: C) Has matured at an equal pace
Turner syndrome results from partial or complete absence of one X chromosome. Ovarian dysgenesis is a common finding, and the associated estrogen deficiency occurs in infancy. In healthy prepubertal girls, ovaries secrete low but measurable amounts of estradiol. It is well known that estrogen has a number of broad physiologic effects on numerous tissues. Researchers have evaluated the effects and potential benefits of introducing estrogen to prepubertal children with Turner syndrome. One of the concerns is the effect on final height as interpreted via bone age evaluations.

In a study of 120 children with Turner syndrome who received GH and either estradiol or placebo, there were no significant effects on bone age maturation by pubertal age based on whether estradiol was started at a prepubertal age or pubertal age. Therefore, Patient 1's bone age is most likely to have matured at a pace equal to that of Patient 2's bone age (thus, Answer C is correct and Answers A, B, D, and E are incorrect). Interestingly, at age 14 years, patients who were started on estradiol at a prepubertal age actually had delayed bone age readings compared with those who started estradiol at a pubertal age of 11 to 12 years, which suggests that the higher dose required to induce puberty (100 ng/kg per day) may advance the bone age faster and that the adjustments to the estradiol dosage based on bone ages had occurred at a younger age in the patients already on estradiol. In the end, there was no difference in final height predicted when comparing both groups.

However, the recent clinical practice guidelines developed by the International Turner Syndrome Consensus Group (2017) do not recommend use of very low-dosage estrogen in prepubertal girls. They note that the study cited above has not been replicated, and that the safety of this intervention has not been evaluated.

The guidelines further describe recommendations for initiation of sex steroid replacement:

- Estrogen should be started at 11 to 12 years of age to assume completion of pubertal development in 2 to 2.5 years
- Use of low-dosage transdermal estrogen is suggested; however, there are limited data to support its advantage over oral estrogen in patients with Turner syndrome
- Estrogen dosages should be increased every 6 months or so to mimic normal puberty; this schedule can be modified depending on the circumstances (may want to progress faster in patients diagnosed at an older age; may want to progress slower in patients trying to gain more height to slow down the progression of growth plate maturation)
- Transdermal patches can be fractionated (cut), although not a recommendation by the manufacturer
- An oral progestin should be added once there is breakthrough bleeding or 2 years after initiation of estrogen
- There are limited data to recommend oral vs transdermal replacement of estrogen with progesterone for long-term maintenance treatment of hypogonadism

The following are the recommended doses of estrogen formulations available in the Unites States, as reported in the clinical guidelines:

Preparation	Suggested Starting Dosage	Adult Dosage
Transdermal E2	3-7 mcg daily*	25-100 mcg daily
Micronized 17β oral E2 (E2)	0.25 mg daily	1-4 mg daily

Educational Objective
Describe the effects of low-dosage estrogen therapy on growth in patients with Turner syndrome.

Reference(s)

Gravholt CH, Andersen NH, Conway GS, et al; International Turner Syndrome Consensus Group. Clinical practice guidelines for the care of girls and women with Turner syndrome: proceedings from the 2016 Cincinnati International Turner Syndrome Meeting. *Eur J Endocrinol.* 2017;177(3):G1-G70. PMID: 28705803

Quigley CA, Wan X, Garg S, Kowal K, Cutler GB Jr, Ross JL. Effects of low-dose estrogen replacement during childhood on pubertal development and gonadotropin concentrations in patients with Turner syndrome: results of a randomized, double-blind, placebo-controlled clinical trial. *J Clin Endocrinol Metab.* 2014;99(9):E1754-E1764. PMID: 24762109

Ruszala A, Wojcik M, Zygmunt-Gorska A, Janus D, Wojtys J, Starzyk JB. Prepubertal ultra-low-dose estrogen therapy is associated with healthier lipid profile than conventional estrogen replacement for pubertal induction in adolescent girls with Turner syndrome: preliminary results. *J Endocrinol Invest.* 2017;40(8): 875-879. PMID: 28397183

21 **ANSWER: C) Adrenal CT**
The boy in this vignette presents with progressive bilateral breast development, pubic hair development, rapid linear growth, and advanced bone age. His testes are prepubertal and small. His laboratory evaluation demonstrates an elevated estradiol level and suppressed gonadotropins, and the rest of the results are normal. It is important to determine the origin of the elevated estradiol. The patient's testes are small and without palpable masses; therefore, an estrogen-producing testicular tumor, which is exceedingly rare in this age group, is unlikely

and testicular ultrasonography (Answer B) would not be the first study of choice. A prolactinoma is unlikely to cause gynecomastia, particularly in a child this young, and it would not cause rapid growth and bone age advancement, although it could suppress gonadotropins. Prolactin measurement (Answer E) is not necessary now.

When a boy has a markedly elevated estradiol level, breast development, pubic hair development, suppressed gonadotropins, and small testes, one must consider the possibility of an estrogen-producing adrenal tumor or a feminizing adrenocortical tumor. While this is the rarest of all adrenal tumors, particularly in women and children (it is most common in men), it is important to diagnose quickly because the tumor may be malignant and carry a poor prognosis. In fact, most feminizing adrenal tumors reported in the literature are carcinomas and metastases are common. Therefore, adrenal imaging (Answer C) should be the next step. Boys with a feminizing adrenocortical tumor present with bilateral breast development that can be painful, but it is not associated with galactorrhea. It is associated with estrogen-driven rapid linear growth, rapid bone age advancement, and pubic hair development. High estradiol levels suppress gonadotropin levels via negative feedback, in turn suppressing testicular testosterone and leading to smaller testicular size over time. Estrogen secretion may be mixed with cortisol and/or androgens or the tumor may be estrogen-secreting only. In this patient, estradiol is the only elevated hormone. However, it is important to rule out Cushing disease and concurrent cortisol overproduction. While his morning cortisol level is normal and he does not have any cushingoid features, hypercortisolism can be subclinical and should be excluded with further testing.

Karyotype analysis (Answer A) may be important when evaluating gynecomastia in a boy. One of the more common chromosomal abnormalities causing gynecomastia is Klinefelter syndrome; however, gynecomastia in this setting may not develop until pubertal age. In addition, while boys with Klinefelter syndrome are tall, they do not exhibit a rapid growth spurt associated with rapid skeletal maturation. Karyotype analysis could be considered, but some of the clinical features described in this patient are not consistent with Klinefelter syndrome, so it is not the most important study to obtain now.

Aromatase excess syndrome due to an autosomal dominant gain-of-function mutation in the *CYP19A1* gene is a rare disorder than can present with prepubertal or peripubertal breast development in boys accompanied by advanced bone age and gonadotropin deficiency. The presentation can be very similar to that of the patient in this vignette, and certainly genetic analysis of the *CYP19A1* gene (Answer D) should be considered. However, an adrenal tumor is a more pressing diagnosis, so adrenal imaging should be done first. Furthermore, because aromatase excess syndrome is autosomal dominant, one would expect a family history of gynecomastia in males, which is absent in this vignette.

Other causes of an elevated estradiol level in males include thyrotoxicosis due to a stimulatory effect of thyroid hormone on aromatase activity, liver disease (particularly cirrhosis), and medications and substances that contain estrogens or have an effect on endogenous estrogen production.

Educational Objective
Suspect a feminizing adrenal tumor on the basis of clinical and laboratory findings.

Reference(s)

Kidd MT, Karlin NJ, Cook CB. Feminizing adrenal neoplasms: case presentations and review of the literature. *J Clin Oncol.* 2011;29(6):e127-e130. PMID: 21115870

Fukami M, Miyado M, Nagasaki K, Shozu M, Ogata T. Aromatase excess syndrome: a rare autosomal dominant disorder leading to pre- or peri-pubertal onset gynecomastia. *Pediatr Endocrinol Rev.* 2014;11(3):298-305. PMID: 24716396

Phornphutkul C, Okubo T, Wu K. Aromatase p450 expression in a feminizing adrenal adenoma presenting as isosexual precocious puberty. *J Clin Endocrinol Metab.* 2001;86(2):649-652. PMID: 11158024

22 ANSWER: A) Obesity

Pseudotumor cerebri (also called idiopathic intracranial hypertension) is an elevation in intracranial pressure that can result in headache, blurred vision, dizziness, and nausea. Pseudotumor cerebri is diagnosed by performing a lumbar puncture and assessing opening pressure, and this procedure can also temporarily relieve symptoms. Another treatment option is acetazolamide, which causes inhibition of carbonic anhydrase, thus decreasing sodium transport across the choroid plexus. While the exact cause is not yet well understood, pseudotumor cerebri is seen most commonly in obese women of childbearing age. There has been increased incidence in the current obesity epidemic. Obesity (Answer A) is the most likely underlying cause of this patient's headaches. Use of oral contraceptive pills (Answer D) also increases risk of pseudotumor cerebri, but not as much as obesity. Retinoid cream (Answer E) is not associated with pseudotumor cerebri. Other endocrine causes include Addison disease, hypoparathyroidism, and treatment with recombinant human GH. Hypothyroidism (Answer C) is not significantly associated with pseudotumor cerebri.

Other causes of headache are also important to consider. Migraines can sometimes be associated with fluctuations in sex hormone levels, and in these cases it may be helpful to discontinue use of oral contraceptives to assess for any potential improvement. However, this patient's headaches started over the past 4 months (after 20 months of oral contraceptive use). In addition, the headaches appear to be similar during menses—a time when estrogen levels are low.

The presence of a tumor itself can also cause increased intracranial pressure and headaches, but the patient's normal MRI is reassuring, making a prolactinoma (Answer B) highly unlikely.

Educational Objective
Explain the association of obesity with an increased risk for pseudotumor cerebri.

Reference(s)

Stevenson SB. Pseudotumor cerebri: yet another reason to fight obesity. *J Pediatric Health Care.* 2008;22(1):40-43. PMID: 18174088

Chen J, Wall M. Epidemiology and risk factors for idiopathic intracranial hypertension. *Int Ophthalmol Clin.* 2014;54(1):1-11. PMID: 24296367

23 ANSWER: A) Serum calcitonin measurement

The association of constipation and peripheral neuropathy with a thyroid nodule should raise concern for multiple endocrine neoplasia type 2B. During the clinic visit, it was apparent that the patient had an elongated face compared with the appearance of his parents, as well as a prominent upper lip. On examination of his tongue, he had multiple fleshy nodules on the tip consistent with mucosal neuromas. His parents reported that he had always had limited tear production when crying. The single laboratory test that would confirm the diagnosis would be calcitonin measurement (Answer A). This child's value was markedly elevated at 6298 pg/mL (0.0-7.5 pg/mL) (SI: 1839 pmol/L [0-2.2 pmol/L]). CT with contrast of the neck, chest, and abdomen was performed for surgical staging because of the 80% risk for regional lymph node metastasis and the 15% to 20% risk of distant metastasis associated with a calcitonin value between 2000 and 10,000 pg/mL. A serum metanephrine panel was also ordered before surgery because of the nearly 50% risk for pheochromocytoma in patients with multiple endocrine neoplasia type 2B (although it is uncommon to develop a pheochromocytoma before age 11 years). *RET* gene analysis was performed and was positive for the codon 918 pathogenic variant.

Thyroglobulin measurement (Answer D) is not informative in the prediction of malignancy and may be elevated because of inflammatory conditions, such as autoimmune or infectious thyroiditis. Thyroid uptake and scan (Answer B) should be performed if the TSH level is low (<0.5 mIU/L) to assess for an autonomously functioning thyroid nodule, most commonly associated with a lower risk for malignancy. In this particular patient, the physical examination features and history were consistent with multiple endocrine neoplasia type 2B, which made calcitonin measurement a more informative option. Axial imaging of the neck (Answer C) can be used to assess for abnormal cervical lymph nodes if there is significant lymphadenopathy on physical examination and ultrasound in an effort to identify lymph nodes in locations that ultrasound has lower sensitivity in detecting (paratracheal, retropharyngeal, subclavicular, and upper mediastinum). For this particular patient without "bulky" lymphadenopathy, however, axial imaging would not be indicated. Lactate dehydrogenase measurement (Answer E), both serum and via FNA, is helpful if there is a concern for primary thyroid lymphoma, although this condition more commonly presents in the fifth to sixth decade of life, with a female predominance, and is associated with a prolonged history of Hashimoto thyroiditis.

Educational Objective
Diagnose multiple endocrine neoplasia type 2B on the basis of clinical findings and describe the association between peripheral neuropathy and this syndrome.

Reference(s)

Carney JA, Bianco AJ Jr, Sizemore GW, Hayles AB. Multiple endocrine neoplasia with skeletal manifestations. *J Bone Joint Surg Am.* 1981;63(3):405-410. PMID: 6110669

Wray CJ, Rich TA, Waguespack SG, Lee JE, Perrier ND, Evans DB. Failure to recognize multiple endocrine neoplasia 2B: more common than we think? *Ann Surg Oncol.* 2008;15(1):293-301. PMID: 17963006

Machens A, Dralle H. Biomarker-based risk stratification for previously untreated medullary thyroid cancer. *J Clin Endocrinol Metab.* 2010;95(6):2655-2663. PMID: 20339026

24 ANSWER: C) Initiate an oral contraceptive

In this patient with clinical and biochemical evidence of hyperandrogenism, as well as oligomenorrhea 2 years after menarche, the generally accepted adult criteria for polycystic ovary syndrome appear to be met. While translation of these criteria to pediatrics may still be considered a work in progress, one need not perform further laboratory or imaging evaluation (Answers A and B) before determining the next steps to address her specific symptoms.

The best therapy for an individual patient with polycystic ovary syndrome may ultimately reflect the patient's specific concerns. The approach to a teenager worried about acne and hirsutism would be quite different from the approach to a woman who presents to the reproductive endocrinologist with fertility concerns. Given that the patient in this vignette has cosmetic concerns (ie, hirsutism and acne), therapy with an oral contraceptive (Answer C), which is generally the first-line therapy in adults, is the best choice. Treatment with an oral contraceptive pill will regulate menstrual cycles, and the suppression of gonadotropin secretion can lead to less ovarian hyperandrogenism. In addition, the estrogen increases sex hormone–binding globulin, leading to a decrease in bioavailable testosterone. Finally, the progestins in some oral contraceptives may have a weak antiandrogen effect, thus decreasing terminal hair growth.

An androgen receptor antagonist such as spironolactone (Answer E) can be used together with an oral contraceptive, a combination that, in some trials, has been shown to have a decreased androgen effect. As spironolactone is a teratogen, it must be used in combination with birth control in girls and women of reproductive age.

Although insulin resistance may be present before clinical signs appear (ie, "lean" polycystic ovary syndrome), this patient does not have findings of hyperinsulinism such as acanthosis nigricans. While metformin (Answer D) increases insulin sensitivity and can improve ovulatory function, it is not a first-line treatment for signs of androgen excess, but it is indicated in women with impaired glucose tolerance or type 2 diabetes mellitus, as defined by an oral glucose tolerance test.

Educational Objective

Explain the role of oral contraceptives in the treatment of hyperandrogenism associated with polycystic ovary syndrome.

Reference(s)

Witchel SF, Oberfield S, Rosenfield RL, et al. The diagnosis of polycystic ovary syndrome during adolescence. *Horm Res Paediatr.* 2015;83:376-389. PMID: 25833060

McCartney CR, Marshal JC. Clinical practice. Polycystic ovary syndrome. *N Engl J Med.* 2016;375(1):54-64. PMID: 27406348

25 ANSWER: E) GH excess, GH deficiency, central precocious puberty, obesity/insulin resistance

Neurofibromatosis type 1 (NF 1) is an autosomal dominant disease affecting approximately 1 in 3000 to 4000 live births. It is caused by pathogenic variants in the *NF1* gene located on chromosome 17q11.2. In roughly half of cases, NF 1 is due to a de novo germline mutation. The clinical diagnosis is established according to United States National Institutes of Health guidelines. At least 2 of the following clinical features must be present to make the diagnosis:

- 6 or more café-au-lait macules (>5 mm in diameter prepuberty or >15 mm postpuberty)
- 2 or more neurofibromas or 1 plexiform neurofibroma
- Inguinal or axillary freckling
- Optic gliomas
- 2 or more Lisch nodules
- Bony lesions (eg, sphenoid dysplasia)
- First-degree relative with NF 1

Individuals with NF 1 have a lifelong increased risk of malignancy, including pheochromocytoma/paraganglioma, which is more commonly seen in adults. Rarely, intraabdominal secretory neoplasms can be present. Hypertension occurs in approximately 4% of individuals with NF 1. The hypertension is usually essential; however, it may be due to renovascular disease, as in this patient, or to pheochromocytoma. Short stature occurs in roughly one-third of individuals with NF 1. Height growth velocity is generally normal, although the pubertal growth spurt is slightly reduced. Children with NF 1 and optic gliomas that involve the optic chiasm or hypothalamus have an increased risk of multiple endocrinopathies. In a recent retrospective study of 36 children with NF 1 and optic glioma who did not receive cranial irradiation, 55.6% had at least 1 endocrinopathy during a mean follow-up of 9.1 years. Transient GH deficiency was the most common endocrinopathy and was found in 36.1% of children. Other endocrinopathies included central precocious puberty in 33.3%, obesity with insulin resistance/impaired glucose tolerance in 11.1%, transient GH excess in 5.5%, reversible ACTH deficiency in 5.5%, hypogonadotropic hypogonadism in 2.7%, and reversible thyrotropin deficiency in 2.7%. Central precocious puberty is most likely due to the tumor's location close to the hypothalamus, interfering with tonic central nervous system inhibition of the hypothalamic-pituitary-gonadal axis. Interestingly, obesity and insulin resistance were found in the patients who also had central precocious puberty or early puberty. Similarly, the GH excess is postulated to occur due to the tumor inhibiting somatostatin tone, allowing unregulated release of GH. Multiple studies suggest the GH excess is transient.

In patients with NF 1, prolactinoma (Answer C), diabetes insipidus (Answer B), hyperthyroidism (Answer A), or Cushing syndrome (Answer D) generally do not occur. The child in this vignette has pubertal levels of LH, FSH, and testosterone with an advanced bone age indicating central precocious puberty, possible GH excess with elevated IGF-1 and IGFBP-3 levels, and signs of obesity and insulin resistance (Answer E best represents this constellation of findings). The high prevalence of endocrinopathies in persons with NF 1 highlights the importance of surveillance in this patient population, especially in the setting of optic pathway tumors involving the chiasm or hypothalamus.

Educational Objective
List the endocrine disorders associated with neurofibromatosis type 1.

Reference(s)

Hersh JH; American Academy of Pediatrics Committee on Genetics. Health supervision for children with neurofibromatosis. *Pediatrics.* 2008;121(3):633-642. PMID: 18310216

Sani I, Albanese A. Endocrine long-term follow-up of children with neurofibromatosis type 1 and optic pathway glioma. *Horm Res Paediatr.* 2017;87(3):179-188. PMID: 28346917

26 **ANSWER: D) Higher proportion of subcutaneous fat than visceral fat**
The patient in this vignette has obesity by virtue of a BMI above the 95th percentile. Her high-normal waist circumference and normal waist-to-hip ratio demonstrate that while she has a high amount of body fat (thus, Answer A is incorrect), her body tends to store this as subcutaneous fat, not visceral fat. Individuals with a high waist circumference and a high waist-to-hip ratio (sometimes referred to as "apple-shaped") most commonly have a high amount of fat in their omentum and surrounding body organs. This fat is more likely to be metabolically active and associated with insulin resistance and the metabolic syndrome. Individuals with a low waist-to-hip ratio (often referred to as "pear-shaped") have a high amount of fat in their subcutaneous fat depots, including those in the gluteofemoral area. These individuals are more likely to be women and are more likely to exhibit characteristics of "healthy obesity," with a lower likelihood of insulin resistance and the metabolic syndrome. The girl in this vignette fits this phenotype and is thus more likely to have a higher proportion of subcutaneous fat than visceral fat (Answer D).

One location where visceral fat is commonly stored is in the liver, contributing to nonalcoholic fatty liver disease (Answer E). This condition is markedly more common in the setting of high visceral adiposity and less so in the setting of predominantly subcutaneous adiposity.

In addition to having an increase in fat mass, obese individuals also have more muscle and bone than normal-weight individuals (thus, Answers B and C are incorrect).

Educational Objective

Counsel families about the characteristic growth pattern and body composition of obese children.

Reference(s)

Cornier MA, Després JP, Davis N, et al. Assessing adiposity: a scientific statement from the American Heart Association. *Circulation*. 2011;124(18):1996-2019. PMID: 21947291

Freedman DS, Sherry B. The validity of BMI as an indicator of body fatness and risk among children. *Pediatrics*. 2009;124(Suppl1):S23-S34. PMID: 19720664

Dâmaso AR, do Prado WL, de Piano A, et al. Relationship between nonalcoholic fatty liver disease prevalence and visceral fat in obese adolescents. *Dig Liver Dis*. 2008;40(2):132-139. PMID: 18082476

Kwiterovich PO. Clinical and laboratory assessment of cardiovascular risk in children: guidelines for screening, evaluation, and treatment. *J Clin Lipidol*. 2008; 2(4):248-266. PMID: 21291741

Avis HJ, Vissers MN, Stein EA, et al. A systematic review and meta-analysis of statin therapy in children with familial hypercholesterolemia. *Atheroscler Thromb Vasc Biol*. 2007;27(8):1803-1810. PMID: 17569881

27 ANSWER: A) Inactivating mutation in the *NPR2* gene

Loss-of-function mutations in the *NPR2* gene (Answer A), encoding the natriuretic peptide receptor B (NPR-B), lead to short stature that may be proportionate or disproportionate. Individuals who have 1 inactivating *NPR2* mutation have been observed to have moderate short stature, sometimes with shortening of the forearms. Thus, inactivating *NPR2* mutations can cause autosomal dominant short stature, and this is the most likely cause in this child's case. He probably inherited the pathogenic variant from his mother, given her short stature. Individuals who have 2 inactivating *NPR2* mutations have acromesomelic dysplasia, Maroteaux type with severe short stature. Gain-of-function mutations in the *NPR2* gene cause tall stature associated with long fingers. The levels of C-type natriuretic peptide and its precursor NTproCNP have been shown to change during growth and in response to GH therapy.

Activating mutations in the *FGFR3* gene (not *inactivating* mutations [Answer B]) cause hypochondroplasia and achondroplasia due to downstream activation of MAP kinase pathways that reduce the proliferation and differentiation of growth plate chondrocytes. Achondroplasia and hypochondroplasia are associated with relative macrocephaly, broad forehead, and disproportionate short stature with near-normal growth of the trunk and head accompanied by short limbs leading to elevated upper-to-lower segment ratio and a short arm span. Milder cases of *FGFR3* activating mutations can be associated with relative macrocephaly and short stature without disproportion.

Cartilage-hair hypoplasia is an autosomal recessive metaphyseal dysplasia caused by homozygous pathogenic variants in the *RMRP* gene (Answer C). The *RMRP* gene is untranslated and encodes an RNA, not a protein, that is imported into the mitochondria to act as a mitochondrial RNA-processing endoribonuclease. *RMRP* pathogenic variants lead to decreased cell growth by impairing ribosomal assembly and by altering cyclin-dependent cell cycle regulation. The degree of functional impairment in vitro correlates with the severity of short stature. Cartilage-hair hypoplasia is also associated with ligamentous laxity, hypoplastic anemia, and immune deficiency.

Mucopolysaccharidosis type VI (Maroteaux-Lamy syndrome) is an autosomal recessive syndrome caused by pathogenic variants in the *ARSB* gene (Answer D), which encodes arylsulfatase B. The growth plates are abnormal in this syndrome due to accumulation of glycosaminoglycans. Short stature in this setting is related to joint abnormalities and dysostosis multiplex. This condition is also associated with corneal clouding, hepatosplenomegaly, cardiac abnormalities, and facial dysmorphism. Intelligence is usually normal.

Metaphyseal chondrodysplasia, Schmid type is caused by heterozygous pathogenic variants in *COL10A1* gene (Answer E) with an autosomal dominant inheritance pattern. This condition is associated with mild to moderate short stature, widened growth plates (especially in the femur) and bowing of the long bones. The described child does not have bowing of the limbs.

Educational Objective
Diagnose skeletal dysplasias.

Reference(s)

Wit JM, Oostdijk W, Losekoot M, van Duyvenvoorde HA, Ruivenkamp CA, Kant SG. Mechanisms in endocrinology: novel genetic causes of short stature. *Eur J Endocrinol.* 2016;174(4):R145-R173. PMID: 26578640

28 ANSWER: C) Restart methimazole at 10 to 20 mg daily (pretreating with diphenhydramine) and repeat thyroid function studies in 2 weeks

This patient presented with severe hyperthyroidism, not thyroid storm. Although she developed a mild reaction to medical treatment, she responded to methimazole, as evidenced by her improved levels, even after holding medication for 6 days. Her previous endocrinologist recommended definitive treatment. She has a strong family history of thyroid storm and her great-grandmother died during thyroidectomy. Her skin reaction to methimazole previously responded to antihistamines, and her hypertension and tachycardia are well controlled on the current dosage of β-adrenergic blocker. Her current thyroid hormone levels, although improved, still put her at high risk to develop thyroid storm if she undergoes radioactive iodine treatment.

Current guidelines addressing the management of hyperthyroidism in children and adolescents recommend starting methimazole before radioactive iodine treatment if the total T_4 concentration exceeds 20 µg/dL (>260 nmol/L) or the free T_4 concentration is higher than 5 ng/dL (>60 pmol/L), in order to decrease the risk of thyroid storm. In addition, radioactive iodine increases the risk of worsening thyroid eye disease.

In this particular patient, it is concerning that she has decreased vision in the left eye. She needs evaluation by an ophthalmologist with expertise in thyroid eye disease to determine whether the decreased vision is secondary to her thyroid eye disease or unrelated to this problem. Although patients must be advised to hold methimazole if they develop a pruritic rash, pending evaluation, the American Thyroid Association recommends the use of antihistamines for the management of mild skin reactions while continuing methimazole. If the problem persists, definitive treatment is needed. Conversely, if the rash is secondary to a severe reaction (ie, vasculitis), treatment with antithyroid medications is contraindicated.

Thus, the best course of action in this patient's management is to restart methimazole at 0.2 to 0.5 mg/kg per day (pretreating with diphenhydramine 30 minutes before administration), closely monitor her, and refer her to an ophthalmologist (Answer C). She would also benefit from consultation with a high-volume thyroid surgeon, as she will most likely need definitive treatment in the near future. Once the ophthalmologist's evaluation is complete, if definitive treatment is pursued, the goal would be to normalize the free T_4 level (or total T_4 level) before surgery. She will also need potassium iodide drops 3 times a day for 10 days before the procedure.

Referring this patient for radioactive iodine treatment within 1 to 2 weeks (Answer A) without pretreatment with antithyroid medications or ophthalmologic evaluation is not appropriate. Steroids (Answer B) are used to treat inflammatory thyroid eye disease or for patients with thyroid storm. This patient does not meet the criteria for thyroid storm and, although she has thyroid eye disease, evaluation by an ophthalmologist is needed to determine whether she has active, inflammatory eye disease that would benefit from steroids before definitive treatment. Starting steroids without completing assessment is incorrect. Potassium iodide should be started 10 days before thyroidectomy and can be used for the treatment of uncontrolled hyperthyroidism in the presence of severe reactions to antithyroid medications while planning for definitive surgical treatment. In addition to antithyroid medications, potassium iodide is also used to treat thyroid storm; however, starting potassium iodide and waiting 4 weeks to repeat thyroid function studies is incorrect as most patients usually escape the effect of iodide treatment after 2 weeks (the Wolf-Chaikoff effect). For the same reason, waiting 6 weeks after starting potassium iodide to perform thyroidectomy (Answer D) is incorrect. The use of potassium iodide or iodinated contrasts before radioactive iodine (Answer E) is contraindicated as these agents block iodine uptake, rendering treatment ineffective.

Educational Objective
Recommend appropriate management for a child with Graves disease for whom thyroidectomy is being considered.

Reference(s)

Bauer AJ. Approach to the pediatric patient with Graves' disease: when is definitive therapy warranted? *J Clin Endocrinol Metab.* 2011;96(3):580-588. PMID: 213783220

Rivkees SA, Stephenson K, Dinauer C. Adverse events associated with methimazole therapy of Graves' disease in children. *Int J Pediatr Endocrinol.* 2010;2010: 176970. PMID: 20224800

Ross DS, Burch HB, Cooper DS, et al. 2016 American Thyroid Association Guidelines for Diagnosis and Management of Hyperthyroidism and Other Causes of Thyrotoxicosis. *Thyroid.* 2016;26(10):1343-1421. PMID: 27521067

29 ANSWER: B) Intravenous calcium gluconate

Hypermagnesemia most commonly arises in the setting of (1) renal failure leading to impaired magnesium excretion and/or (2) response to a large exogenous magnesium load. This patient has severe magnesium toxicity, which was subsequently found to be the result of incorrectly prepared total parenteral nutrition. This rare iatrogenic complication has been reported in neonates, who are particularly prone to develop electrolyte disturbances given their small size and immature renal function. Other potential sources of iatrogenic hypermagnesemia include parenteral infusions in women with preterm labor, laxative abuse, magnesium enemas, and accidental ingestion of Epsom salts (magnesium sulfate).

The most common effects of hypermagnesemia are neuromuscular, arising from decreased transmission across the neuromuscular junction. This results in decreased muscle tone and diminished deep tendon reflexes, which in severe cases may progress to flaccid paralysis with respiratory depression. Cardiovascular effects arise due to a combination of calcium and potassium channel blockade, resulting in conduction defects, hypotension, and bradycardia. Hypocalcemia is common in hypermagnesemia, which activates the calcium-sensing receptor and leads to impaired PTH secretion.

Treatment depends on the severity of hypermagnesemia and the degree of renal function. In patients with normal renal function, cessation of magnesium administration results in relatively rapid correction of serum levels. Patients with renal impairment may have limited excretion of magnesium, and in most cases, levels will improve with administration of isotonic intravenous fluids and loop diuretics. Patients with severe renal impairment require hemodialysis or exchange transfusion to correct hypermagnesemia. Regardless of renal function, patients with severe symptomatic hypermagnesemia should be given intravenous calcium (Answer B), which acts as a magnesium antagonist to reverse the neuromuscular and cardiac effects.

This infant has severe hypermagnesemia in the setting of elevated serum creatinine, indicating either acute or chronic impaired renal function. While intravenous hydration (Answer A) is reasonable, and loop diuretics (Answer D) may be helpful after correction of hypocalcemia, these therapies should be given in combination, and an isotonic solution such as normal saline should be used. This severely affected patient may benefit from hemodialysis (Answer C) or exchange transfusion (Answer E); however, these therapies may take an hour or so to prepare, and intravenous calcium should be given first and may be life-saving.

Educational Objective
Treat a patient with hypermagnesemia.

Reference(s)

Ali A, Walentik C, Mantych GJ, Sadiq HF, Keenan WJ, Noguchi A. Iatrogenic acute hypermagnesemia after total parenteral nutrition infusion mimicking septic shock syndrome: two case reports. *Pediatrics.* 2003;112(1 Pt 1):e70-e72. PMID: 12837909

Abbassi-Ghanavati M, Alexander JM, McIntire DD, Savani RC, Leveno KJ. Neonatal effects of magnesium sulfate given to the mother. *Am J Perinatol.* 2012; 29(10):795-799. PMID: 22773290

30 ANSWER: D) Hyperinsulinism due to a pathogenic variant in the *GLUD1* gene (glutamate dehydrogenase deficiency)

This patient exhibits several clues to suggest that he has hyperinsulinism. A critical sample shows hypoglycemia with measurable insulin levels (in the setting of hypoglycemia, the insulin should be below the lower limit of detection, not less than the normal reference range), low free fatty acids and β-hydroxybutyrate (in the setting of hypoglycemia, free fatty acids should be >1.5 mmol/L and β-hydroxybutyrate should be >2 mmol/L), and a glycemic response to glucagon of greater than 30 mg/dL (>1.7 mmol/L).

This baby boy has a history of seizures occurring during the day and he presented with postmeal hypoglycemia; yet, he was able to fast for 14 hours after a low-protein breakfast. He had postmeal lows during the day in the hospital and had an ammonia level that was just slightly higher than the normal range. Hyperinsulinism due to overactivity of glutamate dehydrogenase is caused by pathogenic variants in *GLUD1* (Answer D) and is characterized by protein-induced hypoglycemia with milder fasting-induced hypoglycemia in addition to a high or high-normal ammonia level. Thus, in this case, *GLUD1* hyperinsulinism, also known as the hyperinsulinism hyperammonemia syndrome, is correct. Although *GLUD1* gene defects are inherited in an autosomal dominant manner, there may not be a positive family history, as pathogenic variants are commonly de novo.

The characteristic feature of K_{ATP} hyperinsulinism (Answer B) is presentation in the newborn period or the first few months of life and severe hypoglycemia that is typically unresponsiveness to diazoxide. Affected children may exhibit some degree of protein sensitivity but not to the extent of patients with *GLUD1* pathogenic variants, and they do not have elevated ammonia.

Glycogen storage disease type 0 due to glycogen synthase deficiency (Answer A) presents with postmeal hyperglycemia and fasting-induced ketotic hypoglycemia and affected patients never—either in the fed or fasted state—have a glycemic response to glucagon because they are unable to make glycogen and have no stores. Likewise, glycogen storage disease type 3 (debrancher enzyme deficiency) (Answer E) manifests with ketotic hypoglycemia after a prolonged fast and those affected have no response to glucagon when hypoglycemia occurs. The characteristic finding is massive firm hepatomegaly with marked elevation of AST and ALT.

Hereditary fructose intolerance due to aldolase B deficiency (Answer C) presents with acute gastrointestinal symptoms after ingesting fructose and is associated with profound hypoglycemia, hepatomegaly, altered liver function tests, metabolic acidosis, and thrombocytopenia after ingesting fructose.

Educational Objective
Differentiate among the various etiologies of hypoglycemia on the basis of clinical features and biochemical testing.

Reference(s)

Flanagan SE, Kapoor RR, Hussain K. Genetics of congenital hyperinsulinemic hypoglycemia. *Semin Pediatr Surg*. 2011;20(1):13-17. PMID: 21185998

Saint-Martin C, Arnoux JB, de Lonlay P, Bellanné-Chantelot C. KATP channel mutations in congenital hyperinsulinism. *Semin Pediatr Surg*. 2011;20(1):18-22. PMID: 21185999

31 ANSWER: E) Before GH (mother's home), 2.5 cm/y; on GH (mother's home), 4.0 cm/y; on GH (grandmother's home), 7.0 cm/y

Psychosocial short stature (dwarfism) is a recognized diagnosis often associated with severe growth failure secondary to emotional deprivation and eating behavior abnormalities that may be characterized by hyperphagia not associated with subsequent obesity. Improvement in growth when a child is removed from the offending environment often confirms the diagnosis. Many such children go undiagnosed and are prescribed GH therapy after borderline GH responses on stimulation testing.

A number of studies have documented that, on average, patients do have an improvement in growth velocity on GH therapy, but they have a more significant response when removed from the home problematic environment (thus, Answer E is correct and Answers A, B, C, and D are incorrect). Gohlke et al studied 65 children with the diagnosis of psychosocial short stature, as determined by a multidisciplinary team. A subset of those patients was started on GH after being determined to be deficient after evaluation by stimulation testing. The rest were followed. All were eventually removed from the offending environment. Once removed from the environment, the GH insufficiency was corrected off GH therapy; thus, it was considered a reversible GH deficiency.

The authors concluded that for those patients who cannot be removed from the environment or do not demonstrate a significant improvement in growth velocity if they are removed, GH may be considered to improve predicted adult height.

Educational Objective
Predict the effects of treatment options for psychosocial short stature.

Reference(s)

Gohlke BC, Frazer FL, Stanhope R. Growth hormone secretion and long-term growth data in children with psychosocial short stature treated by different changes in environment. *J Pediatr Clin Endocrinol Metab*. 2004;17(4):637-643. PMID: 15198295

Albanese A, Hamill G, Jones J, Skuse D, Matthews DR, Stanhope R. Reversibility of physiological growth hormone secretion in children with psychosocial dwarfism. *Clin Endocrinol (Oxf)*. 1994;40(5):687-692. PMID: 8013149

32 ANSWER: A) *KISS1* (KiSS-1 metastasis-suppressor)

This patient has findings consistent with isolated GnRH deficiency, also referred to as isolated hypogonadotropic hypogonadism. The presence of pubic hair without breast development by the age of 16 in this young woman is inconsistent with a diagnosis of simple constitutional delay, as she has undergone what appears to be normal adrenarche.

Pathogenic variants in the *KISS1* gene (Answer A) or in the gene encoding the KISS1 receptor (*KISS1R*) are associated with isolated GnRH deficiency. Autosomal recessive inheritance of pathogenic variants in these genes leads to nonsyndromic, isolated gonadotropin deficiency. Isolated gonadotropin deficiency is not associated with other systemic germline malformations. The *KISS1* gene encodes a protein, kisspeptin, originally described as a suppressor of metastasis, and was noted to be the ligand for the orphan receptor, *GPR54*, now known as *KISS1R*, expressed in GnRH-producing neurons. Kisspeptin is produced in neurons located in the preoptic and infundibular nucleus and it leads to both GnRH release and subsequent LH and FSH production. Infusion of kisspeptin can prompt LH and FSH production in patients with gonadotropin deficiency.

A significant family history of infertility is not mentioned, which therefore points away from autosomal dominant forms of hypogonadism such as pathogenic variants in the *SOX10* gene (Answer E), seen in 2% to 5% of patients with Kallmann syndrome, or X-linked causes of hypogonadism such as pathogenic variants in the *ANOS1* gene (formerly *KAL1*) (Answer D), seen in 5% to 10% of patients with Kallmann syndrome. The lack of anosmia decreases the likelihood of a pathogenic variant in *PROKR2* or *FGFR1*. The aforementioned genes may also be associated with other syndromic findings. *ANOS1* can be associated with digital synkinesia and unilateral renal agenesis. *FGFR1* pathogenic variants are associated with synkinesia, cleft lip/palate, and digital malformations. *SOX10* pathogenic variants are associated with hearing loss and iris hypopigmentation.

Educational Objective

Differentiate among the various genes associated with Kallmann syndrome and isolated gonadotropin deficiency.

Reference(s)

Kim SH. Congenital hypogonadotropic hypogonadism and Kallmann syndrome: past, present, and future. *Endocrinol Metab (Seoul)*. 2015;30(4):456-466. PMID: 26790381

33 ANSWER: D) *STAR* (congenital lipoid adrenal hyperplasia)

The patient in this vignette is a 46,XY female with mildly androgenized genitalia. She was clinically stable in early infancy and even tolerated a surgical procedure with anesthesia without problems. However, at age 5 months she developed an adrenal crisis with hyponatremia and hyperkalemia. The results of the ACTH stimulation test demonstrate low adrenal steroids at baseline, which failed to stimulate with ACTH. While the baseline cortisol level is not undetectable, it is low for a patient who is ill and in a stressed state, and cortisol failed to stimulate appropriately with ACTH. ACTH is markedly elevated, indicating primary adrenal insufficiency. Plasma renin activity is also elevated, indicating mineralocorticoid deficiency. Therefore, this patient has glucocorticoid, mineralocorticoid, and sex steroid deficiency. We know the defect is not only at the adrenal level, but also at the gonadal level as the genitalia are significantly underandrogenized for a patient with a 46,XY karyotype. Looking more carefully, when the initial laboratory testing was conducted at age 6 weeks (at a time approaching mini-puberty), the testosterone level was low for age (for a male), further supporting the fact that gonadal steroidogenesis is deficient in this patient. The first physician who saw the patient considered the diagnosis of androgen insensitivity syndrome, but in that scenario, one would expect a significantly higher testosterone level at that age.

In the setting of glucocorticoid, mineralocorticoid, and sex steroid deficiency, one should think of congenital lipoid adrenal hyperplasia, which is a rare autosomal recessive disorder caused by pathogenic variants in the gene encoding the steroidogenic acute regulatory protein (*STAR*) (Answer D). The StAR protein regulates the delivery of cholesterol from the outer to the inner mitochondrial membrane. Therefore, cholesterol cannot convert to pregnenolone, and all adrenal hormones are deficient. This is the so-called first hit in the pathogenesis of lipoid congenital adrenal hyperplasia. The second hit is thought to be due to excessive cholesterol storage in the adrenal cortex and the gonads, significantly impairing all steroidogenic capacity. Typically, patients with lipoid congenital adrenal hyperplasia present with adrenal crisis in early infancy, and those with a 46,XY karyotype have complete sex reversal with female genitalia because fetal testosterone synthesis is impaired. However, the phenotype can be atypical, as in this patient, where adrenal crisis develops after the newborn period. In addition, in patients with a 46,XY karyotype, the genitalia may be somewhat androgenized, as seen in this vignette where the patient was born with clitoromegaly. Patients have been reported to have been diagnosed with adrenal insufficiency later in life and have normal male genitalia.

Pathogenic variants in the *NR0B1* (*DAX1*) gene (Answer A) cause X-linked adrenal hypoplasia congenita. Patients with this disorder typically exhibit defective glucocorticoid, mineralocorticoid, and androgen production. The genitalia in 46,XY individuals with *NR0B1* pathogenic variants are not quite as underandrogenized as in lipoid congenital adrenal hyperplasia. The main difference is that patients with X-linked adrenal hypoplasia congenita have hypothalamic-pituitary-gonadal axis dysfunction leading to hypogonadotrophic hypogonadism, which is not the case in this patient since the gonadotropins are not low.

Pathogenic variants in the *CYP17A1* gene (Answer B) cause 17α-hydroxylase and 17,20-lyase deficiency, which results in adrenal and gonadal sex-steroid deficiency causing undervirilization of the genitalia in 46,XY individuals. Although there is also cortisol deficiency, there is overproduction of corticosterone, which has glucocorticoid activity, making a life-threatening adrenal crisis unlikely. In addition, there is overproduction of deoxycorticosterone, which causes low renin hypertension with sodium retention and hypokalemia, thus excluding the diagnosis in this patient.

Patients with 17β-hydroxysteroid dehydrogenase type 3 deficiency, caused by pathogenic variants in the *HSD17B3* gene (Answer C), have a defect in conversion from androstenedione to testosterone. Therefore, patients with a 46,XY karyotype have atypical genitalia and inguinal masses at birth, as in this patient, but glucocorticoid and mineralocorticoid production is normal.

Pathogenic variants in the *MC2R* gene (Answer E) cause ACTH resistance and hence glucocorticoid deficiency (commonly knows as familial glucocorticoid deficiency), leading to an adrenal crisis. The ACTH level is markedly elevated, as in this patient, and androgen production may be impaired; however, patients with *MC2R* pathogenic variants do not have deficient mineralocorticoid production.

Educational Objective
Explain the pathophysiology and phenotype variability in StAR protein deficiency.

Reference(s)

Miller WL. Disorders in the initial steps of steroid hormone synthesis. *J Steroid Biochem Mol Biol*. 2017;165(Pt A):18-37. PMID: 26960203

Baker BY, Lin L, Kim CJ, Raza J, Smith CP, Miller WL, Achermann JC. Nonclassic congenital lipoid adrenal hyperplasia: a new disorder of the steroidogenic acute regulatory protein with very late presentation and normal male genitalia. *J Clin Endocrinol Metab*. 2006;91(12):4781-4785. PMID: 16968793

Lekarev O, Mallet D, Yuen T, Morel Y, New MI. Congenital lipoid adrenal hyperplasia (a rare form of adrenal insufficiency and ambiguous genitalia) caused by a novel mutation of the steroidogenic acute regulatory protein gene. *Eur J Pediatr*. 2012;171(5):787-793. PMID: 22083155

34 ANSWER: C) Pathogenic variant in the *ACAN* gene (aggrecan)

Aggrecan, the product of the *ACAN* gene, is a critical component of the extracellular matrix important in the structure and function of the growth plate. Missense mutations in *ACAN* (Answer C) cause secretion of a dysfunctional molecule in a dominant-negative fashion that impairs normal interaction with other proteins in the extracellular matrix leading to poor growth and advanced bone age. However, the bone age may be normal in some affected individuals. Birth weight and birth length tend to be low-normal. The arm span-to-height ratio is normal. The sitting height index is high-normal. Autosomal dominant inheritance in this case is likely given the father's short stature. Osteoarthritis commonly affects the knees of individuals with pathogenic variants in the *ACAN* gene beginning in adolescence.

Children with pathogenic variants in the *COL1A1* gene (Answer A) have osteogenesis imperfecta, which is not associated with advanced bone age.

Activating mutations in the *FGFR3* gene (Answer B) cause hypochondroplasia and achondroplasia due to downstream activation of MAP kinase pathways that reduce the proliferation and differentiation of growth plate chondrocytes. Achondroplasia and hypochondroplasia are associated with relative macrocephaly, broad forehead, and near-normal growth of the trunk and head accompanied by short limbs leading to elevated upper-to-lower segment ratio and a short arm span. The bone age in children with activating *FGFR3* mutations is not advanced.

Mucopolysaccharidosis type II (Hunter syndrome) is caused by pathogenic variants in the gene encoding iduronate-2-sulfatase (*IDS*) (Answer D). The growth plates are abnormal in affected patients due to accumulation of glycosaminoglycans and the bone age is delayed. Short stature in this setting is related to joint abnormalities, contractures, and kyphosis.

Genetic abnormalities causing Russell-Silver syndrome (Answer E) include a methylation defect on chromosome 11p15.5 (65%) and maternal uniparental disomy of chromosome 7 (10%). Affected children have short stature related to early failure to thrive, an increased frequency of relative macrocephaly, frontal bossing, a triangular-shaped face, limb asymmetry, and dental crowding. Children with Russell-Silver syndrome tend to have a delayed bone age that may catch up or become advanced with the onset of premature adrenarche and/or central precocious puberty. These features are not seen in the described child.

Educational Objective

Explain the concept of skeletal age and the nutritional, hormonal, and genetic factors that influence it.

Reference(s)

Gkourogianni A, Andrew M, Tyzinski L, et al. Clinical characterization of patients with autosomal dominant short stature due to aggrecan mutations. *J Clin Endocrinol Metab*. 2017;102(2):460-469. PMID: 27870580

Gibson BG, Briggs MD. The aggrecanopathies; an evolving phenotypic spectrum of human genetic skeletal diseases. *Orphanet J Rare Dis*. 2016;11(1):86. PMID: 27353333

Netchine I, Rossignol S, Dufourg MN, et al. 11p15 imprinting center region 1 loss of methylation is a common and specific cause of typical Russell-Silver syndrome: clinical scoring system and epigenetic-phenotypic correlations [published correction appears in *J Clin Endocrinol Metab*. 2007;92(11):4305]. *J Clin Endocrinol Metab*. 2007;92(8):3148-3154. PMID: 17504900

35 **ANSWER: B) Lymphoid follicular infiltration and epithelial cell destruction with or without fibrosis**

Thyrotoxicosis is a clinical syndrome characterized by an increased amount of T_4 and/or T_3. It can be caused by increased synthesis and secretion of thyroid hormones by the thyroid gland (hyperthyroidism) or other etiologies. The most common causes of primary hyperthyroidism include Graves disease, autonomous thyroid nodules, or multinodular goiter due to somatic gain-of-function mutations in the gene encoding the TSH receptor and familial or sporadic nonautoimmune hyperthyroidism due to germline gain-of-function mutations in the gene encoding the TSH receptor. Thyrotoxicosis that is not secondary to hyperthyroidism is usually caused by thyroiditis or exogenous thyroid hormone.

The diagnostic term *thyroiditis* includes a group of inflammatory or inflammatory-like conditions. Chronic lymphocytic thyroiditis, also known as autoimmune or Hashimoto thyroiditis, is the most common cause of acquired hypothyroidism in children and adolescents and may manifest as an initial hyperthyroid phase secondary to release of thyroid hormones from the thyroid follicular cells being destroyed, similar to subacute thyroiditis. However, the condition is painless and due to chronic T-cell infiltration of the thyroid by still poorly understood defects of immunomodulation. Microscopically, there is a diffuse process consisting of a combination of epithelial cell destruction, lymphoid cellular infiltration, and fibrosis. The patient in this vignette does not have history or symptoms consistent with acute infection of the thyroid or subacute infection. Her condition is also painless. She presents with a suppressed TSH level consistent with thyrotoxicosis, although she is asymptomatic. She is most likely in the thyrotoxic phase of Hashimoto thyroiditis, which is characterized by lymphoid follicular infiltration and epithelial cell destruction with or without fibrosis (Answer B).

Acute, infectious thyroiditis (usually suppurative) is a rare condition caused by infection of the thyroid gland by organisms other than viruses. It can be caused by infiltration of the thyroid by bacteria, mycobacteria, fungi, protozoa, or flatworms, and it is usually associated with risk factors such as pyriform sinus fistula, abnormalities in the development of the third and fourth arches, immunocompromised states, endocarditis, and, rarely, fine-needle aspiration biopsy. This condition is rare, with mostly case reports in the pediatric population usually associated with a pyriform sinus fistula. Pathologic examination shows polymorphonuclear and lymphocytic infiltrate with necrosis and abscess formation in the initial phase and fibrosis as healing occurs. The infectious agent can be identified in material obtained by fine-needle aspiration biopsy to determine the best treatment. Affected patients present with pain in the anterior neck, usually with redness, and they tend to keep the neck extended to avoid pressure in the area. They may also have fever, chills, and a thyroid mass (usually left) and local lymphadenopathy.

Subacute thyroiditis, also known as granulomatous or De Quervain thyroiditis, is presumed to be caused by a viral infection. However, this disease is rare in children. Subacute thyroiditis is also characterized by painful swelling of the thyroid gland, and the thyroid gland is tender to palpation, firm, and sometimes feels nodular. Lymphadenopathy is uncommon. During the acute phase, inflammation leads to follicular destruction and thyrotoxicosis due to release of preformed thyroid hormones. It may be difficult to distinguish subacute thyroiditis from acute suppurative thyroiditis in the early stages of the disease, as both conditions can be associated with preceding upper respiratory infection and elevated erythrocyte sedimentation rate. However, as reviewed by Dr. Allen in 1989, fever, leukocytosis, and a left-sided thyroid mass with normal thyroid function suggest the diagnosis of suppurative thyroiditis. Ultimately, the use of imaging studies (ultrasonography or CT) help in the detection of abscess formation. Pathologic examination reveals granulomatous inflammatory changes with giant cells, associated with zones of parenchymal destruction and fibrosis.

Silent thyroiditis, also known as subacute lymphocytic thyroiditis, is thought to be an autoimmune process, as it is also characterized by lymphocytic infiltrate. However, clinically, patients present with thyrotoxicosis, followed by hypothyroidism and eventual restoration of normal thyroid function, usually within 6 to 12 months. Pathologically, the lymphocytic infiltrate lacks fibrosis.

Riedel thyroiditis is a fixed and usually painless enlargement of the thyroid, a chronic sclerosing thyroiditis, occurring especially in adult women. It tends to progress to destruction of the thyroid gland. This condition usually presents as a painless thyroid mass, usually with compressing symptoms. It is extremely rare and its pathology is characterized by normal tissue that is replaced by inflammatory cells, predominantly lymphocytes in a dense matrix of hyalinized connective tissue. An inflammatory reaction of the venous vascular structures has been described. Granulomatous tissue and malignancy are absent.

Thyroiditis can also occur secondary to medications, most commonly amiodarone.

This patient does not have conditions associated with a painful neck, so acute suppurative thyroiditis (associated with polymorphonuclear infiltrate and necrosis [Answer C]) and De Quervain thyroiditis (associated with granulomas with giant cells and diffuse fibrosis [Answer D]) are incorrect diagnoses. Riedel thyroiditis is rare in pediatrics and she does not have compressing symptoms (thus, Answer A is unlikely). An autonomous nodule is rare and she does not have any palpable masses, which makes a somatic gain-of-function mutation in the gene encoding the TSH receptor (Answer E) less likely than the thyrotoxic phase of Hashimoto thyroiditis. Other possibilities to consider in this patient are early Graves disease and silent thyroiditis.

Educational Objective
Construct a differential diagnosis of thyrotoxicosis and identify the common subtypes of thyroiditis that can cause transient thyrotoxicosis.

Reference(s)

Brown RS. Autoimmune thyroiditis in childhood. *J Clin Res Pediatr Endocrinol.* 2013;5(Suppl 1):45-49. PMID: 23154164

Szabo SM, Allen DB. Thyroiditis. Differentiation of acute suppurative and subacute. Case report and review of the literature. *Clin Pediatr (Phila).* 1989;28(4): 171-174. PMID: 2649297

Farwell AP. Sporadic painless, painful subacute and acute infectious thyroiditis. In: Braverman LE, Cooper DS, eds. *Werner & Ingbar's The Thyroid: A Fundamental and Clinical Text.* 10th ed. Lippincott Williams & Wilkins, Philadelphia PA. 2013.

Samuels MH. Subacute, silent, and postpartum thyroiditis. *Med Clin North Am.* 2012;96(2):223-233. PMID: 22443972

36

ANSWER: C) Measurement of amylase and lipase to assess for pancreatitis

Hypertriglyceridemia is a rare but important cause of recurrent pancreatitis. This is typically seen in settings of very high triglyceride levels (>500 mg/dL [>5.65 mmol/L]). This boy presented with hypertriglyceridemia with only a modest increase in his LDL-cholesterol level. Isolated hypertriglyceridemia can be due to defects in lipoprotein lipase and hepatic lipase. This patient was started on atorvastatin, which can decrease triglycerides by 10% to 20%, and dietary therapy. However, the fact that the family missed their last 2 clinic appointments calls into question their adherence to this regimen. Additionally, while on vacation, there can be a tendency to miss medication doses and eat convenient foods that might significantly raise triglyceride levels, increasing the risk of pancreatitis. Elevated levels of amylase and lipase (Answer C) are diagnostic, although imaging is also important to confirm the diagnosis, assess for ileus, and exclude other causes of abdominal pain. Treatment for pancreatitis is supportive and includes potential hospitalization for initial fluid resuscitation and pain management. Long-term, careful management of triglyceride elevations is important to prevent future episodes of recurrent pancreatitis.

Use of statins has been associated with potential dose-related liver toxicity in adults, although this appears to be a rare occurrence. A systematic review of studies involving almost 800 children followed in placebo-controlled trials of statin therapy revealed no difference in liver toxicity between those on statins and those on placebo. Additionally, hepatotoxicity would not be expected to present with generalized abdominal pain and an otherwise normal physical exam. Thus, assessment of transaminases (Answer E) is not as critical as assessment for pancreatitis in this case.

Similarly, evaluation with endoscopic retrograde cholangiopancreatography (Answer A), abdominal CT (Answer B), and C-reactive protein measurement (Answer D) could be important in the setting of clinical presentations that are more suggestive of the etiologies in the listed answers or in a patient with hypertriglyceridemia and normal amylase and lipase levels.

Educational Objective
Evaluate for pancreatitis in patients with hypertriglyceridemia.

Reference(s)

Kwiterovich PO. Clinical and laboratory assessment of cardiovascular risk in children: guidelines for screening, evaluation, and treatment. *J Clin Lipidol*. 2008;2(4): 248-266. PMID: 21291741

Avis HJ, Vissers MN, Stein EA, et al. A systematic review and meta-analysis of statin therapy in children with familial hypercholesterolemia. *Atheroscler Thromb Vasc Biol*. 2007;27(8):1803-1810. PMID: 17569881

37

ANSWER: C) Iatrogenic cause

This child's presentation with severe, acquired hyperphosphatemia and hypocalcemia is most consistent with exogeneous phosphate administration. Upon further questioning, the family admitted to administering 2 phosphate-containing enemas that morning to try to avoid the bowel cleanout admission. Phosphate-containing enemas act by increasing the osmotic gradient within the bowel, thus increasing fluid absorption into lumen. These agents are intended to act intraluminally; however, after equilibrium is reached, some degree of systemic uptake is likely to occur. Severe and life-threatening instances of hyperphosphatemia have been reported with use of phosphate-containing enemas, particularly in younger children and in those with impaired renal function. This patient's hypocalcemia is a secondary effect of hyperphosphatemia, resulting from formation of complexes between calcium and serum phosphate (thus, Answer C is correct).

Pseudohypoparathyroidism (Answer A) is characterized by hypocalcemia and hyperphosphatemia due to renal resistance to PTH. It most commonly results from pathogenic variants or methylation abnormalities in the *GNAS* gene. Because this patient is presenting acutely, and previously had normal serum calcium and phosphate levels, his current mineral abnormalities are more likely to be the result of an acquired condition as opposed to underlying genetic PTH resistance. Renal failure (Answer B) is a frequent cause of hyperphosphatemia, but given this patient's clinical presentation, phosphate-containing enemas are a more likely etiology. Severe vitamin D deficiency (Answer D) and gastrointestinal malabsorption (Answer E) can lead to hypocalcemia; however, these conditions result in compensatory secondary hyperparathyroidism and hypophosphatemia.

Treatment of severe hypocalcemia due to an excessive phosphate load may require isotonic intravenous hydration and intravenous calcium to ameliorate tetany and seizure. Oral phosphate binders such as sevelamer, as well as gastrointestinal lavage, can be used to decrease intestinal phosphate absorption. Alkalinization of the urine with acetazolamide may be attempted to promote renal phosphate excretion. Treatment with intravenous insulin and glucose can be considered to promote intracellular translocation of phosphate. In severe cases, dialysis is often required to correct electrolyte and mineral abnormalities.

Educational Objective

Explain how acute hyperphosphatemia and hypocalcemia can be caused by phosphate administration (intravenous, oral, or rectal).

Reference(s)

Marraffa JM, Hui A, Stork CM. Severe hyperphosphatemia and hypocalcemia following the rectal administration of a phosphate-containing Fleet pediatric enema. *Pediatr Emerg Care*. 2004;20(7):453-456. PMID: 15232246

Biebl A, Grillenberger A, Schmitt K. Enema-induced severe hyperphosphatemia in children. *Eur J Pediatr*. 2009;168(1):111-112. PMID: 18408952

Ladenhauf HN, Stundner O, Spreitzhofer F, Deluggi S. Severe hyperphosphatemia after administration of sodium-phosphate containing laxatives in children: case series and systematic review of literature. *Pediatr Surg Int*. 2012;28(8):805-814. PMID: 22820833

38 ANSWER: B) *FGFR1* (fibroblast growth factor receptor 1)

The pertinent findings in this case are a history of cleft lip, undescended testes, a diminished sense of smell (hyposmia), dental agenesis, syndactyly, delayed puberty, low gonadotropin and sex steroid hormone levels, hypoplastic olfactory bulbs/tracts on MRI, and absence of other pituitary hormone deficits, which is consistent with isolated GnRH deficiency. This condition is associated with a normal sense of smell (normosmia) in approximately 40% of affected individuals and an absent sense of smell (anosmia) or diminished sense in 60% (Kallmann syndrome). The incidence of Kallmann syndrome is 1 in 30,000 males and 1 in 125,000 females, although this may be an underestimate. Infant boys may present with cryptorchidism and micropenis. Adolescents present with delayed sexual maturation. Skeletal age is delayed. Linear growth is generally normal, but the pubertal growth spurt is absent. The low testosterone or estradiol is due to partial or complete absence of GnRH dependent LH and FSH secretion (hypogonadotropic hypogonadism). The pituitary and hypothalamus appear normal in patients with isolated GnRH deficiency; however, in Kallmann syndrome MRI typically shows aplasia or hypoplasia of the olfactory bulbs, tracts, and sulci. The reason for the absence or hypoplasia of the olfactory bulbs and tracts leading to anosmia is incompletely understood. The embryonic developmental failure occurs between 4 and 10 embryonic weeks. It may involve failure of terminal elongation or targeting of olfactory axons, a primary developmental defect of the olfactory bulbs, and a defect in axonal branching of the olfactory bulb output neurons. During the sixth embryonic week, GnRH cells migrate from the olfactory epithelium to the forebrain, along the olfactory nerve pathway. In a human fetus with a chromosomal deletion at Xp22.3 that included the *ANOS1 (KAL1)* gene, it was shown that the GnRH neurons did not migrate normally and were arrested in the upper nasal region. This proposed defect may be a consequence of early degeneration of the olfactory axons that serve as guiding cues for GnRH migration, or a direct effect on the GnRH cells themselves.

Neuroendocrine genes that control the secretion or action of GnRH may cause normosmic isolated GnRH deficiency. Pathogenic variants in more than 25 genes account for about half of all cases, with the remaining causes currently unknown. Isolated GnRH deficiency can be inherited in an X-linked, autosomal dominant, or autosomal recessive manner; however, almost all known genes associated with isolated GnRH deficiency can be inherited in an oligogenic or indeterminate manner. Of the known genes, pathogenic variants in *FGFR1, CHD7, FGF8, FGF17, HS6ST1, NSMF, PROK2, PROKR2, SEMA7A, NELF, IGSF10, AXL*, and *WDR11* cause Kallmann syndrome and normosmic isolated GnRH deficiency. Pathogenic variants in *ANOS1 (KAL1), CCDC141, FEZF1, SEMA3A, HESX1*, and *SOX10* cause Kallmann syndrome. Pathogenic variants in *GNRH1, GNRHR, KISS1, TAC3*, and *TACR3* are just some of the most commonly identified mutations that cause normosmic isolated GnRH deficiency. Gene testing can be considered based on the mode of inheritance (if known) and the presence of other nonreproductive phenotypes.

Pathogenic variants in the *FGFR1* gene (Answer B) (fibroblast growth factor receptor 1) account for approximately 10% of Kallmann syndrome cases but can also cause normosmic isolate GnRH deficiency. Nonreproductive phenotypes include synkinesia (10%), cleft lip and/or palate, agenesis of more than one tooth, and brachydactyly or syndactyly. While this patient does not have synkinesia, he does have a history of cleft lip, dental agenesis, and syndactyly and an *FGFR1* mutation is the most likely cause of his delayed puberty. Loss-of-function mutations in the *FGFR1* gene were first reported in a kindred with isolated hypogonadotropic hypogonadism inherited in an autosomal dominant fashion. However, *FGFR1* pathogenic variants are associated with marked phenotypic variability and incomplete penetrance.

Pathogenic variants in the *ANOS1* gene *(KAL1)* (anosmin 1) (Answer A) are responsible for 5% to 10% of Kallmann syndrome cases that are inherited in an X-linked manner. Nonreproductive phenotypes include digital synkinesia (in ~80% of males), unilateral renal agenesis (~30% of males), and high-arched palate. However, the boy in this case has no family history suggestive of X-linked inheritance, no evidence of synkinesia, and his renal ultrasonography is normal, so an *ANOS1* mutation is not the most likely cause of Kallmann syndrome.

Pathogenic variants in the *GNRH1* gene (Answer C) (progonadoliberin 1) cause normosmic isolated GnRH deficiency with no other nonreproductive phenotypes. Pathogenic variants in the *CHD7* gene (Answer D) (chromodomain-helicase-DNA-binding protein 7) can cause normosmic or anosmic isolated GnRH deficiency, with the associated phenotype of CHARGE syndrome (*c*oloboma, *h*eart defects, *a*tresia of the choanae, *r*etardation of growth, *g*enital hypoplasia, *e*ar anomalies and deafness). Pathogenic variants in the *MKRN3* gene (Answer E) have been implicated in familial precocious puberty.

Educational Objective
Explain the genetic regulation of the GnRH neuronal migrations and differentiate among the underlying causes of isolated GnRH deficiency.

Reference(s)
Lima Amato LG, Latronico AC, Gontijo Silveira LF. Molecular and genetic aspects of congenital isolated hypogonadotropic hypogonadism. *Endocrinol Metab Clin North Am*. 2017;46(2):283-303. PMID: 28476224

39 **ANSWER: C) Administer stress-dose glucocorticoid therapy during times of illness and other physiologic stress and repeat an ACTH-stimulation test at a later time**

The patient in this vignette developed iatrogenic Cushing syndrome due to dexamethasone drops. He developed suppression of the hypothalamic-pituitary-adrenal axis, yet as the steroids were weaned, there was partial recovery, which included resolution of cushingoid signs and symptoms, and his linear growth improved. The results of the low-dose ACTH-stimulation test demonstrated that while the cortisol level increased, the stimulated level was not in the normal range. There has been some discussion regarding what is considered a normal stimulated cortisol level, but the general consensus is that a stimulated level of 18 µg/dL (500 nmol/L) is consistent with normal adrenal function.

On the basis of the results and the patient's clinical course while off glucocorticoid therapy, one can conclude that the cortisol level is sufficient for daily function and normal growth and development, and yet may not sufficiently rise during times of illness and other stress. Therefore, this patient does not require daily hydrocortisone treatment at physiologic doses (Answer A) or supraphysiologic doses (Answer B). However, because the stimulated cortisol response was not adequate, he should receive hydrocortisone at stress doses during illness or for a significant injury, and the family must be trained in injectable hydrocortisone administration in case of an emergency (Answer C). The patient must also receive glucocorticoid stress dosing during procedures requiring anesthesia.

While the hypothalamic-pituitary-adrenal axis has not completely recovered and the patient requires further follow-up (thus, Answer E is incorrect), his axis should eventually completely recover. Therefore, an ACTH-stimulation test should be repeated. In fact, this patient had another low-dose ACTH-stimulation test 4 and a half months after steroids were discontinued with the following results:

Baseline cortisol = 6.0 µg/dL (165.5 nmol/L)
30-minute stimulated cortisol = 17.9 µg/dL (493.8 nmol/L)
60-minute stimulated cortisol = 19.2 µg/dL (529.7 nmol/L)

These results indicate that the patient's hypothalamic-pituitary-adrenal axis has recovered completely and there is no further need for glucocorticoid stress dosing. Imaging (Answer D) is not necessary because the cause of adrenal insufficiency is iatrogenic, and while the hypothalamic-pituitary-adrenal axis has been altered, one would not anticipate permanent changes in the pituitary gland.

Iatrogenic adrenal insufficiency and Cushing syndrome secondary to oral, inhaled, and topical glucocorticoid therapy is a well-described phenomenon. The clinical scenario has also been described in patients using intranasal steroids. Infants given intranasal steroids may be at greater risk for systemic absorption of the medication because they are supine during administration and may swallow some of the medication and because they have a smaller body surface area than older children and adults. Clinicians must vigilantly monitor for signs and symptoms of Cushing syndrome, as well as for adrenal insufficiency—the indicators of which may be less overt and yet the condition can be life threatening.

Educational Objective
Develop a diagnostic approach to patients with possible secondary adrenal insufficiency due to oral, inhaled, intranasal, and topical steroid treatment.

Reference(s)

Choi IS, Sim DW, Kim SH, Wui JW. Adrenal insufficiency associated with long-term use of inhaled steroid in asthma. *Ann Allergy Asthma Immunol.* 2017;118(1): 66-72.e1. PMID: 27839667

Orton S, Censani M. Iatrogenic Cushing syndrome due to intranasal usage of ophthalmic dexamethasone: a case report. *Pediatrics.* 2016;137(5). PMID: 27244810

Golekoh MC, Hornung LN, Mukkada VA, Khoury JC, Putnam PE, Backeljauw PF. Adrenal insufficiency after chronic swallowed glucocorticoid therapy for eosinophilic esophagitis. *J Pediatr.* 2016;170:240-245. PMID: 26687577

Kapadia CR, Nebesio TD, Myers SE, et al; Drugs and Therapeutics Committee of the Pediatric Endocrine Society. Endocrine effects of inhaled corticosteroids in children. *JAMA Pediatr.* 2016;170(2):163-170. PMID: 26720105

40 ANSWER: D) Placental insufficiency

Infants born to women with diabetes mellitus are at risk for a number of abnormalities at birth. Commonly, infants present large-for-gestational-age due to maternal hyperglycemia (Answer A) and subsequent compensatory fetal insulin hypersecretion (Answer E), leading to overgrowth. In babies born to women with longstanding, poorly controlled diabetes, maternal vasculopathy and nephropathy can result in placental insufficiency (Answer D) leading to poor nutritional transfer to the fetus and subsequent poor fetal growth (small-for-gestational-age infant). Placental insufficiency is the most likely cause of this patient's poor fetal growth.

IGF-2 (Answer B) has been studied in the setting of intrauterine growth retardation. Cordeiro et al documented down-regulation of the *IGF2* gene in RNA analysis of placental tissue extracted from control fetuses and fetuses with intrauterine growth retardation. They also found hypomethylation of the imprinting control centers located in a cluster of genes on chromosome 11p15.5 (genes implicated in growth-restricting Silver-Russell syndrome are co-located in that region in addition to *IGF2* gene). Excess IGF-2 is associated with overgrowth.

Although dysfunctional insulin receptor regulation (Answer C), resulting in lower insulin function, can lead to severe insulin resistance and poor fetal growth, this is not the most likely cause when considering the history in this vignette.

Educational Objective
Explain the effects of poorly controlled maternal diabetes mellitus on fetal growth.

Reference(s)

Holemans K, Aerts L, Van Assche FA. Lifetime consequences of abnormal fetal pancreatic development. *J Physiol.* 2003;547(Pt 1):11-20. PMID: 12562919

Van Assche FA, Holemans K, Aerts L. Fetal growth and consequences for later life. *J Perinat Med.* 1998;26(5):337-346. PMID: 10027128

Cordeiro A, Neto AP, Carvalho F, Ramalho C, Doria S. Relevance of genomic imprinting in intrauterine human growth expression of CDKN1C, H19, IGF2, KCNQ1 and PHLDA2 imprinted genes. *J Assist Reprod Genet.* 2014;31(10):1361-1368. PMID: 24986528

41 ANSWER: E) Fluorodeoxyglucose PET/CT imaging

This patient's presentation with severe, acquired hypophosphatemia is most consistent with tumor-induced osteomalacia, otherwise known as oncogenic osteomalacia. This paraneoplastic syndrome arises from mesenchymal tumors that produce high levels of FGF-23. Patients present with typical symptoms associated with hypophosphatemia, such as muscle weakness, rickets, and fractures. However, unlike genetic forms of FGF-23 excess, these symptoms are usually not present from birth, consistent with an acquired (rather than congenital) condition. The patient in this vignette has a growth curve typical of pediatric-onset tumor-induced osteomalacia, demonstrating normal linear growth velocity until age 9, after which she developed severe growth deceleration, correlating with the onset of her symptoms.

Lesions in tumor-induced osteomalacia are typically benign; however, they are frequently small and difficult to locate. Resection of these lesions is curative, resulting in rapid improvement of serum phosphate and skeletal remineralization. After the diagnosis of tumor-induced osteomalacia has been established, functional imaging with fluorodeoxyglucose PET/CT (Answer E), often in conjunction with octreotide scans, is the best next step to identify the tumor.

This patient's laboratory abnormalities are highly suggestive of FGF-23–mediated hypophosphatemia. The low serum phosphate with inappropriately high urinary phosphate is consistent with renal phosphate wasting. The high PTH with inappropriately low 1,25-dihydroxyvitamin D is also characteristic, secondary to FGF-23–mediated inhibition of 1α-hydroxylase. Additional laboratory studies are appropriate to confirm the diagnosis of FGF-23 excess, including calculation of tubular reabsorption of phosphate ($1 - [$(urinary phosphate × serum creatinine) / (serum phosphate × urine creatinine)$]$) (Answer A) and measurement of serum FGF-23 (Answer C). Genetic forms of rickets are the most common cause of FGF-23 excess in children, and genetic testing (Answer B) is also an appropriate step in establishing the diagnosis. However, the diagnostic test that will have the greatest bearing on future management is functional imaging, because identification of an FGF-23–producing tumor will dictate a potentially curative surgical approach rather than long-term phosphate and calcitriol supplementation. Renal ultrasonography (Answer D) is indicated as part of routine care to evaluate for nephrocalcinosis as a complication of phosphaturia; however, this is unlikely to significantly alter this patient's long-term management.

Educational Objective

Explain the association of hypophosphatemic rickets and mesenchymal tumors of bone and soft tissue (oncogenic osteomalacia) and describe the clinical and pathophysiological similarities between this disorder and X-linked hypophosphatemic rickets.

Reference(s)

Minisola S, Peacock M, Fukumoto S, et al. Tumour-induced osteomalacia. *Nat Rev Dis Primers*. 2017;3:17044. PMID: 28703220

Chong WH, Andreopoulou P, Chen CC, et al. Tumor localization and biochemical response to cure in tumor-induced osteomalacia. *J Bone Miner Res*. 2013;28(6): 1386-1398. PMID: 23362135

42 ANSWER: D) Progressive improvement of height SDS

Activating mutations in the *FGFR3* gene cause hypochondroplasia and achondroplasia, which are associated with relative macrocephaly, broad forehead, near-normal growth of the trunk and head, short limbs, an elevated upper-to-lower segment ratio, and a short arm span. This child's mild short stature is consistent with hypochondroplasia.

Hypochondroplasia is not an FDA-approved indication for GH therapy in children. Meta-analysis of multiple studies of GH therapy in this patient population shows a statistically significant, progressive improvement in height SDS over 3 years of GH therapy from a baseline height of –3.03 to –2.42 SDS (Answer D). Data about adult height outcomes of GH therapy in children with hypochondroplasia are limited. However, one study of 7 children with hypochondroplasia showed that adult height gain was +1.39 ± 0.9 SDS compared with height gain in historical controls. Adverse events described in children with hypochondroplasia receiving GH therapy include worsening of genu varum and development of mild scoliosis. In the existing literature, no cases of intracranial hypertension (Answer E) have been reported and bone age has not been observed to advance more rapidly than expected (Answer A). Although concerns exist about GH treatment aggravating disproportion in children with hypochondroplasia, multiple studies indicate that the height gain is not associated with worsening disproportion (Answer C).

In genome-wide association studies, C-type natriuretic peptide (CNP), encoded by the *NPPC* gene, and its receptor NPR3 have been shown to be associated with adult height. Pharmacologic studies of CNP indicate that it binds to another natriuretic peptide receptor, NPR-B, encoded by the *NPR2* gene, leading to inhibition of FGFR signaling. In children with GH deficiency, idiopathic short stature, hypochondroplasia, and achondroplasia, the levels of CNP and its precursor NTproCNP increase, not decrease (Answer B), during growth and in response to GH therapy.

Educational Objective
Describe the appropriate use of growth hormone in the treatment of disorders including short stature.

Reference(s)

Kubota T, Wang W, Miura K, et al. Serum NT-proCNP levels increased after initiation of GH treatment in patients with achondroplasia/hypochondroplasia. *Clin Endocrinol (Oxf)*. 2016;84(6):845-850. PMID: 26814021

Massart F, Miccoli M, Baggiani A, Bertelloni S. Height outcome of short children with hypochondroplasia after recombinant human growth hormone treatment: a meta-analysis. *Pharmacogenomics*. 2015;16(17):1965-1973. PMID: 26555758

Pinto G, Cormier-Daire V, Le Merrer M, et al. Efficacy and safety of growth hormone treatment in children with hypochondroplasia: comparison with an historical cohort. *Horm Res Paediatr*. 2014;82(6):355-363. PMID: 25323764

43 **ANSWER: A) Glycogen storage disease type 0 (glycogen synthase deficiency)**
The finding of postprandial hyperglycemia and fasting hypoglycemia is a rare combination, but it occurs in several conditions. Many of these conditions have classic features on exam that narrow the diagnosis. Typically, when faced with unusual patterns of glucose levels documented on home glucometers that do not make sense, one tends to blame the testing. However, rare conditions can indeed be associated with the unusual pattern observed in this vignette.

Patients with glycogen storage disease type 0 due to glycogen synthase deficiency (Answer A) present with a combination of postprandial hyperglycemia and fasting-induced hypoglycemia. There is no hepatomegaly on examination, and liver function is normal. If an oral glucose tolerance test is performed, lactate levels should be measured because they rise, in addition to glucose, in the postprandial state, but not enough to cause a clinical lactic acidosis with increased anion gap. This pattern occurs because the patient is unable to make glycogen, so glucose levels rise and that entering the liver must undergo the first steps of glycolysis to lactate. Glycogen storage disease type 0 is the most likely diagnosis in this patient.

GLUT2 deficiency or Fanconi Bickel syndrome (Answer B) results from the absence of the glucose-transporter protein 2 in β cells, liver, and kidneys. Glycogen deposition occurs in the liver (hepatomegaly) and kidney (renomegaly). In addition, aberrant hepatocyte glucose transport results in postprandial hyperglycemia followed by fasting hypoglycemia. Glucose-stimulated insulin release is diminished and contributes to poor glucose control. Hemoglobin A_{1c} in this setting is normal, and fasting hypoglycemia and postprandial hyperglycemia appear to improve with age. Affected patients have Fanconi-like renal tubular acidosis and bone disease, neither of which is evident in this patient's urinalysis and bone markers.

Fructose 1,6-bisphosphatase performs an important step in gluconeogenesis by combining 2 glyceraldehyde-3-phosphate molecules (produced during lipolysis) to make fructose 1,6-bisphosphate, which in turn is converted through several steps to glucose. Deficiency of this enzyme (Answer C) produces fasting hypoglycemia and lactic acidosis and does not result in hyperglycemia. Clinically, affected patients have hepatomegaly. In the most severe form, pathogenic variants in the insulin receptor gene (Answer E) cause Donohue syndrome (also known as leprechaunism), which presents in the prenatal to newborn period. Milder forms of insulin receptor defects cause postprandial hyperglycemia due to insulin resistance. Unlike the insulin resistance associated with type 2 diabetes mellitus, affected patients have fasting hypoglycemia when insulin production finally overcomes insulin resistance. Moreover, by the time the time patients present with hypoglycemia, they have acanthosis nigricans. Older girls often first present with polycystic ovary syndrome (although they are thin), but despite treatment they eventually develop glucose dysregulation with hyperglycemia and hypoglycemia.

Patients with glycogen storage disease IXa due to phosphorylase kinase deficiency (Answer D) are often normal on physical examination, but they occasionally have mild hepatomegaly or short stature. They do not have postmeal hyperglycemia, but have accelerated starvation with ketotic hypoglycemia often occurring after an overnight fast. Deficiency of the phosphorylase kinase enzyme results in an inability to fully break down glycogen at the branch points, so affected persons are able to make some glycogen, release some glucose from glycogen, but not fully empty the liver, which results in a shortened fasting tolerance and early use of ketones for fuel. Patients with what is thought to be recurrent ketotic hypoglycemia should be considered for evaluation of glycogen storage disease IX in addition to types VI or 0, all of which may mimic idiopathic ketotic hypoglycemia. Glycogen storage disease IX is inherited in an X-linked manner (thus, boys are affected), whereas types b and c are autosomal recessive.

Although not offered as an answer choice, it is important to know that patients with Nissen fundoplication who are on G-tube feeds are another group of patients that may present with a combination of hyperglycemia and hypoglycemia. They have a 25% likelihood of having postprandial hyperglycemia followed by rebound hypoglycemia after surgery. The hypoglycemia typically occurs 2 to 5 hours after a meal and is preceded by hyperglycemia, with a postmeal glycemic excursion of more than 50 mg/dL (>2.8 mmol/L). Clinically, such patients have a visible G tube and scars from surgery.

Educational Objective
Identify possible causes of unusual patterns of glucose dysregulation.

Reference(s)

Brown LM, Corrado MM, van der Ende RM, et al. Evaluation of glycogen storage disease as a cause of ketotic hypoglycemia in children. *J Inherit Metab Dis*. 2015; 38(3):489-493. PMID: 25070466

Calabria AC, Charles L, Givler S, De Leon DD. Postprandial hypoglycemia in children after gastric surgery: clinical characterization and pathophysiology. *Horm Res Paediatr*. 2016;85(2):140-146. PMID: 26694545

Santer R, Schneppenheim R, Suter D, Schaub J, Steinmann B. Fanconi-Bickel syndrome--the original patient and his natural history, historical steps leading to the primary defect, and a review of the literature. *Eur J Pediatr*. 1998;157(10):783-797. PMID: 9809815

44 ANSWER: B) Laboratory assay interference

This patient had markedly abnormal laboratory values, consistent with thyrotoxicosis, in the absence of signs or symptoms of hyperthyroidism (confirmed by physical exam during an office visit). The initial action to repeat the laboratory assessment was important to exclude the possibility that the wrong results were reported on the wrong patient. In addition, the second set of lab values allowed for additional hormone levels to aid in determining the etiology.

On repeated testing, the second set of values confirmed the biochemical thyrotoxicosis. The addition of the thyroid-stimulating immunoglobulin, thyroglobulin, and thyroglobulin antibodies was performed to screen for laboratory evidence of thyroiditis, as well as the potential for excess exogenous levothyroxine ingestion, often taken in an attempt to lose weight. The low thyroglobulin with undetectable thyroglobulin antibodies and nonelevated thyroid-stimulating immunoglobulin confirmed the low likelihood of thyroiditis, including Hashitoxicosis (Answer C), Graves disease (Answer A), and silent thyroiditis (Answer D). The normal, nonsuppressed thyroglobulin also decreased the likelihood of excess, exogenous levothyroxine (Answer E), as this would be associated with low or suppressed thyroglobulin. The presence of a goiter was consistent with the underlying history of autoimmune hypothyroidism, and a normal percentage uptake with a scan showing even distribution of ^{123}I throughout the gland ruled out the likelihood of Hashitoxicosis or ingestion of excess exogenous levothyroxine (should have a low percentage uptake with decreased imaging of the radiotracer), Graves disease (should have increased percentage uptake with increased radiotracer throughout the gland), or an autonomously functioning thyroid nodule (should have increased percentage uptake with an area or areas of focal increased radiotracer). These potential results are summarized (*see table*).

Diagnosis	Thyroglobulin	Antithyroglobulin	Thyroid Uptake and Scan (^{123}I)
Hashitoxicosis (Answer C)	Elevated	Elevated	Decreased
Silent thyroiditis (Answer D)	Elevated	Normal or elevated	Decreased
Graves disease (Answer A)	Elevated	Elevated (50%)	Increased
Exogenous ingestion of levothyroxine (Answer E)	Normal	Normal	Decreased
Excess biotin (Answer B)	Normal	Normal	Normal (uniform, <30% at 24 hours)
Autonomously functioning thyroid nodule	Elevated	Normal	Focal increased uptake

With this information, the patient was questioned specifically about over-the-counter supplements, and she reported that she had started taking a supplement to increase the strength of her hair and nails. The patient provided the name of the supplement and the ingredients revealed that each pill contained 5000 mcg of biotin, about 70 to 100 times the daily recommendation. High-dosage biotin can interfere with immunoassays (Answer B) that use biotinylated antibody in a streptavidin "capture" system. Competitive immunoassays are often used to measure small molecules, such as T_3 and T_4, and excess biotin can cause falsely high results. Sandwich immunoassays are often used to measure larger molecules, such as TSH, ACTH, and intact PTH, and excess biotin can displace the biotinylated capture antibody from the biotin-streptavidin complex and yield falsely low measurements. Stopping the biotin supplement for 48 hours before the lab draw avoids the interaction of excess biotin on these immunoassays. Repeating the testing after the patient stopped biotin for 2 days showed normalization of the TSH, free T_4, and T_3.

Educational Objective
Explain the potential for interference of excess biotin ingestion on immunoassays that rely on the use of biotinylated antibody in a streptavidin "capture" system.

Reference(s)

Kummer S, Hermsen D, Distelmaier F. Biotin treatment mimicking Graves' disease. *N Engl J Med*. 2016;375(7):704-706. PMID: 27532849

Trambas CM, Sikaris KA, Lu ZX. More on biotin treatment mimicking Graves' disease. *N Engl J Med*. 2016;375(17):1698. PMID: 27783908

Barbesino G. Misdiagnosis of Graves' disease with apparent severe hyperthyroidism in a patient taking biotin megadoses. *Thyroid*. 2016;26(6):860-863. PMID: 27043844

Elston MS, Sehgal S, Du Toit S, Yarndley T, Conaglen JV. Factitious Graves' disease due to biotin immunoassay interference-A case and review of the literature. *J Clin Endocrinol Metab*. 2016;101(19):3251-3255. PMID: 27362288

45 ANSWER: D) Initiate recombinant leptin

Leptin is a hormone produced primarily by adipocytes in proportion to stored fat; it acts as a signal of long-term energy reserve. This patient has an extremely rare genetic condition resulting from pathogenic variants in the leptin gene (*LEP*). While this condition is rare (thus far identified in fewer than 50 patients worldwide), this case demonstrates 2 important physiologic properties of leptin: (1) leptin has direct action on appetite-regulating centers, with rapid weight gain from infancy when deficient and dramatic weight loss when it is administered to leptin-deficient individuals; (2) leptin is essential for normal reproductive functioning, including menstrual cycles. Thus, the best way to address this patient's secondary amenorrhea is to initiate recombinant leptin (Answer D). This is most likely the medication that she received at the previous institution, resulting in weight loss and normal menses. Leptin exerts a permissive effect on gonadotropin release, which is to say that leptin and its receptor are necessary but not sufficient to stimulate gonadotropin release. The most dramatic demonstration of leptin's role in gonadotropin regulation is in the setting of amenorrhea associated with anorexia nervosa, a state of low physiologic levels of leptin due to low fat mass. A study of young women with amenorrhea due to anorexia nervosa revealed that treatment with leptin for up to 3 months resulted in significant increases in LH levels, ovarian volume, and estradiol levels, as well as resumption of menses. In a study of individuals with genetic leptin deficiency not diagnosed until adulthood, none had progressed through puberty completely; females given recombinant leptin began having regular menstrual periods. Metreleptin is FDA approved for use in congenital and acquired lipodystrophy; use in the setting of leptin deficiency is currently off-label.

Obesity can be associated with dysregulated menstrual periods related to polycystic ovary syndrome. This can be treated with oral contraceptive pills (Answer A) or, because of the role of insulin resistance in this condition, with metformin (Answer B). However, polycystic ovary syndrome is typically associated with hyperandrogenemia and virilizing features, which this girl does not have.

Extreme obesity can contribute to the development of type 2 diabetes, including in cases of leptin deficiency. However, patients with diabetes but without polycystic ovary syndrome typically do not have secondary amenorrhea. Thus, exenatide (Answer D), a treatment for type 2 diabetes, is incorrect.

While lifestyle modification (Answer E) is important in all settings of obesity, leptin replacement produces a much more dramatic effect on weight loss in patients with leptin deficiency. Also, lifestyle modification would not be expected to ameliorate her amenorrhea.

Educational Objective
Explain the physiologic effects of leptin in the setting of leptin deficiency.

Reference(s)

Chou SH, Mantzoros C. 20 years of leptin: role of leptin in human reproductive disorders. *J Endocrinol.* 2014;223(1):T49-T62. PMID: 25056118

Paz-Filho G, Mastronardi CA, Licinio J. Leptin treatment: facts and expectations. *Metabolism.* 2015;64(1):146-156. PMID: 25156686

Welt CK, Chan JL, Bullen J, et al. Recombinant human leptin in women with hypothalamic amenorrhea. *N Engl J Med.* 2004;351(10):987-997. PMID: 15342807

46 ANSWER: B) Adamantinomatous craniopharyngioma

The pertinent facts in this child's case are a suprasellar mass with solid and cystic components and evidence of hypothalamic-pituitary axis abnormalities (slow growth with low IGF-1, weight gain, low TSH, and diabetes insipidus). Craniopharyngiomas are rare intracranial tumors, with an overall incidence of 0.5 to 2 cases per million persons per year. However, they account for 6% to 9% of all childhood brain tumors. There is a peak incidence in children aged 5 to 14 years and in adults aged 50 to 70 years. While craniopharyngiomas are histologically benign, their location near the pituitary stalk, hypothalamus, and optic chiasm and their adherence to critical brain structures can lead to significant morbidity. They also have a high rate of recurrence. Affected children may present with signs of increased intracranial pressure, endocrine deficits (52%-87%), and vision impairment (62%-84%). Involvement of the hypothalamus is common in pediatric craniopharyngiomas, and this poses significant challenges for surgical resection and subsequent quality of life (pituitary dysfunction, hypothalamic obesity, somnolence, memory deficits, and emotional changes). Therefore, surgeons often opt for partial resection, leaving residual tumor that is invasive to the hypothalamus, and treat with subsequent adjuvant radiotherapy.

Nearly all childhood craniopharyngiomas are of the adamantinomatous type (Answer B). They arise from the neoplastic transformation of embryonal remnants of the hypophyseal duct through which the Rathke pouch migrates to form the anterior pituitary gland. The tumors have both solid and cystic components, with calcifications and viscous cholesterol-rich fluid in the cysts. Occasionally teeth can be present. MRI and CT typically reveal a multicystic suprasellar mass with calcification. Most adamantinomatous craniopharyngioma tumors harbor activating mutations in the *CTNNB1* gene, which encodes β-catenin. This results in overactivation of the WNT signaling pathway. Craniopharyngiomas of the papillary type (Answer E), which harbor *BRAF* V600E pathogenic variants, occur nearly exclusively in adult patients.

This child has only a minimal prolactin elevation, most likely due to the stalk effect (pituitary stalk compression or damage to dopaminergic neurons). A large prolactinoma (Answer A) would be expected to be associated with a much higher prolactin level, typically greater than 250 ng/mL. Germinomas (Answer C) account for less than 5% of all intracranial tumors. They arise from germ cells in midline, diencephalic structures. They are most commonly located in the pineal region; however, they can also be suprasellar, arising from the hypothalamus. Diabetes insipidus is a common presenting feature. Emaciation, precocious puberty, visual symptoms, and increased intracranial pressure can also occur. On MRI, germinomas appear as homogeneous, well-rounded, solid masses. The lack of cystic and calcified components distinguish germinomas from craniopharyngiomas. Rathke cleft cysts (Answer D) are benign cystic lesions derived from remnants of the Rathke pouch and arise in the region of the pars intermedia. They typically have an intrasellar location with suprasellar extension. These cysts are usually found incidentally, although rarely they cause symptoms related to mass effect. MRI of a Rathke cleft cyst shows a round, sharply defined intrasellar or suprasellar mass located anterior to the infundibular stalk between the anterior and posterior pituitary. In contrast to childhood craniopharyngiomas, Rathke cleft cysts do not calcify.

Educational Objective

Diagnose craniopharyngioma in children on the basis of clinical signs, symptoms, and laboratory findings and explain the classification, histology, and etiology of different types of craniopharyngioma.

Reference(s)

Müller HL, Merchant TE, Puget S, Martinez-Barbera JP. New outlook on the diagnosis, treatment and follow-up of childhood-onset craniopharyngioma. *Nat Rev Endocrinol.* 2017;13(5):299-312. PMID: 28155902

Cohen LE. Update on childhood craniopharyngiomas. *Curr Opin Endocrinol Diabetes Obes.* 2016;23(4):339-344. PMID: 27258775

Yildiz AE, Oguz KK, Fitoz S. Suprasellar masses in children: characteristic MR imaging features. *J Neuroradiol.* 2016;43(4):246-259. PMID: 27131616

47 **ANSWER: D) Maternal TSH receptor–blocking antibodies**
The most common etiology for congenital hypothyroidism is thyroid dysgenesis, accounting for 85%, followed by thyroid dyshormonogenesis, accounting for 10% to 15%. For patients with thyroid dysgenesis, up to two-thirds have thyroid ectopy (abnormal migration) with significant variation in the location of ectopic tissue, as well as the amount of normal tissue that is found in a normal location (thyroid bed). For patients with profound congenital hypothyroidism, defined as a TSH value greater than 100 mIU/L on a confirmatory sample, the most likely diagnoses are thyroid dysgenesis, thyroid dyshormonogenesis, or maternally derived factors that have the capacity for transplacental transmission, including iodine excess and maternally derived TSH receptor–blocking antibodies (TRAb).

For this patient, the initial laboratory values were consistent with several possible etiologies. However, the decreasing need for levothyroxine replacement is consistent with a transient, maternally derived explanation rather than a permanent abnormality in thyroid gland formation or migration (Answer A) or thyroid hormone production defect (Answer C).

Thyroid ultrasonography was performed and revealed a eutopic thyroid with normal echotexture (*see image*). TRAb were documented to be elevated (2.5 IU/L [reference range ≤ 1.75 IU/L]) (Answer D). With data confirming the etiology, a thyroid scan was not performed; however, one would anticipate decreased radioisotope uptake secondary to elevated TRAb levels. Excess maternal iodine ingestion during pregnancy and during lactation can result in laboratory values consistent with congenital hypothyroidism, but iodine was measured in a spot urine sample and was normal. Interestingly, the mother had no known history of autoimmune thyroid disease, but was referred back to her primary care physician for screening and Hashimoto thyroiditis was subsequently diagnosed.

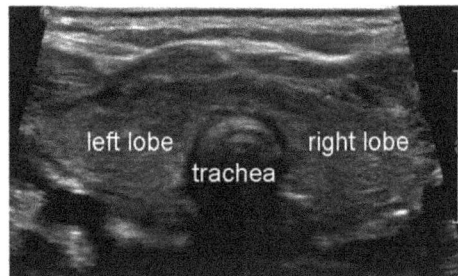

left lobe   right lobe
trachea

Both central hypothyroidism (Answer E) and thyroxine-binding globulin deficiency (Answer B) can be associated with low total T_4; however, TSH should be normal, not elevated as in this case.

Transient congenital hypothyroidism secondary to maternally derived TRAb affects between 1.5% and 2% of newborns, although there is concern that this may be an underestimate of the true prevalence. For many infants, normal thyroid gland development and function are likely. However, there is concern over potential negative impact neurocognitive development in infants born to mothers who have undiagnosed autoimmune hypothyroidism, as well as the potential for altered fetal thyroid gland development and function due to maternal TRAb. In infants with a normal thyroid gland on ultrasonography, the levothyroxine dosage may be decreased before 3 years of age if the TSH is suppressed or it can be trialed off at 3 years if the TSH level is stable despite no increase in levothyroxine dosage over the same time frame.

Educational Objective
Explain how maternal TSH receptor–blocking antibodies can cause transient congenital hypothyroidism.

Reference(s)
Brown RS, Alter CA, Sadeghi-Nejad A. Severe unsuspected maternal hypothyroidism discovered after the diagnosis of thyrotropin receptor-blocking antibody-induced congenital hypothyroidism: failure to recognize and implications to the fetus. *Horm Res Paediatr.* 2015;83(2):132-135. PMID: 25427793

Evans C, Gregory JW, Barton J, et al. Transient congenital hypothyroidism due to thyroid-stimulating hormone receptor blocking antibodies: a case series. *Ann Clin Biochem.* 2011;48(Pt 4):386-390. PMID: 21606073

Connelly KJ, Boston BA, Pearce EN, et al. Congenital hypothyroidism caused by excess prenatal maternal iodine ingestion. *J Pediatr.* 2012;161(4):760-762. PMID: 22841183

48 **ANSWER: B) 9α-fludrocortisone and sodium chloride**
This patient has hyponatremia, hyperkalemia, acidosis, and failure to thrive accompanied by an inappropriately low aldosterone level and elevated plasma renin activity level. This is consistent with mineralocorticoid deficiency. Salt-wasting congenital adrenal hyperplasia (CAH) due to 21-hydroxylase deficiency is the most common inherited cause of adrenal insufficiency that presents with salt-wasting in infancy, and the

clinical presentation is similar to that of this patient. The findings that are inconsistent with the diagnosis of 21-hydroxylase deficiency are her normal genital examination without evidence of androgenization (although mild genital atypia can be missed) and, more strikingly, that the baseline and stimulated 17-hydroxyprogesterone, androstenedione, and testosterone are normal. Cortisol, which is typically low in classic CAH, is also normal here at baseline and after stimulation. 3β-Hydroxysteroid dehydrogenase deficiency is a more rare form of CAH in which salt-wasting occurs; however, in this form, androgens are elevated and there is genital atypia in both sexes. StAR protein deficiency is a rare form of CAH, the hallmark of which is glucocorticoid, mineralocorticoid, and sex steroid deficiency. Therefore, the clinical presentation in the vignette is not consistent with this diagnosis either. This patient has no evidence of glucocorticoid deficiency or androgen excess or deficiency, so the presentation appears to be consistent with an isolated mineralocorticoid pathway defect.

When thinking about an isolated mineralocorticoid pathway defect, the 2 main diagnoses, particularly in this age group, are pseudohypoaldosteronism and isolated aldosterone deficiency. Pseudohypoaldosteronism type 1 is the more common form in which there is apparent unresponsiveness or resistance to the action aldosterone at the renal tubules. The aldosterone level is typically elevated, which excludes the diagnosis in this patient. Her aldosterone level is inappropriately low; therefore, her clinical presentation is consistent with isolated primary hypoaldosteronism.

Isolated primary hypoaldosteronism is a rare autosomal recessive disorder caused by loss-of-function mutations in the *CYP11B2* gene, which encodes the aldosterone synthase enzyme (P450c11AS). Two forms of aldosterone synthase deficiency have been recognized: corticosterone methyloxidase deficiency (CMO) type 1 and type 2. A typical laboratory profile for each type of CMO is as follows:

CMO type	Aldosterone	18-Hydroxycorticosterone	Urine Steroid Profile
Type 1	Undetectable	Low or normal	• Undetectable tetrahydroaldosterone* • Corticosterone metabolites elevated in comparison with cortisol metabolites • Low 18-hydroxycorticosterone metabolites
Type 2	Subnormal or normal	Elevated	• Subnormal or normal tetrahydroaldosterone • Elevated 18-hydroxycorticosterone metabolites

*Tetrahydroaldosterone is a major metabolites of aldosterone

It should be noted that while hyponatremia and hyperkalemia are typically seen in combination, there are reported cases of aldosterone synthase deficiency where potassium levels are normal.

Regarding treatment, an aldosterone analogue 9α-fludrocortisone has a crucial role in normalizing sodium and potassium levels. In infancy, because breast milk and formula are low in sodium, sodium chloride supplementation several times a day is important. This can be discontinued once the patient is on table food with a sufficient amount of salt (thus, Answer B is correct and Answer E is incorrect).

While a combination of sodium chloride, sodium bicarbonate, and potassium-binding resins (Answer A) may normalize the electrolytes, several reports have indicated that treatment with fludrocortisone is necessary for normal linear growth. While this treatment combination is frequently used in pseudohypoaldosteronism, it is not the treatment of choice in aldosterone synthase deficiency. Because glucocorticoid production in aldosterone synthase deficiency is normal and there is no androgen excess that would require ACTH suppression and in turn suppression of androgens, treatment with glucocorticoids (Answers C and D) is not needed.

The condition improves with age because of the improvement of the metabolic function of the renin-angiotensin system and the aldosterone activities on the renal tubules. Some have advocated discontinuing treatment in adulthood, although there is evidence to suggest that electrolyte abnormalities can still occur during times of dehydration, illness, and other stressors and patients may develop orthostatic hypotension. In addition, recent studies suggest that even with absence of electrolyte abnormalities but with elevated plasma renin activity and elevated angiotensin levels, patients can develop glomerulosclerosis.

Educational Objective
Construct a differential diagnosis for hypoaldosteronism and develop a diagnostic approach.

Reference(s)

Li N, Li J, Ding Y, et al. Novel mutations in the CYP11B2 gene causing aldosterone synthase deficiency. *Mol Med Rep.* 2016;13(4):3127-3132. PMID: 26936515

Collinet E, Pelissier P, Richard O, et al. Four cases of aldosterone synthase deficiency in childhood. *Arch Pediatr.* 2012;19(11):1191-1195. PMID: 23062999

Pela I, Capirchio L, Menchini C, Anzilotti G, Seminara S. Isolated aldosterone deficiency in two infants: mistakes and dilemmas in the diagnosis and treatment of a rare disease. *Open J Pediatr.* 2013;3(4):391-396.

49 ANSWER: A) Perform retinal exam, assess for microalbuminuria, order lipid panel, and assess for hypertension

In this vignette, an African American adolescent presents with the combination of obesity, acanthosis nigricans, and severe diabetic ketoacidosis. Although most episodes of diabetic ketoacidosis that occur in new-onset diabetes are in patients with type 1 diabetes, 5% to 10% of patients with type 2 diabetes present with diabetic ketoacidosis. This rate is higher in individuals of nonwhite ethnicity (up to 25%). Given the current epidemic of obesity in the pediatric population, it is not uncommon to see obese patients with type 1 diabetes with evidence of insulin resistance. Because the long-term treatment and risk of complications are different for type 1 vs type 2 diabetes, it is important to distinguish between these 2 entities. The acute treatment of diabetic ketoacidosis in type 1 and type 2 diabetes is similar, but one must be very careful to identify those patients with type 2 diabetes who present with nonketotic hyperosmolar hyperglycemia, as the acute treatment is very different and the risk of morbidity and mortality due to poor treatment is very high. In the long term, patients with type 2 diabetes might be able to discontinue insulin therapy after a few months of combined insulin, metformin, and successful implementation of lifestyle changes. However, as long as the hemoglobin A_{1c} level is above 8.5% (>69 mmol/mol), the patient should remain on insulin.

Surveillance for comorbid conditions and disease complications is different in type 1 and type 2 diabetes. In childhood, type 2 diabetes may be far more severe than in adulthood, with a significant number of patients having disease complications at diagnosis and a proportion developing complete insulin deficiency at a far earlier stage than an adult might. Therefore, retinal exam, lipid screening, urine microalbuminuria screening, and careful examination for the presence of hypertension should be performed immediately after diagnosis once the patient is out of metabolic crisis (Answer A). Any surveillance plan that delays or does not include these critical assessments is inadequate (Answers B, C, D, and E). Patients with type 2 diabetes do not have an increased risk of thyroid disease or celiac disease, both of which are autoimmune-mediated conditions.

Educational Objective
Explain the differences in disease surveillance between patients with type 1 and type 2 diabetes mellitus.

Reference(s)

American Diabetes Association. 12. Children and adolescents. *Diabetes Care.* 2017;40(Suppl 1):S105-S113. PMID: 27979899

Copeland KC, Zeitler P, Geffner M, et al; TODAY study group. Characteristics of adolescents and youth with recent onset type 2 diabetes: the TODAY cohort at baseline. *J Clin Endocrinol Metab.* 2011;96(1):159-167. PMID: 20962021

50 ANSWER: B) LH level

Klinefelter syndrome, a chromosomal aneuploidy characterized by a 47,XXY karyotype (and mosaic variations), occurs in approximately 1 in 500 males. It is among the most common etiologies of male-factor infertility and frequently remains undiagnosed through childhood and adolescence. Pathognomonic findings include small testes with a generous phallus inconsistent with the stage of puberty, tall stature, and learning differences. It can be diagnosed prenatally, when children are of school age (when undergoing evaluation for learning and developmental issues, possibly associated with clinical features), or, most commonly, in fertility clinics.

With increasing use of laboratory genetics to complement clinical evaluation, more patients will most likely be referred at a younger age, and questions of fertility preservation will arise. Although infertility is the rule, the exception of fertility, often associated with 47,XXY/46,XY mosaicism, is reported. To predict, and hence preserve, future fertility is part of the routine clinical care of peripubertal children. Testicular microdissection has an approximately 30% yield in obtaining viable spermatozoa; therefore, methods to predict the best candidates for this invasive technique are imperative.

Interestingly, LH (Answer B) and testosterone levels, markers of Leydig-cell function, and not other biochemical or clinical findings that are associated with Sertoli-cell function (eg, FSH [Answer E], testicular volume [Answer C], or antimullerian hormone [Answer D]), correlate best with the presence of spermatozoa in patients who undergo testicular microdissection. In men with a 46,XY karyotype, FSH, inhibin B, and testosterone levels are predictors of fertility. However, this does not hold true for men with a 47,XXY karyotype. The progressive hyalinization of the Sertoli cells seen in Klinefelter syndrome suggests that Leydig-cell function best predicts the possibility of fertility.

Educational Objective
Counsel patients with Klinefelter syndrome regarding the best predictors of fertility.

Reference(s)

Rohayem J, Fricke R, Czeloth K, et al. Age and markers of Leydig cell function, but not of Sertoli cell function predict the success of sperm retrieval in adolescents and adults with Klinefelter's syndrome. *Andrology*. 2015;3(5):868-875. PMID: 26235799

Aksglaede L, Juul A. Testicular function and fertility in men with Klinefelter syndrome: a review. *Eur J Endocrinol*. 2013;168(4):R67-R76. PMID: 23504510

51 ANSWER: D) Heterophile antibodies

Heterophile antibodies (Answer D) are naturally occurring antibodies induced by external antigens that may cross-react with self-antigens and cause interference with immunoassays. Two-site, noncompetitive "sandwich" assays are particularly vulnerable to interference from heterophile antibodies, which may lead to falsely elevated values by bridging between the capture and signal antibody, or falsely low levels by blocking them. Heterophile antibodies are common, occurring in 30% to 40% of all serum samples; however, they result in assay interference in less than 0.05%.

Serial dilution is a technique that can be applied if an interfering agent is suspected. Serially diluting a sample typically leads to a linear decrease in the amount of analyte, while heterophile antibody interference does not typically change in a linear fashion. Heterophile antibody interference can be eliminated by removing immunoglobulins and extracting the analyte through gel chromatography or precipitation with polyethylene glycol.

In this patient, the isolated PTH elevation, lack of additional mineral disturbances, and lack of clinical abnormalities are suggestive of assay interference. His history of excessive exercise is the most likely etiology of his recurrent stress fractures. The patient's serum was subjected to serial dilutions (1/2, 1/4, 1/8), which showed a minimal and nonlinear decrease in PTH levels, suggesting the presence of assay interference. The patient's serum was then subjected to precipitation with polyethylene glycol to remove interfering antibodies, and the PTH level was subsequently documented to be normal (59 pg/mL).

Primary hyperparathyroidism (Answer A) is associated with hypercalcemia and hypophosphatemia, while PTH resistance (Answer C) is associated with hypocalcemia and hyperphosphatemia. This patient's mineral markers, however, are within the normal range. 25-Hydroxyvitamin D deficiency (Answer B) can be associated with secondary hyperparathyroidism due to insufficient dietary calcium absorption. However, this patient's level of vitamin D is minimally decreased and is unlikely to be associated with this severe apparent PTH elevation. In addition, his 1,25-dihydroxyvitamin D level is discordantly normal given his PTH elevation. Excessive dietary protein intake (Answer E) can lead to increased urinary calcium excretion due to an increased renal acid load. However, this is unlikely to result in PTH elevation to this degree, and this patient's urinary calcium is normal.

Educational Objective
Explain the uses and limitations of assays for PTH and vitamin D metabolites and other calciotropic hormones.

Reference(s)

Tate J, Ward G. Interferences in immunoassay. *Clin Biochem Rev*. 2004;25(2):105-120. PMID: 18458713

Gulbahar O, Konca Degertekin C, Akturk M, et al. A case with immunoassay interferences in the measurement of multiple hormones. *J Clin Endocrinol Metab*. 2015;100(6):2147-2153. PMID: 25897621

52 ANSWER: D) Constitutional tall stature

This child most likely has constitutional tall stature (Answer D). This is a condition that mirrors constitutional short stature. Children with constitutional tall stature are taller than expected for their genetic potential and, while their skeletal maturation is advanced and their pubertal development tends to occur at an earlier than average age, their adult height prediction falls within their genetic potential (target height or midparental height range). Their growth velocity is not abnormally rapid, but it is robust as is the case for typical tall children compared with typical short children.

Onset of normal puberty in boys can happen as early as age 9 years. The first clinical sign of activation of the hypothalamic-pituitary-gonadal axis in boys (true puberty) is testicular growth (testicular volume of ≥4 mL). The boy in this vignette is approaching this testicular volume at age 9 and 5/12 months. While on the early side, this is not considered precocious (Answer A). In addition, his LH, testosterone, and free testosterone levels are clearly prepubertal.

Premature adrenarche (Answer B) is the term used for early activation of the adrenal production of androgens before age 9 years in boys. The child in this vignette has Tanner stage 2 pubic hair and a DHEA-S level consistent with adrenarche; however, it is not premature given his age. Random levels of 17-hydroxyprogesterone, 17-hydroxypregnenolone, and androstenedione are not elevated and do not support a diagnosis of congenital adrenal hyperplasia.

The patient's IGF-1 level is within the normal range for age and his prolactin level is normal. These analytes would be expected to be elevated in the setting of gigantism (GH excess) (Answer E).

Educational Objective
Diagnose constitutional tall stature and differentiate it from precocious puberty and gigantism.

Reference(s)

Papadimitriou A, Nicolaidou P, Fretzayas A, Chrousos GP. Clinical review: constitutional advancement of growth; a.k.a. early growth acceleration, predicts early puberty and childhood obesity. *J Clin Endocrinol Metab.* 2010;95(10):4535-4541. PMID: 20610589

Laron Z. To be or not to be "TALL"? *Pediatr Endocrinol Rev.* 2012;9(4):696-697. PMID: 23304805

Baron J, Savendahl L, DeLuca F, et al. Short and tall stature: a new paradigm emerges. *Nat Rev Endocrinol.* 2015;11(12):735-746. PMID: 26437621

53 ANSWER: C) TSH measurement

When evaluating prematurely developing breast buds in girls (before age 8 years), one must distinguish between gonadotropin-independent precocious puberty vs central precocious puberty vs pseudoprecocious puberty. Exposure to estrogen or a compound that can act as an estrogen, such as lavender or tea tree essential oil, should be considered, but the estradiol level in such patients remains prepubertal, which is not the case here.

Her growth pattern suggests primary hypothyroidism. Severe primary hypothyroidism has been known to be associated with pseudoprecocious puberty, also termed Van Wyk-Grumbach syndrome. Bone age can also be frankly delayed in affected patients, which is consistent with this patient's presentation. Therefore, the best next step is to measure her TSH level (Answer C). The exact mechanism underlying this association is not entirely clear. Some evidence supports direct effect of thyrotropin-releasing hormone on the pituitary resulting in FSH and prolactin elevations, and other evidence points to high TSH levels acting on the FSH receptor (less effect on the LH receptor). Girls with severe hypothyroidism can present in a similar way to this patient (with a predominantly FSH effect), so that estradiol is elevated. However, in boys, the testicular volume is enlarged (FSH effect), while testosterone levels are prepubertal.

In early puberty, LH pulses occur at night, so it is common to have prepubertal LH levels during the day, even with the currently available ultrasensitive assays. Therefore, if central precocious puberty is suspected, one may consider repeating the LH measurement (Answer D), or performing a leuprolide-stimulation test (Answer A) to confirm the diagnosis.

Pelvic ultrasonography (Answer B) is helpful in documenting ovarian cysts that are often seen in McCune-Albright syndrome, a well-known form of gonadotropin-independent precocious puberty associated with café-au-lait spots with irregular margins and/or fibrous dysplasia bony lesions that can be noted on x-rays or a bone scan (Answer E). However, one of the hallmarks of puberty is an increase in height velocity, which is absent in this case. Because her height velocity was only at the 10th percentile, the likelihood of either central precocious puberty or

McCune-Albright syndrome is not high. Patients with Van Wyk-Grumbach syndrome can also have large ovarian cysts, but ultrasonography would not be the diagnostic test for this condition.

Educational Objective

Suspect primary hypothyroidism as a cause of pseudoprecocious puberty.

Reference(s)

Cabrera SM, DiMeglio LA, Eugster EA. Incidence and characteristics of pseudoprecocious puberty because of severe primary hypothyroidism. *J Pediatr*. 2013; 162(3):637-639. PMID: 23196132

Zhang H1, Geng N, Wang Y, Tian W, Xue F. Van Wyk and Grumbach syndrome: two case reports and review of the published work. *J Obstet Gynaecol Res*. 2014; 40(2):607-610. PMID: 24118179

54   ANSWER: D) Pathogenic variant in the transcription factor *HNF1A* or *HNF4A* genes

Pathogenic variants in the hepatocyte nuclear factor-1 alpha gene (*HNF1A*) (Answer D) are the most common cause of monogenic diabetes (maturity-onset diabetes of the young type 3 [MODY 3]), but affected patients are often misdiagnosed as having type 1 diabetes and started on insulin treatment. Patients with *HNF1A*-related diabetes (MODY 3) are particularly sensitive to the glucose-lowering effect of sulfonylureas, which are the pharmacologic treatment of choice. Sulfonylurea responsiveness progressively diminishes in the third and fourth decades. Pathogenic variants in the *HNF4A* gene (MODY 1) are rare, but the clinical presentation of affected patients is similar to that of patients with *HNF1A* mutations with milder features. Normal fasting glucose is a key feature in this case. MODY 1 and MODY 3 are progressive conditions with worsening glycemic control over time. Affected patients may require insulin therapy in addition to oral agents.

The *GCK* gene encodes the pancreatic glucose sensor, glucokinase, a rate-limiting enzyme that catalyzes the phosphorylation of glucose. Heterozygous loss-of-function mutations result in mild fasting hyperglycemia throughout life. Persons with *GCK*-related MODY (MODY 2) have a defect in glucose sensing. Hence, glucose homeostasis is maintained at a higher set point, resulting in mild, asymptomatic fasting hyperglycemia and hemoglobin A_{1c} values in the range of 5.8% to 7.0% (40 to 53 mmol/mol). The condition is present from birth and shows slight deterioration with age. Pharmacologic treatment is rarely required and does not appear to alter glycemic control. The patient in this vignette has normal fasting glucose with a higher hemoglobin A_{1c} value than patients who present with *GCK*-related MODY. His family members' diabetes progression is also not consistent with *GCK*-related MODY.

The major histocompatibility complex on chromosome 6 is the main susceptibility region for type 1 diabetes. Polymorphisms in the *HLA-DRB1* and *HLA-DQB1* class II loci encoding DR and DQ molecules (Answer B) are most strongly associated with disease risk or protection, but there is evidence that other loci within the HLA gene area contribute to disease susceptibility as well. However, in this setting, the inheritance pattern of type 1 diabetes is not autosomal dominant as observed in this vignette.

The *PDX1* gene (Answer C) encodes a transcriptional activator of several genes, including insulin, somatostatin, glucokinase, islet amyloid polypeptide, and glucose transporter type 2. The encoded nuclear protein is involved in the early development of the pancreas and has a major role in glucose-dependent regulation of insulin gene expression. Homozygous defects in *PDX1* are a cause of pancreatic agenesis and neonatal diabetes, as well as heterozygous pathogenic variants leading to MODY 4. The clinical features resemble those of type 2 diabetes, including obesity and insulin resistance. The *INS* gene is also a protein-coding gene that is essential in insulin transcription. Pathogenic variants in these genes can result in a variety of defects in glucose homeostasis, but they are not consistent with the clinical presentation in this vignette.

Transcription factor 7-like 2 encoded by the *TCF7L2* gene is a key element of the Wnt signaling pathway. Genome-wide association studies have shown that *TCF7L2* is the most important locus predisposing to type 2 diabetes. At the individual level, carrying the *TCF7L2* risk allele increases the risk of type 2 diabetes by 50%. However, at the population level, the attributable risk is lower than 25% and varies with the allele frequency. The *TCF7L2* gene is expressed in β cells, and defects possibly impair GLP-1–induced insulin secretion and/or the production of new mature β cells. Although this is a possible etiology in this vignette, the autosomal dominant inheritance pattern and lack of type 2 diabetes phenotype make this choice unlikely.

Educational Objective

Differentiate among monogenic forms of diabetes on the basis of clinical presentation, laboratory values, and family history.

Reference(s)

Scott RA, Scott LJ, Magi R, et al; DIAbetes Genetics Replication And Meta-analysis (DIAGRAM) Consortium. An expanded genome-wide association study of type 2 diabetes in Europeans. *Diabetes*. 2017;66(11):2888-2902. PMID: 28566273

Shields BM, Shepherd M, Hudson M, et al; UNITED study team. Population-based assessment of a biomarker-based screening pathway to aid diagnosis of monogenic diabetes in young-onset patients. *Diabetes Care*. 2017;40(8):1017-1025. PMID: 28701371

Noble JA, Erlich HA. Genetics of type 1 diabetes. *Cold Spring Harb Perspect Med*. 2012;2(1):a007732. PMID: 22315720

Cauchi S, Froguel P. TCF7L2 genetic defect and type 2 diabetes. *Curr Diab Rep*. 2008;8(2):149-155. PMID: 18445358

Chakera AJ, Steele AM, Gloyn AL, et al. Recognition and management of individuals with hyperglycemia because of a heterozygous glucokinase mutation. *Diabetes Care*. 2015;38(7):1383-1392. PMID: 26106223

Fajans SS, Bell GI, Paz VP, et al. Obesity and hyperinsulinemia in a family with pancreatic agenesis and MODY caused by the IPF1 mutation Pro63fsX60. *Transl Res*. 2010;156(1):7-14. PMID: 20621032

55 ANSWER: B) Prolactinoma

The pertinent findings in this case are secondary amenorrhea, galactorrhea, and hyperprolactinemia. Prolactin synthesis and secretion by pituitary lactotroph cells is under tonic inhibition from hypothalamic dopamine, which traverses the portal venous system onto the lactotroph D2 receptors. Several factors induce prolactin synthesis and secretion, including estrogen, thyrotropin-releasing hormone, epidermal growth factor, and dopamine receptor antagonists. Prolactin functions to induce and maintain lactation of the primed breast. Nonpregnancy hyperprolactinemia is most often caused by prolactinomas (lactotroph adenomas) (Answer B). Prolactinomas account for approximately 40% of all pituitary tumors. Prolactinomas are rare in children, but account for 50% of all pediatric pituitary adenomas and 2% of all pediatric intracranial tumors. Hyperprolactinemia can also be idiopathic or result from pharmacologic interruptions of hypothalamic-pituitary-dopaminergic pathways, or pathologic interruptions. Hyperprolactinemia can cause galactorrhea, hypogonadism, infertility, and reduced bone mineral density, although it can also be asymptomatic. The prolactin level most often correlates with the size of the adenoma. Macroprolactinomas (>10 mm) are typically associated with prolactin levels greater than 250 ng/mL (>10.9 nmol/L). When levels are not as high as expected, it is important to repeat the measurement after a 1:100 serum sample dilution to overcome the possible hook effect that can occur with 2-site immunoradiometric assays. The most likely diagnosis in this patient is a prolactinoma.

One must rule out medication usage, hypothyroidism, renal failure, and parasellar tumors as possible causes of nonphysiologic hyperprolactinemia. The most common physiologic cause of hyperprolactinemia is pregnancy. This patient has been taking oral contraceptive pills with excellent adherence, as well as condoms, so pregnancy (Answer E) is highly unlikely.

Interruption of hypothalamic dopaminergic inhibition of prolactin by disruption or compression of the pituitary stalk ("stalk effect") due to a nonsecreting pituitary tumor or parasellar mass can cause prolactin elevations (eg, large nonfunctioning pituitary tumors, craniopharyngioma, granulomatous infiltration of the hypothalamus). In a study of 226 patients with histologically confirmed nonfunctioning pituitary adenomas, prolactin levels greater than 94 ng/mL (>4.1 nmol/L) reliably distinguished prolactinomas from nonfunctioning pituitary adenomas. This patient's prolactin level of 112 ng/mL (4.9 nmol/L) is higher than one would expect from stalk effect caused by a craniopharyngioma (Answer D).

The most common cause of nontumoral hyperprolactinemia is medications, most often antipsychotic and neuroleptic agents. Hyperprolactinemia due to medications is generally associated with prolactin levels between 25 and 100 ng/mL (1.1 and 4.3 nmol/L), although some medications, including risperidone, phenothiazines, and metoclopramide, can cause prolactin levels greater than 200 ng/mL (>8.7 nmol/L). While some antidepressant medications (Answer C) can cause hyperprolactinemia, they are not likely to cause such a high degree of elevation as is observed in this patient. Twelve to thirty percent of women taking higher dosage estrogen-containing oral contraceptives (Answer A) have mild increases in prolactin. This patient, however, has a markedly elevated prolactin level.

A summary of the etiologies of hyperprolactinemia is shown (*see table*).

Physiologic
Pregnancy
Lactation
Stress
Sleep
Coitus
Exercise
Pathologic
Systemic disorders
Primary hypothyroidism
Renal insufficiency
Cirrhosis
Polycystic ovary syndrome
Epileptic seizures
Pseudocyesis
Hypothalamic disorders
Tumors: craniopharyngioma, dysgerminoma, meningioma, extension of suprasellar mass
Infiltrative or granulomatous disease: histiocytosis, sarcoidosis
Cranial irradiation
Rathke cleft cyst
Trauma: suprasellar surgery
Pituitary disorders
Prolactinoma
Acromegaly
Lymphocytic hypophysitis
Thyrotropinoma
Cushing disease
Macroprolactinemia
Trauma
Surgery
Neurogenic
Chest wall lesions: burns, breast surgery, herpes zoster, thoracotomy, nipple rings
Spinal cord injury: cervical ependymoma, tabes dorsalis, intrinsic tumor
Breast stimulation
Idiopathic
Ectopic prolactin production
Renal cell carcinoma
Ovarian teratoma
Gonadoblastoma
NonHodgkin lymphoma
Uterine cervical carcinoma
Pharmacologic
Neuroleptics/antipsychotics
Anticonvulsants: phenytoin
Antidepressants: tricyclic, MAO inhibitors, SSRIs
Antihistamines (H2)
Antihypertensives
Dopamine synthesis inhibitor
Opioids and opiod antagonists
Anesthetics
Estrogens: oral contraceptives
Prokinetic agents: metoclopramide, domperidone

Educational Objective
Distinguish between prolactin-secreting tumors and hyperprolactinemia due to other causes.

Reference(s)

Melmed S, Casanueva FF, Hoffman AR, et al; Endocrine Society. Diagnosis and treatment of hyperprolactinemia: an Endocrine Society clinical practice guideline. *J Clin Endocrinol Metab*. 2011;96(2):273-288. PMID: 21296991

Hoffmann A, Adelmann S, Lohle K, Claviez A, Müller HL. Pediatric prolactinoma: initial presentation, treatment, and long-term prognosis. *Eur J Pediatr*. 2018; 177(1):125-132. PMID: 29168011

56 ANSWER: C) Elevated deoxycorticosterone

This patient has a 46,XX karyotype, primary amenorrhea, minimal pubertal development (Tanner stage 2 breasts and no pubic or axillary hair development), hypertension, mild hypokalemia, and a low plasma renin activity. In the clinical scenario of a 46,XX karyotype, a disorder of pubertal development, and low renin hypertension, one must consider 17α-hydroxylase/17,20-lyase deficiency. This is a rare autosomal recessive condition caused by pathogenic variants in the *CYP17A1* gene. Affected patients with a 46,XY karyotype present with female or slightly atypical genitalia due to undervirilization, cryptorchidism, elevated blood pressure, low renin, and hypokalemia. Individuals with a 46,XX karyotype, such as this patient, have normal external and internal female genitalia. However, due to deficient 17α-hydroxylase and 17,20-lyase enzymatic activity, both in the adrenal glands and in the gonads, production of androgens (ie, testosterone and androstenedione) is low and production of ovarian estrogen is low. Because of ovarian dysfunction, affected patients have amenorrhea and little to no breast development. There is little to no pubic or axillary hair development due to low androgens. The steroidogenic blockade also affects cortisol production.

The steroidogenic blockade in androgen production in the zona reticularis of the adrenal cortex and cortisol production in the zona fasciculata in turn leads to overproduction of precursors with mineralocorticoid activity at the zona glomerulosa. Therefore, serum levels of deoxycorticosterone (DOC), corticosterone, and 18-deoxycorticosterone become elevated, leading to suppression of renin levels and causing hypertension (*see figure*). It should be noted, however, that depending on the degree of the steroidogenic deficiency, some patients may be normotensive, so absence of hypertension should not rule out *CYP17A1* deficiency. Hypokalemia is variable as well, and some affected patients have normal potassium levels. Because of the location of the blockade, pregnenolone and progesterone levels can also be elevated.

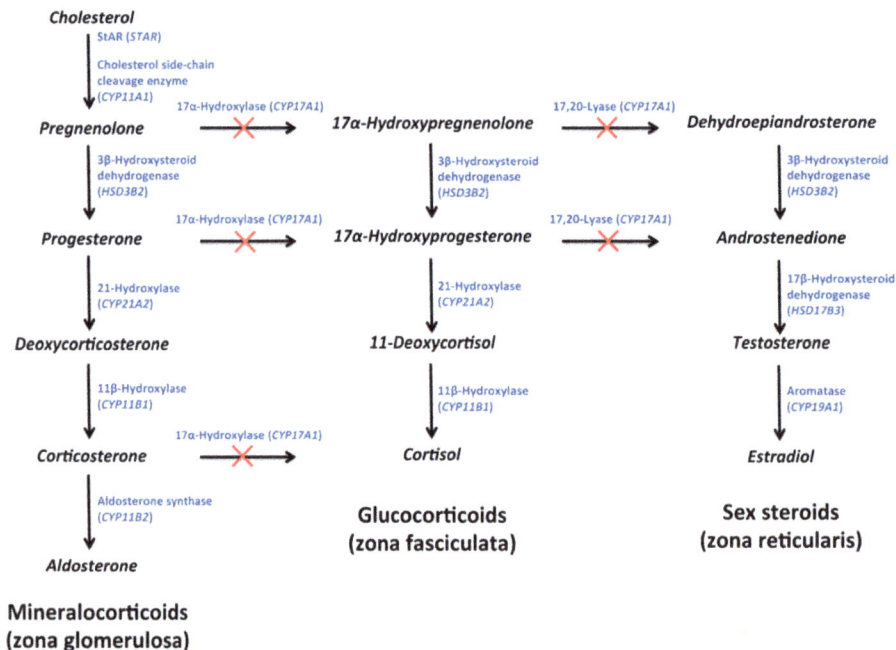

Elevated DOC (Answer C) is one of the markers of 17α-hydroxylase/17,20-lyase deficiency. In this setting, androgens such as testosterone are low, not high (Answer A). Because of gonadal insufficiency, gonadotropin levels are expected to be elevated, not low (Answer B). Interestingly, most patients with this disorder have ovarian enlargement or ovarian cysts and are at risk for ovarian torsion. Because of little to no estrogen exposure, the uterus is small for age and even hypoplastic. ACTH levels are often elevated because of cortisol deficiency and are rarely in the normal range (Answer D). Finally, corticosterone production is elevated, not low (Answer E).

The aim of treatment is to lower ACTH levels, in turn suppressing the levels of precursors with mineralocorticoid activity (such as DOC, corticosterone, and 18-deoxycorticosterone), increasing renin production, and normalizing blood pressure. This can be achieved with glucocorticoid therapy such as hydrocortisone in children or dexamethasone in fully grown adolescents and adults. Female patients with 17α-hydroxylase/17,20-lyase deficiency also require hormone replacement therapy to progress through puberty and achieve menses. A recent report documented that patients with *CYP17A1* deficiency have higher incidence of anxiety and depression, and it is speculated that reduced *CYP17A1* expression in the central nervous system has a role.

Educational Objective

Explain the pathophysiology of patients with pathogenic variants in the *CYP17A1* gene.

Reference(s)

Carvalho LC, Brito VN, Martin RM, et al. Clinical, hormonal, ovarian, and genetic aspects of 46,XX patients with congenital adrenal hyperplasia due to CYP17A1 defects. *Fertil Steril*. 2016;105(6):1612-1619. PMID: 26920256

Costa-Santos M, Kater CE, Auchus RJ; Brazilian Congenital Adrenal Hyperplasia Multicenter Study Group. Two prevalent CYP17 mutations and genotype-phenotype correlations in 24 Brazilian patients with 17-hydroxylase deficiency. *J Clin Endocrinol Metab*. 2004;89(1):49-60. PMID: 14715827

Young WF. Endocrine hypertension. In: Melmed S, Polonsky KS, Larsen PR, Kronenberg HM. *Williams Textbook of Endocrinology*. 13th ed. Elsevier. 2016: 556-588.

57 ANSWER: B) Surgical referral for gonadectomy

Additional testing revealed a 46,XY karyotype; thus, this patient was diagnosed with complete androgen insensitivity syndrome. This condition is caused by mutations in the gene encoding the androgen receptor (*AR*) and affects up to 1 in 20,000 persons with a male karyotype.

The risk of a malignant germ-cell tumor in persons with complete androgen insensitivity is very low in childhood, so there is no need for prophylactic gonadectomy at an early age. Deferring gonadectomy until late adolescence allows for spontaneous breast development, as well as bone mass accrual during puberty through peripheral aromatization of testosterone to estrogens. Tumor incidence increases in adulthood, with low risk of progression to invasive disease. However, adequate tools do not currently exist that can detect a noninvasive tumor. Therefore, the current recommendation is for gonadectomy at completion of puberty (Answer B).

Malignant testicular germ-cell tumors are thought to occur in approximately 10% of individuals with androgen insensitivity syndrome. The risk for germ-cell tumors is increased in individuals with disorders of sexual development who have Y-chromosome material. Loci that may be involved in the pathogenesis of malignant germ-cell proliferation include the gonadoblastoma on Y (GBY) region and testis-specific protein, Y-linked (TSPY). Deferring gonadectomy beyond adolescence would result in increased risk of tumor development. Thus, simply providing counseling (Answer C) is incorrect.

Currently, no satisfactory diagnostic tools are available to allow for serial monitoring of in situ neoplastic lesions. Ultrasonography does not allow for adequate visualization of intra-abdominal gonads, and this vignette demonstrates that structures can be misidentified on ultrasound. Although MRI (Answer D) is preferred for visualization of intra-abdominal gonads, it has poor ability to detect germ-cell neoplasia in situ. MRI can be useful in the workup after an invasive germ-cell tumor has developed.

Likewise, tumor markers such as β-hCG and α-fetoprotein (Answer A) are useful in evaluation of certain germ-cell malignancies, including choriocarcinomas and yolk sack tumors, but not in seminomas, which are the most common malignancy in complete androgen insensitivity syndrome or germ-cell neoplasia in situ. Detection of microRNAs belonging to the miR-371 and miR-302/367 clusters shows promise in detecting invasive testicular germ-cell tumors; however, it is less likely that germ-cell neoplasia in situ tumors would secrete these microRNAs.

Postpubertal individuals with complete androgen insensitivity syndrome would be expected to have total testosterone levels in the adult male range. There is some overlap in this patient's testosterone levels with androgen-secreting tumors of the ovaries and adrenal glands; however, these tumors would be expected to cause significant virilization. Thus, additional evaluation for an adrenal tumor with CT (Answer E) is unlikely to be helpful in this case.

Educational Objective
Counsel families on management of complete androgen insensitivity syndrome, taking into account the risk of malignancy.

Reference(s)

Cools M, Looijenga L. Update on the pathophysiology and risk factors for the development of malignant testicular germ cell tumors in complete androgen insensitivity syndrome. *Sex Dev.* 2017;11(4):175-181. PMID: 28719895

Mendoza N, Motos MA. Androgen insensitivity syndrome. *Gynecol Endocrinol.* 2013;29(1):1-5. PMID: 22812659

58 ANSWER: E) Order screening lab tests including free T_4, TSH, IGF-1, LH, FSH, and testosterone and consider stimulation studies

Childhood cancer survivors are at risk for multiple endocrinopathies based on their cancer diagnosis and treatment history. About 50% of childhood cancer survivors develop 1 or more endocrine disorder in their lifetime. Risk of endocrine late effects is directly related to the underlying cancer diagnosis and treatment. A comprehensive cancer treatment summary is crucial in assessing the need for appropriate screening for endocrine late effects. Patients with brain tumors close to the hypothalamus/pituitary are at risk for acute pituitary dysfunction due to mass effect and/or surgery. Hypopituitarism is a potential late effect observed years after cranial radiation therapy, the prevalence of which increases with increasing radiation dose and duration after radiation therapy. Typically, patients with brain tumors are treated with high doses of radiation (>30 Gy), putting them at highest risk for hypopituitarism among all childhood cancer survivors. GH deficiency is the most common pituitary dysfunction noted after cranial irradiation, although hypothyroidism (primary or central), central precocious puberty, and hypogonadotropic hypogonadism can also occur and affect growth. Testicular size may be misleading in the assessment of pubertal status in childhood cancer survivors, as relatively smaller testicular volume can be seen despite advanced or completed puberty due to differential effects of gonadal toxicity of alkylating agent chemotherapy and radiation on testicular germ cells vs Leydig cells. Spinal radiation can have a direct effect on the growth of the spine and cause disproportionate short stature as evidenced by more compromised sitting height vs standing height measurement. However, this patient needs to be screened for hypopituitarism (Answer E). Careful consideration should also be given to conducting stimulation studies to assess adrenal cortisol sufficiency.

Performing no further evaluation (Answers A and B) is not appropriate for a child with a history of a brain tumor who presents with poor growth and short stature. Although screening for celiac disease (Answer C) should be considered in any patient presenting with poor growth or short stature, a patient with a history of high-dose cranial radiation therapy and short stature should be tested for hypopituitarism regardless of celiac screening results. TSH measurement without also measuring T_4 (Answer D) is not an adequate screen for central hypothyroidism. Although a low IGF-1 level could be indicative of severe GH deficiency, documenting a normal IGF-1 value is not enough to rule out GH deficiency since it is a poor marker of GH status in these patients. GH-stimulation testing should be considered in childhood cancer survivors who are at high risk for GH deficiency even if their IGF-1 level is normal.

Educational Objective
Assess childhood cancer survivors for endocrine late effects, including hypopituitarism.

Reference(s)

Chemaitilly W, Cohen LE, Mostoufi-Moab S, et al. Endocrine late effects in childhood cancer survivors. *J Clin Oncol.* 2018;36(21):2153-2159. PMID: 29874130

Sklar CA, Antal Z, Chemaitilly W, et al. Hypothalamic-pituitary and growth disorders in survivors of childhood cancer: an Endocrine Society clinical practice guideline. *J Clin Endocrinol Metab.* 2018;103(8):2761-2784. PMID: 29982476

Chemaitilly W, Armstrong GT, Gajjar A, Hudson MM. Hypothalamic-pituitary axis dysfunction in survivors of childhood CNS tumors: importance of systematic follow-up and early endocrine consultation. *J Clin Oncol.* 2016;34(36):4315-4319. PMID: 27998231

59 ANSWER: B) GH-stimulation test

The patient in this vignette has abnormal weight gain, a common sequela following resection of a craniopharyngioma. This weight gain potentially occurs as a result of disruption in appetite-regulating centers such as the infundibular or arcuate nucleus in the hypothalamus, although it is not common to visualize the damage to individual hypothalamic nuclei on MRI (Answer A). Unfortunately in this scenario, even with the knowledge of dysregulation of appetite centers, no additional steps can be taken beyond usual approaches to unhealthy weight gain, including recommendations to increase in physical activity and decrease food intake.

The most common pituitary abnormality following craniopharyngioma removal is GH deficiency. In contrast to the pattern of linear growth failure typically seen with other causes of GH deficiency, following craniopharyngioma removal, linear growth may be normal and IGF-1 levels can also be in the normal range, both potentially in part related to the excess weight gain. Nevertheless, values on GH-stimulation testing (Answer B) are low. Treatment of GH deficiency results in a decrease of 4 to 6 kg in fat mass and an increase in lean mass, which is better than durable changes seen following many approaches to obesity treatment. Therefore, the best diagnostic assessment to perform now is a GH-stimulation test. While there may be theoretical risks of stimulating neoplasms with GH therapy, studies have shown that GH treatment does not increase the risk of craniopharyngioma recurrence.

Although assessment of beverage consumption (Answer E) and recommendations to decrease intake of calorie-dense drinks such as sugar-sweetened beverages and juice should certainly be undertaken to decrease this patient's total caloric intake, elimination of sugar-sweetened beverages has led to only a small decrease in weight gain in randomized controlled trials. These changes are modest in comparison to changes in fat mass that occur with GH replacement among GH-deficient individuals.

Other pituitary deficiencies also frequently occur, including TSH deficiency, which may contribute to decreased linear growth and increased BMI. Excess production of pituitary hormones such as ACTH is not expected, so measurement of 24-hour urinary free cortisol (Answer C) is incorrect.

Craniopharyngiomas can recur, but this could be observed on MRI. Second operations (Answer D) only increase the risk for sequelae.

Educational Objective
Assess for growth hormone deficiency as the most common pituitary abnormality after craniopharyngioma removal.

Reference(s)

Tiulpakov AN, Mazerkina NA, Brook CG, Hindmarsh PC, Peterkova VA, Gorelyshev SK. Growth in children with craniopharyngioma following surgery. *Clin Endocrinol (Oxf)*. 1998;49(6):733-738. PMID: 10209560

Carroll PV, Christ ER, Bengtsson BA, et al. Growth hormone deficiency in adulthood and the effects of growth hormone replacement: a review. Growth Hormone Research Society Scientific Committee. *J Clin Endocrinol Metab*. 1998;83(2):382-395. PMID: 9467546

60 **ANSWER: E) TSH is low for age; the newborn may be discharged and TSH and free T$_4$ should be measured in 2 to 4 days, or sooner if symptomatic**

This newborn's TSH level is inappropriately low for age. Normally after birth there is a TSH surge, when TSH levels may be as high as 86 ± 6.8 mIU/L. Peak TSH surge occurs at 30 minutes; however, elevated TSH levels may persist up to 48 hours. The classic study by Delbert Fisher in 1969 showed that at 24 hours of life, TSH levels average 17.1 ± 3 mIU/L. This has been the basis to draw samples for newborn screening at 48 hours of life. Therefore, this newborn's TSH level, although normal for an older child, is suspiciously low for this newborn (thus, Answers A, B, and C are incorrect).

The baby has hyperthyroidism secondary to neonatal Graves disease. TSH measured on day 4 of life showed suppressed TSH (0.1 mIU/L) and elevated free T$_4$ (3.09 ng/dL [39.8 pmol/L]). The prevalence of transient hyperthyroidism in babies born to women with Graves disease (neonatal Graves disease) varies from 1% to 5% and is associated with TSH receptor antibodies in the second trimester. There are 2 main types of TSH receptor antibodies: the type that stimulates the TSH receptor (thyroid-stimulating immunoglobulins) and the type that binds the receptor and blocks TSH binding (TSH receptor–blocking inhibiting immunoglobulins). Both are IgG antibodies and cross the placenta. Therefore, infants of mother with Graves disease are also at risk for transient congenital hypothyroidism, depending on whether the mother is also making TSH receptor–blocking antibodies. Antibodies usually clear in 3 to 6 months.

Results of thyroid function studies performed at birth do not predict whether an infant will develop hyperthyroidism. Most affected infants develop hyperthyroidism between 1 and 29 days of life. Most experts agree with measuring levels between 3 and 5 days of life, or sooner if the newborn has signs or symptoms of hyperthyroidism. Most recently, it has been noted that a TSH value of 0.9 mIU/L or less between days 3 and 7 is a strong predictor of neonatal Graves disease. Algorithms have been developed for newborns at risk for thyrotoxicosis.

This patient is asymptomatic and doing well clinically. Although she could be kept for observation, she can be discharged with outpatient follow-up in 1 to 4 days (Answer E). Most importantly, there is no need to start methimazole (Answer D), as she is asymptomatic and doing well clinically. Thyroid function studies can be obtained in the outpatient setting and antithyroid medications can be started, if needed, on the basis of results and clinical status.

Although it is true that this newborn with a maternal history of autoimmune thyroid disease may develop hyperthyroidism or hypothyroidism, it is not appropriate to wait 2 weeks to reassess her thyroid function for hyperthyroidism (Answer A) or 4 weeks to assess for hypothyroidism (Answer B). In this newborn, TSH and free T_4 levels should be obtained in the first 3 to 5 days of life and should be followed closely.

Educational Objective
Describe the occurrence of the immediate TSH surge in the first hours of postnatal life and interpret TSH levels in the first 48 hours of life.

Reference(s)
Banige M, Polak M, Luton D; Research Group for Perinatal Dysthyroidism (RGPD) Study Group. Prediction of neonatal hyperthyroidism. *J Pediatr*. 2018;197: 249-254. PMID: 29605392

Fisher DA, Odell WD, Hobel CJ, Garza R. Thyroid function in the term fetus. *Pediatrics*. 1969;44(4):526-535. PMID: 4981401

Samuels SL, Namoc SM, Bauer AJ. Neonatal thyrotoxicosis. *Clin Perinatol*. 2018;45(1):31-40. PMID: 29406005

61 ANSWER: C) Crohn disease

Approximately one-third of pediatric patients with Crohn disease (Answer C) present with growth failure before therapy is initiated. Glucocorticoid therapy is well known to negatively affect linear growth. A state of chronic inflammation in Crohn disease has a direct effect on growth by inhibiting cell proliferation in the process of chondrogenesis. Chronic inflammation also leads to GH resistance through impairment of GH signal transduction in the liver, mainly induced by interleukin 6 and tumor necrosis factor. Low energy intake and nutritional deficiency also contribute to growth failure in these individuals. Genetic factors associated with Crohn disease (eg, genes that confer susceptibility to the disease) do not seem to be related to poor linear growth.

Although this patient's TSH level is slightly above the upper normal limit, his free T_4 value is within the reference range. These results do not support hypothyroidism (Answer A) as an explanation for the degree of growth failure.

His symptoms and laboratory evaluation do suggest the presence of inflammatory bowel disease. However, Crohn disease—not ulcerative colitis (Answer B)—is most often associated with growth failure in children.

Inflammation leads to GH resistance, and this is the most likely explanation for this patient's low IGF-1 value. In addition, poor nutritional status contributes to subnormal IGF-1 levels. For both of these reasons, GH deficiency (Answer D) is unlikely.

Juvenile idiopathic arthritis (Answer E) could be considered given the elevated erythrocyte sedimentation rate. However, the patient's history does not point toward this condition, as there is no report of fevers, arthritis, rash, or lymphadenopathy. In addition, short stature associated with juvenile idiopathic arthritis is more frequently related to decreased growth of the lower limbs, which would be manifested by an increased upper-to-lower segment ratio.

Educational Objective
Diagnose Crohn disease as a cause of poor growth and identify clinical and laboratory clues to support this diagnosis.

Reference(s)
Ley D, Duhamel A, Behal H, et al. Growth pattern in paediatric Crohn disease is related to inflammatory status. *J Ped Gastroenterol Nutr*. 2016;63(6):637-643. PMID: 26925610

Gasparetto M, Guariso G. Crohn's disease and growth deficiency in children and adolescents. *World J Gastroenterol*. 2014;20(37):13219-13233. PMID: 25309059

Sanderson IR. Growth problems in children with IBD. *Nat Rev Gastroenterol Hepatol*. 2014;11(10):601-610. PMID: 24957008

Umlawska W, Prusek-Dudkiewicz A. Growth retardation and delayed puberty in children and adolescents with juvenile arthritis. *Arch Med Sci*. 2010;6(1):19-23. PMID: 22371715

62 ANSWER: D) *IGSF1* genetic testing

This adolescent boy was initially evaluated for short stature, and his phenotype evolved over time to reveal what appeared to be central hypothyroidism with a normal TSH level and low-normal free T_4 level. Free T_4 does not need to be below the reference range to make the diagnosis. He was determined to be GH sufficient. His normal neurocognitive status does not suggest a pathogenic variant in the *SLC16A2* gene (alias *MCT8*) (an X-linked condition associated with mental retardation) or the thyroid hormone receptor α gene, two conditions for which T_3 measurement is important. In both conditions, the TSH level is usually normal and measuring free T_4 and TSH alone may lead one to assume that the patient has central hypothyroidism. If total or free T_3 and reverse T_3 (Answer C) are going to be measured, it is best to order them together with TSH and total or free T_4 measurements before starting levothyroxine, so total or free T_4-to-T_3 ratios can be assessed as well. In patients with a pathogenic variant in *MCT8*, T_3 is elevated, reverse T_3 is low, and T_4 is low-normal. Patients with a pathogenic variant in the thyroid hormone receptor α gene have a low T_4-to-T_3 ratio and a low reverse T_3 level. Measuring total T_3 and reverse T_3 is therefore not the best next step.

Central hypothyroidism is often associated with other pituitary deficiencies, most commonly GH deficiency. This is either due to tumors or infiltrative diseases of the pituitary/hypothalamic area (or radiation effects) or pathogenic variants in genes encoding transcription factors that affect pituitary development. In those circumstances, central hypothyroidism is rarely isolated. In most patients with central hypothyroidism, performing a pituitary MRI with and without contrast (Answer A) is important. However, in this vignette, this is not the best answer, as his phenotype has additional unusual features—large testicular volume and delayed production of testosterone. As there is no suspicion of hypogonadism, measuring FSH and LH (Answer B) is also incorrect.

At age 14.5 years, this patient's testicular volume was larger than one would expect for a testosterone level of 16 ng/dL (0.56 nmol/L). Eventually, his testes became very large (macroorchidism). While the macroorchidism might prompt one to consider testing for fragile X syndrome (Answer E), his adequate school performance argues against this approach.

His presentation raises suspicion that he may have a pathogenic variant in the gene encoding immunoglobulin superfamily member 1 (*IGSF1*) (Answer D). Such pathogenic variants cause an X-linked condition that manifests in males as central hypothyroidism and, in most, development of macroorchidism by adulthood. Indeed, testing confirmed that this boy has a pathogenic variant in *IGSF1*. After initiating levothyroxine therapy, his height velocity improved to 11.2 cm/y, more consistent with what one would expect during a pubertal growth spurt. This is now considered to be the most common genetic cause of central hypothyroidism. The pathophysiology is not comprehensively understood, but decreased responsiveness to thyrotropin-releasing hormone may have a role in central hypothyroidism. Although central hypothyroidism is observed in all boys and men with pathogenic variants in *IGSF1*, a recent review by Bernard et al describes that males also display other common characteristics with variable prevalence, including hypoprolactinemia (61%); GH dysregulation (with deficiency in some children and increased or high-normal IGF-1 values in most adults); and disharmonious pubertal development. This boy's prolactin level was high-normal, and findings on a subsequent pituitary MRI were normal. Females with *IGSF1* pathogenic variants are less severely affected, but they can have central hypothyroidism (18%), delayed menarche (31%), and low prolactin levels (22%).

Educational Objective

Suspect pathogenic variants in the *IGSF1* gene as the cause of central hypothyroidism, especially if associated with macroorchidism.

Reference(s)

Bernard DJ, Brûlé E, Smith CL, Joustra SD, Wit JM. From consternation to revelation: discovery of a role for IGSF1 in pituitary control of thyroid function. *J Endocr Soc*. 2018;2(3):220-231. PMID: 29594256

Joustra SD, Heinen CA, Schoenmakers N, et al; IGSF1 Clinical Care Group. IGSF1 deficiency: lessons from an extensive case series and recommendations for clinical management. *J Clin Endocrinol Metab*. 2016;101(4):1627-1636. PMID: 26840047

63
ANSWER: D) Initiate a low-fat, low-cholesterol diet and start medication if cholesterol is still high after 3 months

The patient in this vignette most likely has heterozygous familial hypercholesterolemia (FH). This is the most common familial dyslipidemia, which is inherited in an autosomal dominant manner with a prevalence of 1 in 500 individuals. This condition results from a pathogenic variant or deletion in one of an individual's 2 alleles for the LDL receptor gene, causing a significant decrease in the liver's ability to re-absorb LDL from the circulation. This in turn results in an increase in cholesterol synthesis within hepatocytes and high levels of circulating LDL molecules. Affected children and adolescents have elevations in LDL-cholesterol and total cholesterol levels, while triglycerides are not significantly affected and HDL-cholesterol levels are only mildly reduced. Individuals with heterozygous FH often have myocardial infarctions before age 50 years. Individuals with homozygous FH have LDL-cholesterol levels typically greater than 500 mg/dL (>12.95 mmol/L), can have xanthomas by age 5 years, and often experience myocardial infarctions in their second decade of life.

Previous research has demonstrated that lipid abnormalities in childhood affect formation of atherosclerosis and long-term risk of adult cardiovascular disease. Longstanding guidelines for the management of pediatric hyperlipidemia revolve around LDL-cholesterol levels and family history. For individuals with LDL-cholesterol levels greater than 190 mg/dL (>4.92 mmol/L) or for individuals with levels of 160 to 189 mg/dL (4.14 to 4.90 mmol/L) with a family history of early cardiovascular disease, the recommendation is to initiate a diet very low in saturated fat and cholesterol for 3 to 6 months. If the BMI is at the 85th percentile or higher, additional lifestyle changes are recommended. If the LDL-cholesterol levels remain elevated despite this diet (as is likely in the case of FH) and the child is 10 years or older, treatment with statins (and likely other agents) should be initiated (thus, Answer D is correct and Answers B and C are incorrect). The treatment goal is an LDL-cholesterol level less than 130 mg/dL (<3.37 mmol/L), which in the case of FH usually requires both dietary changes and multiple medications. Low-carbohydrate diets have been used with mixed success to encourage weight loss. From a lipid perspective, these diets usually result in an increase in HDL-cholesterol, but in some individuals, these diets can increase LDL-cholesterol levels. Low-carbohydrate diets (Answer E) are not recommended for children with cholesterol abnormalities.

Nonfasting laboratory studies can result in artificially higher triglyceride levels, which can in-turn lower the calculated LDL-cholesterol level. Since this patient's triglycerides were not severely elevated and her LDL-cholesterol level is far above the cut-off to induce dietary changes, rechecking a fasting lipid panel in 3 to 6 months (Answer A) is not going to change this child's need for treatment. If rechecking is performed, this should be done sooner in a case like this, given the extreme LDL-cholesterol elevations.

Educational Objective
Diagnose and manage familial hypercholesterolemia in a child.

Reference(s)

Kwiterovich PO Jr. Recognition and management of dyslipidemia in children and adolescents. *J Clin Endocrinol Metab.* 2008;93(11):4200-4209. PMID: 18697860

Expert Panel on Integrated Guidelines for Cardiovascular Health and Risk Reduction in Children and Adolescents; National Heart, Lung, and Blood Institute. Expert panel on integrated guidelines for cardiovascular health and risk reduction in children and adolescents: summary report. *Pediatrics.* 2011;128(Suppl 5): S213-S256. PMID: 22084329

64
ANSWER: C) Malnutrition—risk for unhealed osteomalacia

Bisphosphonates are analogues of inorganic pyrophosphate and have potent inhibitory effects on bone resorption. They act by incorporating into hydroxyapatite and selectively inhibiting osteoclast activity. Osteoblast activity is less affected, leading to proportionally greater bone formation and increased bone mass. Bisphosphonates are used most frequently for treatment of postmenopausal osteoporosis and adults with metastatic bone disease; however, they have also been shown to increase bone density in children with a variety of skeletal disorders.

Rigorous controlled trials of bisphosphonate use in children are lacking, although findings from observational studies and small randomized controlled trials suggest they are well-tolerated. The most common adverse effect is an acute phase reaction, consisting of a nonspecific physiologic response associated with increased inflammatory cytokines, fever, and flu-like symptoms. These reactions are typically limited to the first 1 to 2 infusions and are generally mild and manageable with nonsteroidal anti-inflammatory drugs and supportive care. Inhibition of osteoclast activity decreases release of skeletal calcium into the circulation and places patients at risk for hypocalcemia, particularly in the setting of concomitant vitamin D deficiency. This can be mitigated by ensuring adequate vitamin D and calcium levels before treatment, and by supplementing calcium and vitamin D analogues in patients at high risk. Osteonecrosis of the jaw is a rare, serious event reported in adults where progressive bone destruction occurs in the maxillofacial region, particularly after invasive oral procedures. The etiology of osteonecrosis of the jaw is unknown; however, it appears to occur in the setting of extensive treatment with high-dosage, potent intravenous bisphosphonates. Atypical femoral fractures are an extremely rare form of femoral stress fracture associated with long-term bisphosphonate treatment, which has been reported primarily in adults.

The patient in this vignette is malnourished, suggesting she has not received adequate dietary calcium and protein to support bone health. Many children with malnutrition develop osteomalacia, where bone is poorly mineralized due to inadequate dietary calcium. Placement of a gastrostomy tube and introduction of alimentary formula will most likely result in increased bone mineralization and improved bone density. Bisphosphonates should be avoided in patients with osteomalacia because they may negatively affect the increase in bone modeling/remodeling that occurs during this healing phase (thus, Answer C is correct). While she may potentially still benefit from bisphosphonate therapy, the most prudent course is to correct her nutritional deficiencies and then reassess.

This patient's malabsorption decreases the availability of dietary calcium and vitamin D, placing her at increased risk for hypocalcemia with bisphosphonate therapy. However, this can most likely be mitigated with supplemental calcium, vitamin D analogues, and close laboratory monitoring. It is a lesser concern than her malnutrition (thus, Answer A is incorrect).

The prevalence of osteonecrosis of the jaw is well below 1% in observational studies of adults with osteoporosis, and only rare cases have been reported in children (thus, Answer B is incorrect). Nonetheless, the possibility of osteonecrosis of the jaw as a complication of oral surgery should certainly be discussed with the family and the craniofacial team, and she should be encouraged to maintain excellent dental hygiene.

Respiratory distress has been rarely reported with pamidronate treatment in infants with osteogenesis imperfecta who had preexisting pulmonary disease and is not likely to be a concern in this patient (thus, Answer D is incorrect).

Acute phase reactions are common after initial bisphosphonate infusions, affecting approximately 20% to 30% of patients, and are typically manageable with supportive care. No specific clinical features have been clearly correlated with the risk of acute phase reactions (thus, Answer E is incorrect).

Educational Objective
Counsel patients about the primary adverse effects of bisphosphonates for the treatment of juvenile osteoporosis and explain the mechanism of action of these drugs.

Reference(s)
George S, Weber DR, Kaplan P, Hummel K, Monk HM, Levine MA. Short-term safety of zoledronic acid in young patients with bone disorders: an extensive institutional experience. *J Clin Endocrinol Metab*. 2015;100(11):4163-4171. PMID: 26308295

Ward LM, Konji VN, Ma J. The management of osteoporosis in children. *Osteoporos Int*. 2016;27(7):2147-2179. PMID: 27125514

Munns CF, Rauch F, Mier RJ, Glorieux FH. Respiratory distress with pamidronate treatment in infants with severe osteogenesis imperfecta. *Bone*. 2004;35(1):231-234. PMID: 15207762

65 **ANSWER: C) Add an aromatase inhibitor to his medication regimen**
The pertinent findings in this case are marked hyperprolactinemia; low GH, cortisol, free T_4, gonadotropin, and testosterone levels; and evidence of a macroprolactinoma on MRI. Upon presentation, the patient already had evidence of hypopituitarism and neurologic deficits (visual field cut). Treatment with cabergoline resulted in marked lowering of his prolactin level and resolution of his visual field cut. However, escalating doses of cabergoline did not normalize his prolactin level and he continued to show evidence of hypogonadism. After starting treatment with testosterone, his prolactin level more than doubled. The goals of treating prolactinoma are to suppress excessive prolactin secretion and its clinical consequences, including infertility, sexual dysfunction, and osteoporosis; to control tumor mass and relieve visual field defects, cranial nerve dysfunction, and possibly hypopituitarism; to preserve or improve any residual pituitary function; and lastly, to prevent disease recurrence or progression. While most prolactinomas are responsive to cabergoline, approximately 11% demonstrate resistance to this therapy.

However, roughly 24% of patients demonstrate resistance to bromocriptine, so switching to bromocriptine (Answer A) would be incorrect. While this patient had a marked reduction in prolactin levels with cabergoline (from greater than 5000 ng/mL to 424 ng/mL), escalating to very high cabergoline doses did not result in a further reduction, so increasing the cabergoline dosage even higher (Answer B) is unlikely to have any effect on his prolactin level. In addition, long-term use of high-dosage cabergoline may be associated with a risk of cardiac valvular regurgitation.

As in this patient, hypogonadism persists in up to 50% of men with macroprolactinomas. Treatment with cabergoline alone did not resolve this patient's hypogonadism, so decreasing his testosterone dosage (Answer D) is not indicated.

Estrogen is known to stimulate prolactin synthesis and secretion. It does this by disrupting the inhibitory effect of dopamine. Chronic exposure to estrogen functionally uncouples the D2 receptor in the anterior pituitary from its G protein–coupled receptor. In vitro, estrogen stimulates prolactin gene transcription and prevents dopamine agonists from inhibiting prolactin synthesis and secretion. In vivo, large doses of estrogen have induced prolactinomas. It is likely that treatment of this patient with testosterone caused the increase in prolactin due to aromatization of testosterone to estrogen. Although still experimental, off-label use of an aromatase inhibitor (anastrozole) (Answer C) along with exogenous testosterone and high-dosage cabergoline may restore normal sexual function without further elevating prolactin levels. It would be worthwhile to consider a trial of this treatment before embarking on another more aggressive therapy, such as surgical resection. Long-term effects of aromatase inhibitors are uncertain; therefore, this therapeutic approach should be considered only in specific situations that are not amenable to standard therapy.

Transsphenoidal surgery (Answer E) is generally reserved for those who are unresponsive or cannot tolerate high cabergoline dosages. Unfortunately, 7% to 50% of surgically resected prolactinomas recur. This patient did have resolution of his visual field cut and some reduction in his prolactin level with cabergoline, so it would be wise to first offer a trial of an aromatase inhibitor.

Educational Objective
Describe the effects of sex steroids, especially estradiol, on prolactin secretion.

Reference(s)

Melmed S, Casanueva FF, Hoffman AR, et al; Endocrine Society. Diagnosis and treatment of hyperprolactinemia: an Endocrine Society clinical practice guideline. *J Clin Endocrinol Metab*. 2011;96(2):273-288. PMID: 21296991

Gillam MP, Middler S, Freed DJ, Molitch ME. The novel use of very high doses of cabergoline and a combination of testosterone and an aromatase inhibitor in the treatment of a giant prolactinoma. *J Clin Endocrinol Metab*. 2002;87(10):4447-4451. PMID: 12364416

Gillam MP, Molitch ME, Lombardi G, Colao A. Advances in the treatment of prolactinomas. *Endocr Rev*. 2006;27(5):485-534. PMID: 16705142

66 ANSWER: D) Defer sperm retrieval/extraction into adulthood

Klinefelter syndrome affects approximately 1 in 660 males, but it is estimated that only about 25% of affected individuals are diagnosed before puberty given that signs and symptoms can be subtle. Approximately 10% of patients are identified by prenatal testing. The clinical hallmarks of Klinefelter syndrome are small testes, hypergonadotropic hypogonadism, infertility, gynecomastia, and learning difficulties. Parents of boys with Klinefelter syndrome often have questions about fertility preservation and the effects of testosterone on success rate of fertility treatments.

Men with Klinefelter syndrome are almost always infertile, and spontaneous pregnancy in partners of individuals with Klinefelter syndrome remains extremely rare. While there is some evidence to suggest that sperm retrieval may be less successful after age 34 years, current studies show no decrease in successful sperm retrieval rates from age 16-19 to 34 years. There appears to be no benefit of early testicular sperm extraction, and studies suggest that most adolescents with Klinefelter syndrome are not psychologically prepared to make decisions on future fertility. Thus, deferring sperm retrieval/extraction into adulthood (Answer D) is the best advice for this patient.

There are some concerns that early testosterone treatment could negatively impact future fertility; however, studies do not show a benefit of attempting sperm retrieval in adolescence (before starting testosterone treatment) vs retrieval at the time of desired fertility (thus, Answers C and E are incorrect). Four studies have been published reporting sperm recovery attempts by ejaculation in adolescents and young men with Klinefelter syndrome; no normal spermatozoa were found in any of the 27 participants. Studies of testicular sperm extraction in adolescents with Klinefelter syndrome found spermatogonia in some of the boys (aged 10 to 16 years), but only one instance of spermatozoa. Another study found a spermatozoa retrieval rate of 49% in boys aged 15 to 19 years, but only 10% in boys aged 13 to 14 years. An analysis of 22 studies investigating testicular sperm extraction in adults with Klinefelter syndrome showed a comparable overall sperm retrieval rate of 50%.

Some advocate for initiating testosterone treatment at the beginning of puberty, with goals of normal masculinization and preservation of bone mineral density. While individuals with Klinefelter syndrome appear to have inherently unfavorable body composition and higher risk of metabolic syndrome, well-controlled studies of the effects of testosterone treatment on body composition are lacking and currently there is no clear benefit to testosterone therapy in asymptomatic adolescents with Klinefelter syndrome who have normal testosterone levels (Answer A).

Boys with Klinefelter syndrome typically experience a normal testosterone increase at the onset of puberty, with normal adult development of the penis and pubic hair. Up to 35% do not experience low testosterone levels, even into adulthood. By current standards, treatment is indicated if testosterone is below the reference range or if the patient is experiencing symptoms of hypoandrogenism (lack of energy, decreased libido, pubertal arrest), independent of gonadotropin levels. Thus, waiting to start testosterone treatment until gonadotropin levels become elevated (Answer B) is incorrect.

While there remains some controversy over the timing of testosterone therapy and attempts at fertility preservation in individuals with Klinefelter syndrome, the current evidence indicates that testosterone treatment should be initiated in the setting of either low testosterone levels or symptoms. Testosterone dosages should be titrated to midnormal serum testosterone levels to reduce the risk of hyalinization of the testes. With current sperm retrieval techniques, testosterone replacement does not appear to impair chances of future fertility and should not be deferred for this reason.

Educational Objective
Identify pros and cons of testosterone treatment and timing of therapy initiation in Klinefelter syndrome.

Reference(s)

Groth KA, Skakkebæk A, Høst C, Gravholt CH, Bojesen A. Clinical review: Klinefelter syndrome--a clinical update. *J Clin Endocrinol Metab*. 2013;98(1):20-30. PMID: 23118429

Radicioni AF, Ferlin A, Balercia G, et al. Consensus statement on diagnosis and clinical management of Klinefelter syndrome. *J Clin Invest*. 2010;33(11):839-850. PMID: 21293172

Gies I, Unuane D, Velkeniers B, De Schepper J. Management of Klinefelter syndrome during transition. *Eur J Endocrinol*. 2014;171(2):R67-R77. PMID: 24801585

67 ANSWER: B) Endoscopic biopsy

Celiac disease should be considered in the differential diagnosis of poor growth and short stature in any child. Malabsorption due to small intestine villous atrophy can lead to abdominal pain, diarrhea, weight loss, and poor growth. Iron deficiency anemia is prevalent in patients with celiac disease with or without symptoms of malabsorption. Other features associated with celiac disease include rash, low bone mineral density or osteopenia, and neuropsychiatric symptoms such as headache or anxiety/depression. Patients with celiac disease are at a higher risk for developing other autoimmune diseases. In a large multinational study comparing data on more than 52,000 patients with type 1 diabetes from pediatric registries across 3 continents, biopsy-proven celiac disease was noted in about 3.5% of patients. More than 80% were diagnosed within the first 5 years of type 1 diabetes diagnosis. Overall glycemic control as measured by hemoglobin A_{1c} was not different between patients with and without celiac disease in this study; however, patients with celiac disease did have a lower height SD score.

Endoscopic biopsy (Answer B) is the gold standard test to diagnose celiac disease, but results can be normal in a patient who is on a gluten-free diet for longer than 12 months. This patient has been following a gluten-free diet for less than 12 months, so endoscopic biopsy may still be used to diagnose celiac disease. Appropriate gluten challenge with 4 to 8 slices of bread per day for 2 months before further testing can increase the chances of positive test results in a patient with celiac disease. However, 1 to 2 slices of wheat bread a day for 2 weeks (Answer E) is not sufficient.

HLA genotyping (Answer A) to look for *HLA-DQ2* and *HLA-DQ8* is helpful for its negative predictive value. Less than 1% of all patients with celiac disease are negative for *HLA-DQ2* and *HLA-DQ8*. However, the positive predictive value of HLA genotyping is poor, as 30% to 40% of the general population has *HLA-DQ2* and 5% to 10% has *HLA-DQ8*. Thus, HLA genotyping can be used to exclude celiac disease (if negative for *HLA-DQ2* and *HLA-DQ8*) in several scenarios, including when patients are already on a gluten-free diet for more than 12 months in whom serologic testing and biopsy may be less accurate. In children who have highly positive serologic tests (>10 times upper normal limit), HLA genotyping can be used to avoid invasive endoscopy. Also, HLA genotyping can be used to rule out celiac disease in first-degree relatives of patients with celiac disease to avoid further invasive testing.

Serologic testing with tissue transglutaminase antibody IgA, endomysial antibody IgA, and gliadin-derived peptide IgA and IgG antibodies (Answers C and D) can be falsely negative in a patient adherent to a gluten-free diet for more than 6 months. When testing patients who eat a gluten-containing diet, these tests have high specificity and sensitivity (>90%). Also, serologic testing with IgA antibodies can be falsely negative in patients with IgA deficiency. Selective IgA deficiency (with normal IgG and IgM levels) is the most common immunodeficiency in humans and is 10 to 15 times more common in patients with celiac disease than in the general population. Patients with IgA deficiency can have recurrent sinusitis/pneumonia and intestinal giardiasis and are at high risk for other autoimmune diseases. Anaphylactic reaction to transfusions with blood products containing IgA have been reported in patients with severe IgA deficiency (total IgA <7 mg/dL) who also have IgA antibodies; this can be averted by the use of IgA-depleted blood products for transfusion.

Educational Objective
Identify celiac disease as a cause of poor growth in children and explain the advantages and limitations of available celiac screening and diagnostic tests.

Reference(s)

Shannahan S, Leffler DA. Diagnosis and updates in celiac disease. *Gastrointest Endosc Clin N Am*. 2017;27(1):79-92. PMID: 27908520

Fasano A, Catassi C. Clinical practice. Celiac disease. *N Engl J Med*. 2012;367(25):2419-2426. PMID: 23252527

Singh P, Sharma PK, Angihotri A, et al. Coeliac disease in patients with short stature: a tertiary care centre experience. *Natl Med J India*. 2015;28(4):176-180. PMID: 27132724

Craig ME, Prinz N, Boyle CT, et al; Australasian Diabetes Data Network (ADDN); T1D Exchange Clinic Network (T1DX); National Paediatric Diabetes Audit (NPDA) and the Royal College of Paediatrics and Child Health; Prospective Diabetes Follow-up Registry (DPV) initiative. Prevalence of celiac disease in 52,721 youth with type 1 diabetes: international comparison across three continents. *Diabetes Care*. 2017;40(8):1034-1040. PMID: 28546222

68 **ANSWER: D) Reduce the metformin dosage to the previously tolerated dosage**
Metformin's most common adverse effects are related to the gastrointestinal tract and include abdominal pain, nausea, metallic taste, bloating, and diarrhea. In clinical trials, up to 35% of patients developed gastrointestinal intolerance and 5% needed to discontinue the medication. Thus, simply reassuring the family and continuing the same metformin dosage for another 2 weeks (Answer B) is incorrect. Adverse effects can often be minimized by starting metformin at a low dosage and increasing the dosage gradually as tolerated. If a patient begins experiencing gastrointestinal symptoms, the first step is to reduce the metformin dosage to that previously tolerated without any adverse effects (Answer D). Simply discontinuing metformin (Answer A) is incorrect. Extended-release formulations of metformin seem to have better gastrointestinal tolerability than immediate-release formulations. Switching to the immediate-release formulation (Answer C) at the same dosage will not improve the reported symptoms.

No serious adverse effects were noted with long-term metformin use (18 months) in clinical trials. A rare but life-threatening adverse effect of metformin is lactic acidosis. The risk of lactic acidosis with metformin is known to be low when it is prescribed correctly. There are reported cases of lactic acidosis in adolescents who have overdosed on metformin. In adults, lactic acidosis has been reported primarily in patients with diabetes who have significant renal insufficiency. When renal function is impaired, the plasma half-life of metformin is prolonged and its renal clearance is decreased in proportion to the decrease in creatinine clearance. In such patients, the metformin dosage should be adjusted based on the glomerular filtration rate. Metformin-associated lactic acidosis is considered to be one of the complications caused by intravascular contrast media administration in patients with diabetes, especially in those with coexisting renal or cardiac impairment. Symptoms of lactic acidosis include exhaustion, muscle cramps, weakness, headache, decreased appetite, and abdominal pain. While it is important to determine whether the patient has been exposed to any intravenous contrast or alcohol (Answer E) these are less likely factors given the reported symptoms.

Metformin treatment has also been associated with clinically significant vitamin B_{12} deficiency in some patients. It has been associated with an almost 3-fold increased risk of severe B_{12} deficiency (<150 pg/mL) and a 2-fold increased risk of moderately low vitamin B_{12} levels (150-220 pg/mL). Almost one-fifth to one-third of patients with type 2 diabetes who take metformin have low vitamin B_{12} levels. A meta-analysis of 29 studies that included 8089 patients found that metformin increased the risk of vitamin B_{12} deficiency, with an odds ratio of 2.45 vs the risk in non–metformin-exposed individuals. Monitoring vitamin B_{12} levels, and supplementing when necessary, may be useful in all patients on long-term metformin therapy (>1 year).

Educational Objective
Identify potential adverse effects of metformin therapy and recommend a strategy to address these symptoms.

Reference(s)

Florez H, Luo J, Castillo-Florez S, et al. Impact of metformin-induced gastrointestinal symptoms on quality of life and adherence in patients with type 2 diabetes. *Postgrad Med.* 2010;122(2):112-120. PMID: 20203462

Owen MR, Doran E, Halestrap AP. Evidence that metformin exerts its anti-diabetic effects through inhibition of complex 1 of the mitochondrial respiratory chain. *Biochem J.* 2000;348(Pt 3):607-614. PMID: 10839993

Feher MD, Al-Mrayat M, Brake J, et al. Tolerability of prolonged-release metformin (Glucophage SR) in individuals intolerant to standard metformin--results from four UK centres. *Br J Diabetes Vasc Dis.* 2007;7(5):225-228.

Singh AK, Kumar A, Karmakar D, Jha RK. Association of B12 deficiency and clinical neuropathy with metformin use in type 2 diabetes patients [published correction appears in *J Postgrad Med.* 2014;60(1):99]. *J Postgrad Med.* 2013;59(4):253-257. PMID: 24346380

69 ANSWER: B) Perform CT of the neck and chest

Multiple endocrine neoplasia type 2B is almost always due to the *RET* M918T pathogenic variant. Because of the high risk for medullary thyroid cancer, it is recommended that patients with this pathogenic variant have a total thyroidectomy in infancy. Early thyroidectomy is the best way to achieve cure.

In this particular case, the doubling time for both calcitonin and CEA is quite rapid. It can be calculated using the tool provided by the American Thyroid Association (https://www.thyroid.org/professionals/calculators/thyroid-cancer-carcinoma/). Four measurements are required within a 2-year period, although doubling times less than 6 months can be reliably estimated within the first 12 months postoperatively. Following her calcitonin or CEA levels (Answers C and D) would not change recommended management and would not provide additional prognostic information. However, serially following those levels after removal of neck metastases would be important.

In the American Thyroid Association 2015 guidelines, the 5- and 10-year survival rates in patients with serum calcitonin doubling times less than 6 months are noted to be 25% and 8%, respectively, compared with 92% and 37% in those with doubling times between 6 and 24 months. Despite the fact that this patient's actual calcitonin levels are not extremely high, her prognosis is not good on the basis of the doubling time data. The preoperative neck metastases add to that assessment. Her calcitonin level is still less than 500 pg/mL (<146 pmol/L), which most likely reflects neck metastases, as distant metastases are expected to cause much higher calcitonin levels. Removing metastatic neck lymphadenopathy can favorably affect her prognosis.

The 2015 American Thyroid Association guidelines recommend the following: "If the postoperative serum calcitonin level exceeds 150 pg/mL patients should be evaluated by imaging procedures, including neck US, chest CT, contrast-enhanced MRI or three-phase contrast-enhanced CT of the liver, and bone scintigraphy and MRI of the pelvis and axial skeleton." Because neck ultrasonography revealed a focus in this patient in 2 ultrasounds over a 6-month interval, the best next step is CT of the neck and chest (Answer B), which may give better definition or identify additional lesions not detected on neck ultrasonography. Chest CT often provides a good image of the liver, with little additional radiation exposure. If one opted to repeat neck ultrasonography, waiting a year (Answer A) is too long.

In patients with multiple endocrine neoplasia type 2B, screening for pheochromocytoma (Answer E) is recommended at age 11 years, although this tumor has been reported to occur in such patients as early as age 8 years.

The extra precaution of screening for pheochromocytoma was taken before this patient's thyroidectomy, and it was negative.

Educational Objective
Manage elevated calcitonin levels postoperatively in patients with multiple endocrine neoplasia type 2B.

Reference(s)
Wells SA Jr, Asa SL, Dralle H, et al; American Thyroid Association Guidelines Task Force on Medullary Thyroid Carcinoma. Revised American Thyroid Association guidelines for the management of medullary thyroid carcinoma. *Thyroid*. 2015;25(6):567-610. PMID: 25810047

Waguespack SG, Rich TA, Perrier ND, Jimenez C, Cote GJ. Management of medullary thyroid carcinoma and MEN2 syndromes in childhood. *Nat Rev Endocrinol*. 2011;7(10):596-607. PMID: 21862994

Laure Giraudet A, Al Ghulzan A, Auperin A, et al. Progression of medullary thyroid carcinoma: assessment with calcitonin and carcinoembryonic antigen doubling times. *Eur J Endocrinol*. 2008;158(2):239-246. PMID: 18230832

70 ANSWER: C) Obesity
The child in this vignette has obesity, with a BMI of 24 kg/m^2 (>97th percentile for age). While contributors to obesity are varied, significant life changes (such as this boy's move to a new environment) can be associated with changes in eating and activity patterns, contributing to weight gain. This boy will require careful counseling towards lifestyle modification for weight loss (Answer C).

The boy's obesity is the most likely cause of his low response to a GH-stimulation test. Obesity is frequently accompanied by high levels of insulin and IGF-1 (relative to values observed in lean individuals), but low basal and stimulated GH levels. GH deficiency (Answer A) is unlikely given the boy's steady growth over time.

His slightly elevated TSH level in the face of a high-normal free T$_4$ level could be due to either early autoimmune thyroiditis or, more likely, due to the obesity, which is associated with mild elevations in TSH and T$_3$, both of which normalize after weight loss. Either way, such a mild TSH elevation (Answer B) would not be expected to contribute to problems of weight gain or growth.

His cortisol value was in the normal range, so hypercortisolism (Answer D) is unlikely. Additionally, he does not have growth suppression to raise suspicion of hypercortisolism. Similarly, while brain tumors are potential causes of GH deficiency, pituitary suppression from a brain tumor (Answer E) would still be expected to result in poor linear growth and low IGF-1, as well as central symptoms, including headache and vomiting.

Educational Objective
Identify the effects of obesity on growth hormone and insulinlike growth factors.

Reference(s)
Nam SY, Lee EJ, Kim KR, et al. Effect of obesity on total and free insulin-like growth factor (IGF)-1, and their relationship to IGF-binding protein (BP)-1, IGFBP-2, IGFBP-3, insulin, and growth hormone. *Int J Obes Relat Metab Disord*. 1997;21(5):355-359. PMID: 9152736

Reinehr T, Andler W. Thyroid hormones before and after weight loss in obesity. *Arch Dis Child*. 2002;87(4):320-323. PMID: 12244007

Williams T, Berelowitz M, Joffe SN, et al. Impaired growth hormone responses to growth hormone–releasing factor in obesity. A pituitary defect reversed with weight reduction. *N Engl J Med*. 1984;311(22):1403-1407. PMID: 6436706

71 ANSWER: D) Reassure the family, adjust levothyroxine to keep TSH between 0.5 and 1.0 mIU/L, and measure nonstimulated thyroglobulin and thyroglobulin antibodies in 3 to 6 months
In the past, most pediatric patients with differentiated thyroid carcinoma were treated with radioactive iodine, with the goal to treat any remnant disease, decrease the risk for recurrence, and improve survival. However, in view of new awareness of the adverse effects of radioactive iodine therapy, efforts are being made to better identify which patients will benefit from adjuvant therapy.

Adjuvant ^{131}I therapy has been shown to improve disease-free survival in young adults; however, the value of radioactive iodine treatment for small stage I differentiated thyroid carcinoma has not been elucidated. The main argument in favor of using therapeutic ^{131}I in all children and adolescents with thyroid carcinoma is that the presence of remnant thyroid may affect the ability to monitor patients for recurrent or metastatic disease via serum thyroglobulin measurement or whole-body scan. However, arguments against universal treatment include the following: (1) [131]I treatment is associated with short- and long-term complications, including a higher risk of developing second malignancies; (2) there is a lack of data showing benefit for small, localized differentiated thyroid carcinoma; and (3) data show overall decreased survival in patients receiving radioactive iodine treatment.

There are short- and long-term adverse effects associated with exposure to [131]I. Short-term adverse effects result from damage to tissues that incorporate iodine and include xerostomia, sialoadenitis, stomatitis, ocular dryness, nasolacrimal duct obstruction/dysfunction, nausea and vomiting, and thyroiditis. Gonadal damage has also been reported with elevated FSH levels following exposure to ^{131}I with defects in spermatogenesis and transient amenorrhea. Acute suppression of the bone marrow may also occur, although cell counts usually recover. Long-term adverse effects include permanent sialoadenitis, permanent nasolacrimal dysfunction, permanent bone marrow suppression, lung fibrosis, secondary malignancies, and fertility alterations. Late adverse effects, except for fertility alterations, have been shown to be associated with the number of treatments and cumulative activities of radioactive iodine. Therapy with ^{131}I is indicated for the treatment of iodine-avid, nodal persistent disease that cannot be surgically resected and for the management of known or suspected iodine-avid distant metastases.

This patient has stage I papillary thyroid carcinoma (T1a, N0, Mx disease). She is at low risk for recurrence on the basis of current American Thyroid Association pediatric risk level. Radioactive iodine treatment would pose more risk than benefit for this patient and it is not recommended. In addition, postoperative staging can be done by measuring thyroglobulin levels and obtaining additional imaging studies, as indicated. The TSH goal is 0.5 to 1.0 mIU/L and surveillance is recommended with neck ultrasonography and thyroglobulin measurement (Answer D). One important consideration is that this patient was diagnosed with autoimmune thyroid disease. She may, therefore, have thyroglobulin antibodies, which could affect the thyroglobulin tumor marker levels. It is very important to measure thyroglobulin antibodies together with thyroglobulin levels as part of her follow-up. Although this may limit the value of the thyroglobulin level, following thyroglobulin antibody titers in antibody-positive patients is a valuable tool in following up patients with thyroid carcinoma. Different assays have varying sensitivities, and the same assay should be used when monitoring thyroglobulin antibodies. Recently, assessment of thyroglobulin by liquid chromatography–tandem mass spectrometry has been advocated for thyroglobulin antibody–positive patients; however, this method has been shown to have less sensitivity and may need additional validation.

She has very low risk for local metastases and treating any iodine uptake noted on whole-body scan (Answer A), including remnant ablation, is not recommended. Although it is true that ablation of remnant thyroid tissue could facilitate follow-up of thyroglobulin levels, exposing this patient to radioactive iodine provides small benefit and puts her at risk for acute and long-term complications. Therefore, [131]I (Answer C) is not recommended. The universal use of adjuvant [131]I (Answer B) is not recommended based on current guidelines. Currently, risk stratification is the preferred approach. Lastly, although reassuring the family about low recurrence risk is appropriate, this patient still needs to be followed closely with neck ultrasonography and thyroglobulin measurement. She also needs to be under mild TSH suppression to keep TSH between 0.5 and 1.0 mIU/L. Therefore, providing no further treatment (Answer E) is incorrect.

Educational Objective
Determine whether it is appropriate to use ^{131}I in the treatment of thyroid carcinoma in children and adolescents.

Reference(s)

Albano D, Bertagna F, Panarotto MB, Giubbini R. Early and late adverse effects of radioiodine for pediatric differentiated thyroid cancer. *Pediatr Blood Cancer.* 2017;64(11). PMID: 28436606

Azmat U, Porter K, Senter L, Ringel MD, Nabhan F. Thyroglobulin liquid chromatography-tandem mass spectrometry has a low sensitivity for detecting structural disease in patients with antithyroglobulin antibodies. *Thyroid.* 2017;27(1):74-80. PMID: 27736322

Francis GL, Waguespack SG, Bauer AJ, et al. Management guidelines for children with thyroid nodules and differentiated thyroid cancer. *Thyroid.* 2015;25(7): 716-759. PMID: 25900731

Jindal A, Khan U. Is thyroglobulin level by liquid chromatography tandem-mass spectrometry always reliable for follow-up of DTC after thyroidectomy: a report on two patients. *Thyroid.* 2016;26(9):1334-1335. PMID: 27277116

Matrone A, Latrofa F, Torregrossa L, et al. Changing trend of thyroglobulin antibodies in patients with differentiated thyroid cancer treated with total thyroidectomy without ^{131}I ablation. *Thyroid.* 2018;28(7):871-879. PMID: 29860933

Spencer CA. Clinical review: clinical utility of thyroglobulin antibody (TgAb) measurements for patients with differentiated thyroid cancers (DTC). *J Clin Endocrinol Metab.* 2011;96(12):3615-3627. PMID: 21917876

Wassner AJ, Della Vecchia M, Jarolim P, Feldman HA, Huang SA. Prevalence and significance of thyroglobulin antibodies in pediatric thyroid cancer. *J Clin Endocrinol Metab.* 2017;102(9):3146-3153. PMID: 28398507

72 ANSWER: E) *HSD3B2* (3β-hydroxysteroid dehydrogenase deficiency)

To approach the diagnosis in this vignette, one must consider what could cause undervirilization in a newborn with a 46,XY karyotype. Without even looking at the laboratory data, one of the answer choices (11β-hydroxylase deficiency [Answer C]) can be eliminated. While patients with a 46,XX karyotype with 11β-hydroxylase deficiency are born with atypical genitalia, patients with a 46,XY karyotype are born with typical male genitalia.

Patients with 17α-hydroxylase/17,20-lyase deficiency (Answer A) can certainly have undervirilization, but the hormonal profile would look different. Because the conversion of pregnenolone to 17-hydroxypregnenolone and the conversion of progesterone to 17-hydroxyprogesterone is affected, 17-hydroxypregnenolone and 17-hydroxyprogesterone levels would be low, unlike in this vignette.

Patients with P450 oxidoreductase deficiency (Answer B) who have a 46,XY karyotype have undervirilized genitalia. However, patients with severe pathogenic variants in the *POR* gene also typically have severe skeletal findings consistent with Antley-Bixler skeletal malformation syndrome (craniosynostosis, radioulnar or radiohumeral synostosis, and other variable skeletal disorders). Patients with less severe pathogenic variants do not exhibit skeletal malformations. To make a biochemical diagnosis of P450 oxidoreductase deficiency, an ACTH-stimulation test is very helpful. However, even without the stimulation test, the diagnosis can be excluded in this patient based on the biochemical profile. In patients with P450 oxidoreductase deficiency, 17-hydroxyprogesterone is typically mildly elevated at baseline and is modestly hyperresponsive to ACTH. 17-Hydroxypregnenolone and DHEA are normal in this setting, unlike in this patient. Mineralocorticoid deficiency has not been described in P450 oxidoreductase deficiency and plasma renin activity and electrolytes are generally normal.

Patients with X-linked adrenal hypoplasia congenita (Answer D) can have a variable clinical presentation, ranging from the most severe phenotype of adrenal insufficiency in infancy, undervirilization of the genitalia, and hypogonadotropic hypogonadism, to only mild adrenal insufficiency diagnosed in adulthood. Patients with this disorder typically exhibit defective glucocorticoid, mineralocorticoid, and androgen production, as well as hypothalamic-pituitary-gonadal axis dysfunction leading to hypogonadotrophic hypogonadism. One can expect to see normal or, more likely low, levels of 17-hydroxypregnenolone, 17-hydroxyprogesterone, and DHEA in patients with a more severe presentation, unlike in the patient in this vignette. Testosterone and androstenedione levels would be low as well.

This patient has 3β-hydroxysteroid dehydrogenase deficiency (Answer E). This is an autosomal recessive condition and a rare form of congenital adrenal hyperplasia. The phenotype varies from the severe salt-wasting form with gonadal dysfunction and atypical genitalia in both males and females to a nonclassic form without genital atypia and with premature pubarche in young children and hirsutism and menstrual dysfunction in older women. 3β-Hydroxysteroid dehydrogenase, encoded by the *HSD3B2* gene in humans, is essential for the formation of progesterone, the precursor hormone for aldosterone, 17-hydroxyprogesterone, the precursor hormone for cortisol, as well as for the formation of androstenedione, testosterone, and estrogen in the adrenal glands and the gonads. Because of the enzymatic deficiency, certain hormones are deficient while others are in excess, including 17-hydroxypregnenolone and DHEA as observed in this patient. Older studies demonstrated that 3β-hydroxysteroid dehydrogenase deficiency could be diagnosed if ACTH-stimulated values of 17-hydroxypregnenolone, DHEA, ratios of 17-hydroxypregnenolone to cortisol, 17-hydroxypregnenolone to 17-hydroxyprogesterone, and DHEA to androstenedione were 2 standard deviations above the mean. New data, however, fail to demonstrate a consistent phenotype-genotype correlation when using these hormonal criteria, and new criteria have been proposed using baseline and ACTH-stimulated 17-hydroxypregnenolone levels and 17-hydroxypregnenolone-to-cortisol ratios. Although this vignette does not provide ACTH-stimulated values and a random cortisol level in a newborn is not entirely useful, the diagnosis can be made because of the significantly elevated 17-hydroxypregnenolone level.

Educational Objective

Diagnose 3β-hydroxysteroid dehydrogenase deficiency on the basis of the clinical presentation and laboratory values.

Reference(s)

Lutfallah C, Wang W, Mason JI, et al. Newly proposed hormonal criteria via genotypic proof for type II 3beta-hydroxysteroid dehydrogenase deficiency. *J Clin Endocrinol Metab.* 2002;87(6):2611-2622. PMID: 12050224

Benkert AR, Young M, Robinson D, Hendrickson C, Lee PA, Strauss KA. Severe salt-losing 3β-hydroxysteroid dehydrogenase deficiency: treatment and outcomes of HSD3B2 c.35G>A homozygotes. *J Clin Endocrinol Metab.* 2015;100(8):E1105-E1115. PMID: 26079780

73

ANSWER: A) Change to low-calcium infant formula

This patient has subcutaneous fat necrosis of the newborn, an unusual form of transient panniculitis that may lead to hypercalcemia. Affected newborns are typically born at term and may have associated risk factors, including meconium aspiration, preeclampsia, maternal diabetes, and therapeutic cooling. Nodular lesions appear anytime between birth and age 6 weeks and are often associated with edema, erythema, and pain. Typical biopsy findings include lobular panniculitis with fat necrosis, inflammatory granulomas with multinucleated giant cells, and fibrosis. Nodules typically self-resolve within 6 months, although most babies continue to show cutaneous atrophy in affected regions. Hypercalcemia occurs in approximately 25% of affected infants, and it ranges in severity from mild and asymptomatic to severe and life-threatening. Hypercalcemia arises due to increased production of 1α-hydroxylase from lesional macrophages, leading to increased gastrointestinal calcium absorption. The onset of hypercalcemia occurs anytime between the initial emergence of the lesions to near resolution; it is therefore important to monitor calcium levels in all infants with subcutaneous fat necrosis.

This baby has mild, asymptomatic hypercalcemia. The initial step in management is to decrease dietary calcium intake, which can be achieved through low-calcium formula preparations (Answer A). In patients with severe forms that are not controlled through dietary changes alone, steroids (Answer B) may be used to inhibit the excess calcitriol synthesis and thus inhibit gastrointestinal calcium absorption. Bisphosphonates (Answer E) inhibit osteoclast release of skeletal calcium and are another option for second-line therapy. Hydration is an important component of management in hypercalcemia because hypercalciuria induces urinary salt wasting and hypovolemia can exacerbate hypercalcemia. This child has mild hypercalcemia and probably does not require intravenous hydration (Answer D) at this time. In addition, although furosemide can increase urinary calcium excretion, it is likely to exacerbate hypovolemia, particularly in infants. Increasing formula feeds without changing to a low-calcium formula (Answer C) will increase dietary calcium.

Educational Objective

Develop an approach to treatment of an infant with subcutaneous fat necrosis of the newborn and subsequent hypercalcemia.

Reference(s)

Farooque A, Moss C, Zehnder D, Hewison M, Shaw NJ. Expression of 25-hydroxyvitamin D3-1alpha-hydroxylase in subcutaneous fat necrosis. *Br J Dermatol.* 2009;160(2):423-425. PMID: 18811689

Shumer DE, Thaker V, Taylor GA, Wassner AJ. Severe hypercalcaemia due to subcutaneous fat necrosis: presentation, management and complications. *Arch Dis Child Fetal Neonatal Ed.* 2014;99(5):F419-F421. PMID: 24907163

Wiadrowski TP, Marshman G. Subcutaneous fat necrosis of the newborn following hypothermia and complicated by pain and hypercalcaemia. *Australas J Dermatol.* 2001;42(3):207-210. PMID: 11488718

74

ANSWER: E) Lower his insulin-to-carbohydrate ratio to 1:6 for breakfast and dinner intervals to deliver more insulin bolus to avoid postprandial hyperglycemia

Diabetes technology has progressed in the past decade from separate continuous subcutaneous insulin infusion pumps and continuous glucose monitors (CGMs) to integrated systems that use continuous glucose feedback from CGMs and historical insulin delivery information to calculate insulin dosing to be delivered by the pump. The first commercial hybrid closed-loop system for management of type 1 diabetes uses a proprietary proportional-integral-derivative controller with insulin feedback to calculate insulin doses continually based on CGM data. The system works in 2 modes: open-loop "manual mode" (insulin pump with or without sensor) and hybrid closed-loop "auto mode" in which the system algorithmically calculates background "auto-basal" insulin delivery based on CGM glucose values, with predefined insulin delivery limits adapted daily. When the system operates in manual mode, all insulin dosing parameters common to continuous subcutaneous insulin infusion are modifiable, including programmed basal rates, insulin-to-carbohydrate ratios, insulin sensitivity factors, active insulin time, and glucose targets. When the auto mode feature is enabled, the system automates insulin delivery, although it still requires user-initiated boluses for carbohydrates and optional correction doses. The user can modify the auto mode system only by adjusting insulin-to-carbohydrate ratios, active insulin time, and the rate of bolus insulin delivery (standard or quick bolus). The glucose target can be temporarily increased from 120 to 150 mg/dL (6.7 to 8.3 mmol/L) for exercise or driving. All other parameters are system-determined based on the previous days of total daily insulin and fasting glycemic control.

Setting a temporary basal rate when he is physically active to avoid hypoglycemia while in auto mode (Answer A) is incorrect because basal rates cannot be programmed when in auto mode; only the temporary target glucose can be altered.

Increasing the manual basal rate to 1.1 units per hour to match the total daily auto basal in delivering adequate basal insulin if he is not in auto mode (Answer B) is something that should be considered for patients who are spending a significant amount of time in manual mode. For this patient, it is not the best next step in management.

Decreasing active insulin time to 1:45 hours to help avoid postprandial hyperglycemia late in the evening (Answer C) is incorrect because active insulin time cannot be less than 2 hours.

In auto mode, the pump sets the sensitivity factor automatically by an algorithm derived from the previous days of total insulin use and therefore cannot be altered. Thus, lowering his sensitivity to deliver more insulin bolus for correction of hyperglycemia in the evening when he is in auto mode (Answer D) is incorrect.

Of the listed options, lowering his insulin-to-carbohydrate ratio to 1:6 for breakfast and dinner intervals to deliver more insulin bolus (Answer E) is the best approach, as this will reduce postprandial hyperglycemia.

Educational Objective
Make insulin dose adjustments in patients with type 1 diabetes mellitus using home glucose monitoring.

Reference(s)

Kowalski A. Pathway to artificial pancreas systems revisited: moving downstream. *Diabetes Care*. 2015;38(6):1036-1043. PMID: 25998296

Thabit H, Hovorka R. Coming of age: the artificial pancreas for type 1 diabetes. *Diabetologia*. 2016;59(9):1795-1805. PMID: 27364997

Ruiz JL, Sherr JL, Cengiz E, et al. Effect of insulin feedback on closed-loop glucose control: a crossover study. *J Diabetes Sci Technol*. 2012;6(5):1123-1130. PMID: 23063039

Messer LH, Forlenza GP, Sherr JL, et al. Slover optimizing hybrid closed-loop therapy in adolescents and emerging adults using the MiniMed 670G system. *Diabetes Care*. 2018;41(4):789-796. PMID: 29444895

75 ANSWER: C) Educational assessment for learning disability

The girl in this vignette has Turner syndrome, confirmed with testing that revealed a 45,X karyotype. Recommended preventive health care for all children in the United States includes annual developmental and behavioral screenings. In patients with Turner syndrome, this should be augmented by neuropsychologic assessments specific to the neurocognitive profile of Turner syndrome at preschool age, school entry, transition to high school, and any other time that difficulties may arise.

Women with Turner syndrome demonstrate characteristic neurocognitive profiles of intact verbal abilities and impaired visuospatial skills despite preserved ovarian function or adequate estrogen replacement. Learning disabilities (Answer C) have a high prevalence in Turner syndrome, estimated at approximately 50%, and characteristically affect nonverbal abilities. This is the most likely factor affecting her school performance.

Girls with Turner syndrome do not experience global intellectual disability (Answer A) at rates higher than that in the general population.

Studies of early low-dosage estrogen treatment in prepubertal girls with Turner syndrome suggest that there may be improvements in areas such as motor speed, nonverbal processing time, and memory. While estrogen replacement (Answer E) should certainly be considered in a 12-year-old girl with Turner syndrome, deficits that are most closely associated with Turner syndrome such as visuospatial and visual motor processing appear to persist despite estrogen replacement. Current recommendations are to start estrogen replacement at age 11 to 12 years (as long as gonadotropins are elevated) and titrate up to the adult dosage over the course of 2 to 3 years.

Impaired executive function and attention-deficit/hyperactivity disorder have been observed at a higher rate in individuals with Turner syndrome. Affected persons are noted to have greater risk of problems with hyperactivity and impulsivity and may have more social difficulties related to impairments in processing facial expression and emotions. This suggests that autism may be more common in girls with Turner syndrome, but this is controversial, and neither attention-deficit/hyperactivity disorder nor autism has been reported to occur as frequently as visuospatial deficits in this population. Thus, neither stimulant therapy (Answer B) nor evaluation for autism spectrum disorder (Answer D) is correct.

Educational Objective
Identify behavioral and psychological problems that can be present in girls with Turner syndrome.

Reference(s)

Gravholt CH, Andersen NH, Conway GS, et al; International Turner Syndrome Consensus Group. Clinical practice guidelines for the care of girls and women with Turner syndrome: proceedings from the 2016 Cincinnati International Turner Syndrome Meeting. *Eur J Endocrinol.* 2017;177(3):G1-G170. PMID: 28705803

Kesler SR. Turner syndrome. *Child Adolesc Psychiatr Clin N Am.* 2007;16(3):709-722. PMID: 17562588

76 ANSWER: B) Measure erythrocyte sedimentation rate, perform thyroid iodine uptake scan, and prescribe propranolol

This child has mild hyperthyroidism on the basis of her mild tachycardia and mild elevations of free T_4 and total T_3. The history of jaw pain and a small tender goiter on examination are strongly suggestive of subacute thyroiditis. In subacute thyroiditis, the erythrocyte sedimentation rate is expected to be elevated and the iodine uptake is low during the hyperthyroid phase. A thyroid uptake scan is also indicated and is helpful if a hot nodule is suspected. A thyroid uptake scan is usually not indicated if Graves disease is suspected. However, lack of eye findings or negative thyroid-stimulating immunoglobulin antibodies does not exclude Graves disease. Propranolol, a nonselective β-adrenergic blocker, would provide immediate relief of the tachycardia and help reduce the conversion of T_4 to T_3. A selective β-1 blocker should be used if the patient had asthma. The best next step in this patient's management is to measure the erythrocyte sedimentation rate, perform a thyroid iodine uptake scan, and prescribe propranolol (Answer B). Prescribing propranolol but not pursuing further evaluation to confirm subacute thyroiditis (Answer A) is inadequate.

This child had subacute thyroiditis confirmed by an elevated erythrocyte sedimentation rate and very low uptake on thyroid scan. As the hyperthyroid phase in subacute thyroiditis is brief, usually lasting a few weeks up to 2 months at most, methimazole (Answer C) would only become effective when the hyperthyroid phase is already starting to resolve. In the United States, methimazole is now the recommended thionamide. Propylthiouracil (PTU) can be considered in the first trimester of pregnancy or for short-term use during thyroid storm. Methimazole is indicated in patients with Graves disease and it is not usually used in transient cases of hyperthyroidism. Methimazole can be considered in severe thyrotoxicosis, which is not the case here. It is important to monitor thyroid function during the second phase, which is a hypothyroid phase that may warrant temporary levothyroxine replacement until the patient becomes euthyroid. Because TPO and thyroglobulin antibodies can be transiently elevated in subacute thyroiditis, it is important to confirm that there is no true autoimmune thyroiditis by repeating the titers at least 3 months after presentation. In this girl, the titers indeed became negative.

Repeating the thyroid-stimulating immunoglobulin antibody assessment (Answer D) is not indicated, especially because there is not a strong suspicion of Graves disease. TSH-receptor antibodies (Answer E) are also not indicated for that same reason, and that assay measures both blocking and stimulating antibodies.

Educational Objective
Diagnose and manage subacute thyroiditis.

Reference(s)

Radfar N, Kenny FM, Larsen PR. Subacute thyroiditis in a lateral thyroid gland: evaluation of the pituitary-thyroid axis during the acute destructive and the recovery phases. *J Pediatr.* 1975;87(1):34-37. PMID: 807695

Szabo SM1, Allen DB. Thyroiditis. Differentiation of acute suppurative and subacute. Case report and review of the literature. *Clin Pediatr (Phila).* 1989;28(4): 171-174. PMID: 2649297

77 ANSWER: C) Arginine-insulin tolerance test preceded by administration of 50 mg of testosterone intramuscularly 1 week before the test

The differential diagnosis for this patient includes constitutional delay of growth and puberty, GH deficiency, and suboptimal nutrition. The factors favoring constitutional delay of growth and puberty are the family history of relative delay of pubertal development in both parents, the presence of delayed skeletal maturation, and a previously adequate growth velocity inferred from the description of his growth pattern provided by the parents. The factor supporting the diagnosis of suboptimal nutrition is the greater compromise of weight compared with height and the low IGF-1 level at initial presentation. Aspects that favor GH deficiency include his height being below the 3rd percentile, the delayed skeletal maturation, and the low IGF-1 level. Low IGF-1 levels, however, can also be explained by delayed puberty and poor weight gain. Nevertheless, the poor growth velocity and the persistently low IGF-1 level despite nutritional recovery for 6 months should increase suspicion for GH deficiency. A GH-stimulation test should be performed to exclude GH deficiency. In the United States, 2 stimuli are required to perform this test, which may include a combination of insulin, arginine, clonidine, L-dopa, and glucagon. Exercise (a burst of intense physical activity) can also stimulate GH secretion, but this is not standardized for use in a clinical setting with reliable results. This patient has some delay in pubertal maturation as manifested by his Tanner stage and his testicular volume in the prepubertal range. Priming with sex steroids is recommended to avoid a false-positive diagnosis of GH deficiency in a prepubertal male older than 11 years who may only have constitutional delay of growth and puberty. Therefore, an arginine-insulin tolerance test preceded by administration of 50 mg of testosterone intramuscularly 1 week before the test (Answer C) is preferred over an arginine-insulin tolerance test with no priming. Different protocols for sex-steroid priming have been proposed, including the one mentioned in this vignette or the use of β-estradiol at a dose of 2 mg orally per night for the 2 nights immediately preceding the GH-stimulation test.

While it is clear that this patient has some delay in pubertal maturation, the administration of exogenous testosterone for several months to "jump start" puberty (Answer B) is usually recommended at a later age, typically around 14 or 14.5 years.

In the past, measurement of overnight spontaneous GH secretion (Answer A) was proposed to diagnose GH neurosecretory defects, but this is no longer recommended. Due to the pulsatile pattern of GH secretion, random measurement of GH (Answer D) should never be used to confirm a diagnosis of GH deficiency. Brain MRI (Answer E) is appropriate once a diagnosis of GH deficiency has been confirmed to rule out organic causes of GH deficiency such as suprasellar tumors. However, ordering MRI at this stage would be inappropriate, as it is not intended to confirm or exclude the diagnosis of GH deficiency.

Educational Objective
Explain the importance of sex-steroid priming in the performance of GH-stimulation tests and identify the more commonly used strategies for sex-steroid priming.

Reference(s)
Grimberg A, DiVall SA, Polychronakos C, et al; Drug and Therapeutics Committee and Ethics Committee of the Pediatric Endocrine Society. Guidelines for growth hormone and insulin-like growth factor-I treatment in children and adolescents: growth hormone deficiency, idiopathic short stature, and primary insulin-like growth factor-I deficiency. *Horm Res Paediatr.* 2016;86(6):361-397. PMID: 27884013

Cole TJ, Hindmarsh PC, Dunger DB. Growth hormone (GH) provocation tests and the response to GH treatment in GH deficiency. *Arch Dis Child.* 2004;89(11): 1024-1027. PMID: 15499055

Carel JC, Tresca JP, Letrait M, et al. Growth hormone testing for the diagnosis of growth hormone deficiency in childhood: a population register-based study. *J Clin Endocrinol Metab.* 1997;82(7):2117-2121. PMID: 9215281

Martinez AS, Domene HM, Ropelato MG, et al. Estrogen priming effect on growth hormone (GH) provocative test: a useful tool for the diagnosis of GH deficiency. *J Clin Endocrinol Metab.* 2000;85(11):4168-4172. PMID: 11095449

78 **ANSWER: E) Congenital hypopituitarism**
The pertinent findings in this case are a full-term baby with mild hepatomegaly, hypoglycemia, hyponatremia, and direct hyperbilirubinemia, born to a mother with severe preeclampsia. GH and cortisol are important counter-regulatory hormones. Hypoglycemia in infants with congenital pituitary deficiencies generally occurs due to GH deficiency, ACTH deficiency, or both. In the setting of hypoglycemia, GH stimulates lipolysis and cortisol stimulates gluconeogenesis. Absence of these hormones would be expected to result in hypoglycemia. ACTH deficiency (as well as hypothyroidism) has been associated with hyponatremia due to compromised free water clearance. Additionally, some studies suggest increased vasopressin activity in the setting of glucocorticoid deficiency. Furthermore, congenital GH deficiency has been associated with giant-cell hepatitis and direct

hyperbilirubinemia. In this case, the baby has hypoglycemia, hyponatremia, and direct hyperbilirubinemia. Congenital hypopituitarism (Answer E) is the most likely diagnosis.

Congenital hyperinsulinism (Answer A) is the most common cause of persistent hypoglycemia in infants. Congenital hyperinsulinism is most often associated with inactivating pathogenic variants in 1 of 2 adjacent genes, *ABCC8* and *KCNJ11*, encoding the sulfonylurea receptor 1 and Kir6.2 proteins, which together form the ATP-sensitive plasma membrane potassium (KATP) channel in pancreatic β cells. Pathogenic variants in *GLUD1*, *GCK*, *HADH*, *UCP2*, *HNF4A*, *HNF1A*, and *SLC16A1* can also cause congenital hyperinsulinism. However, in addition to hypoglycemia, this infant has hyponatremia and direct hyperbilirubinemia, neither of which is associated with congenital hyperinsulinism.

Congenital adrenal hyperplasia (Answer B) can be associated with hypoglycemia and hyponatremia; however, hyponatremia due to salt-wasting would not be expected immediately following delivery. In addition, if hyponatremia were present due to salt-wasting, hyperkalemia would also be expected due to mineralocorticoid deficiency. It is also important to consider neonatal sepsis in any newborn with hypoglycemia and poor temperature regulation, but it is not generally associated with direct hyperbilirubinemia or hyponatremia.

Glycogen storage disease type 1a (Answer C) is the most common glycogen storage disease and is due to deficiency of glucose-6-phosphatase. Affected infants have hepatomegaly and liver dysfunction but would not be expected to have hyponatremia.

Hypoglycemia can occur in some neonates exposed to perinatal stress (Answer D) such as intrauterine growth retardation, maternal preeclampsia, birth asphyxia, or prematurity. The cause appears to be transient hyperinsulinism, causing an inability to mobilize glycogen or oxidize fatty acids. While this baby was born to a mother with severe preeclampsia and could have hypoglycemia due to transient hyperinsulinism, she would not be expected to have hyponatremia or hyperbilirubinemia.

Educational Objective
List the metabolic abnormalities associated with neonatal hypopituitarism.

Reference(s)

Parks JS. Congenital hypopituitarism. *Clin Perinatol*. 2018;45(1):75-91. PMID: 29406008

Snider KE, Becker S, Boyajian L, et al. Genotype and phenotype correlations in 417 children with congenital hyperinsulinism. *J Clin Endocrinol Metab*. 2013;98 (2):E355-E363. PMID: 23275527

Karnsakul W, Sawathiparnich P, Nimkarn S, Likitmaskul S, Santiprabhob J, Aanpreung P. Anterior pituitary hormone effects on hepatic functions in infants with congenital hypopituitarism. *Ann Hepatol*. 2007;6(2):97-103. PMID: 17519832

79 **ANSWER: B) Complete neck ultrasonography and FNA biopsy of the thyroid nodule, the right inferior lymph node, and other suspicious lymph nodes (if found)**

Children and young adult cancer survivors who were treated with radiation therapy are a high-risk population for the development of thyroid cancer. The patients at highest risk are survivors of leukemia, Hodgkin lymphoma, and brain tumors. Among survivors who received radiation to the thyroid gland, incidence ratios for developing differentiated thyroid cancer range from 5- to 69-fold, depending on the radiation dose.

The American Thyroid Association guidelines for the management of thyroid nodules in children and adolescents, inaugurated in 2015, highlight that thyroid nodules develop in cancer survivors at a rate of 2% annually, and seem to peak 15 to 25 years after radiation exposure. Patients who received radiation at a younger age and those who received radiation doses up to 20 to 29 Gy are considered to be at highest risk. However, currently, there are no specific guidelines on screening this population with neck ultrasonography, as there are no data to determine whether early detection of nonpalpable thyroid nodules affects quality of life or improves survival. Current guidelines recommend an annual physical examination for children at high risk of developing thyroid neoplasia and to pursue additional imaging if the patient has palpable nodules, abnormal lymphadenopathy, or thyroid asymmetry.

Recently, an international panel of 33 experts (Clement and colleagues) attempted to develop guidelines for thyroid cancer surveillance in survivors of cancer in childhood, adolescence, and young adulthood. After they enumerated the possible benefits and harms of surveillance, they attempted to answer the following: (1) who needs screening, (2) which surveillance method should be used, (3) how frequently and for how long thyroid cancer surveillance should be performed, and (4) what to do if abnormalities are identified. They confirmed that childhood and young adult cancer survivors treated with radiotherapy or ^{131}I-meta-iodobenzylguanidine (MIBG) that accidentally exposes the thyroid gland are at increased risk for the development of thyroid cancer. Exposure to anthracyclines also increases the risk of developing thyroid cancer. No data have shown that chemotherapy alone is associated with a higher risk. The dose-response curve describing the relationship between external radiation and the risk of developing differentiated thyroid cancer is linear up to 10 Gy and then plateaus and declines. However, differentiated thyroid cancer occurs in survivors receiving as low as 1 Gy and as high as 40 Gy to the thyroid field. Therefore, the authors recommend counseling childhood and young adult cancer survivors regarding their risk of developing thyroid cancer. The authors also recommend counseling about the advantages of surveillance (detecting cancer earlier and potentially decreasing rates of recurrence and improving surgical outcomes) vs the disadvantages of surveillance (increasing the use of unnecessary tests and/or detecting indolent disease, benign nodules, or other incidental findings). However, the authors are unable to provide recommendations regarding the preferred surveillance method to detect a thyroid nodule (neck palpation vs thyroid ultrasonography). They suggest that commencing surveillance 5 years after exposure is reasonable. The panel suggests that if periodic thyroid palpation is chosen, repeating surveillance every 1 to 2 years is reasonable, while if using thyroid ultrasound, repeating surveillance every 3 to 5 years is reasonable. Referral to a thyroid specialist is recommended if a thyroid nodule is found by either method of surveillance.

The best approach for this patient is complete neck ultrasonography and FNA of the thyroid nodule, the right inferior lymph node, and other suspicious lymph nodes (if found) (Answer B).

Although this patient is at high risk for differentiated thyroid cancer, counseling the family to proceed with total thyroidectomy and central neck dissection (Answer A) is not appropriate, as differentiated thyroid cancer has not been diagnosed yet.

She has been in remission and has been followed closely by her oncology team. Although she could certainly develop other malignancies such as lymphoma (Answer C) or recurrent leukemia, this is less likely in this setting given her age, lack of symptoms, lack of other findings on examination, and the presence of a thyroid nodule identified on neck ultrasonography.

The thyroid nodule is highly suspicious for malignancy as it has microcalcifications and some border irregularities. The lymph node is also highly suspicious for malignancy (round, lack of hilum, peripheral vascularity). Therefore, although the thyroid nodule is smaller than 1 cm, it does indeed have suspicious features and should be aspirated. Thus, neck ultrasonography in 4 to 6 months (Answer D) is insufficient. For the same reasons, follow-up with palpation (Answer E) is even more inappropriate in this case.

This patient underwent complete neck ultrasonography and no suspicious lymph nodes were noted on the left side of her neck. She underwent FNA of the thyroid nodule and the right suspicious lymph node and both were diagnostic of papillary thyroid carcinoma. She underwent total thyroidectomy with central neck and right neck dissection. Pathologic examination revealed multifocal papillary thyroid cancer in the right lobe, with a maximum extension of 3.5 cm. There was extrathyroidal extension to adipose tissue and to the anterior soft-tissue margin, with lymphovascular and perineural invasion. The left lobe has multifocal papillary thyroid cancer, 1.5 cm in the largest dimension, with extrathyroidal invasion and extensive lymphatic invasion. All central neck lymph nodes showed metastatic disease and she had 2 positive lymph nodes in the lateral neck. She was treated with radioactive iodine, and the posttreatment scan showed uptake in thyroid bed and bilateral neck lymph nodes, without distant metastases.

Educational Objective
Recommend appropriate surveillance for thyroid cancer in children who have undergone neck radiation and evaluate thyroid nodules in this setting.

Reference(s)

Clement SC, Kremer LCM, Verburg FA, et al. Balancing the benefits and harms of thyroid cancer surveillance in survivors of childhood, adolescent and young adult cancer: recommendations from the international late effects of childhood cancer guideline harmonization group in collaboration with the PanCareSurFup Consortium. *Cancer Treat Rev.* 2018;63:28-39. PMID: 29202445

Francis GL, Waguespack SG, Bauer AJ, et al; American Thyroid Association Guidelines Task Force. Management guidelines for children with thyroid nodules and differentiated thyroid cancer. *Thyroid.* 2015;25(7):716-759. PMID: 25900731

Langer JE, Mandel SJ. Sonographic imaging of cervical lymph nodes in patients with thyroid cancer. *Neuroimaging Clin N Am.* 2008;18(3):479-489. PMID: 18656029

80

ANSWER: C) LH, 6.1 mIU/mL; FSH, 14.5 mIU/mL; testosterone, 628 ng/dL

Aromatase inhibitors limit the conversion of androgens such as androstenedione and testosterone to estrone and estradiol. Third-generation nonsteroidal aromatase inhibitors such as anastrozole (1 mg daily) and letrozole (2.5 mg daily) are highly effective in blocking greater than 95% activity of this cytochrome P450 enzyme. As a result, these medications can delay epiphyseal fusion and prolong the duration of linear growth.

Safety data show that children have a significant increase in LH, FSH, and testosterone levels while on aromatase inhibitors, most likely due to the release of feedback inhibition on gonadotropins by the reduction in estradiol levels. These increases are observed in patients of any age and pubertal stage, but those in advanced puberty have more robust increases. Therefore, the most likely set of test results to be observed in this patient is depicted in Answer C. Increased testosterone levels could lead to potential adverse effects such as worsening acne and polycythemia. These observed elevations return to the normal range within 6 months of stopping aromatase inhibitor therapy.

Investigators of a few studies have examined the safety and effectiveness of these agents to improve growth velocity and final height prediction/attainment in children with short stature of several etiologies (eg, idiopathic short stature, constitutional delay of growth and puberty, and GH deficiency), either as a standalone treatment or in combination with other agents such as testosterone or GH. A Cochrane review in 2015 concluded that there are insufficient data on clinical efficacy of aromatase inhibitors in improving final height or near-final height due to the limited number of randomized controlled trials. However, retrospective chart review studies have documented contradictory results—some supporting the positive effect and others not. A randomized open-label study of 76 pubertal boys with idiopathic short stature treated under 1 of 3 arms (aromatase inhibitors only, GH only, aromatase inhibitors + GH) for 24 to 36 months showed highest height gain in the combination group. Patients treated with only aromatase inhibitors did have a higher height gain than what would have been expected on the basis of Centers for Disease Control growth charts (there was no control group in the study). Although a previous study raised concern for possible risk of vertebral anomalies with the use of aromatase inhibitors, this particular study of the 76 patients showed no significant difference among the 3 groups.

At this time, aromatase inhibitors continue to be used only off-label in children with short stature. These agents have also been studied in other conditions such as familial male-limited precocious puberty, McCune-Albright syndrome, congenital adrenal hyperplasia, and pubertal gynecomastia. While the potential risk for decreased bone mineral density due to blocking estradiol production is a concern, limited data on bone health parameters have not shown this to be the case. There are also other concerns such as their effect on spermatogenesis/fertility and carbohydrate/lipid metabolism that have not yet been fully studied. Long-term, well-designed studies are needed to carefully document the safety and efficacy of aromatase inhibitors in pediatric endocrine practice.

Educational Objective

Describe the observation that aromatase inhibitors significantly increase gonadotropin levels and testosterone levels when used in pubertal-aged boys.

Reference(s)

McGrath N, O'Grady MJ. Aromatase inhibitors for short stature in male children and adolescents. *Cochrane Database Syst Rev.* 2015;(10):CD010888. PMID: 26447646

Mauras N, Ross JL, Gagliardi P, et al. Randomized trial of aromatase inhibitors, growth hormone, or combination in pubertal boys with idiopathic, short stature. *J Clin Endocrinol Metab.* 2016;101(12):4984-4993. PMID: 27710241

Pedrosa LF, de Oliveira JM, Thomé PRV, Kochi C, Damiani D, Longui CA. Height increment and laboratory profile of boys treated with aromatase inhibitors with or without growth hormone. *Horm Metab Res.* 2017;49(10):778-785. PMID: 28859208

Ferris JA, Geffner ME. Are aromatase inhibitors in boys with predicted short stature and/or rapidly advancing bone age effective and safe? *J Pediatr Endocrinol Metab.* 2017;30(3):311-317. PMID: 28207416

81

ANSWER: D) Precocious puberty

In an infant with hyperthyroidism, neonatal Graves disease is the first diagnosis on the differential. There is a maternal history of a thyroid disorder, and it is possible that the mother has an undisclosed history of Graves disease for which she was treated with radioactive iodine or surgery or perhaps she simply became hypothyroid with time. However, the infant has additional findings on physical exam—facial plethora and hypertrichosis, which are strongly suggestive of Cushing syndrome. The constellation of findings including hyperthyroidism and hypercortisolism in an infant should make one consider McCune-Albright syndrome. Hypercortisolism is very rare in patients with McCune-Albright syndrome, but when it is present, it occurs only in infancy. It is always ACTH-independent and has been described as primary bimorphic adrenocortical disease. It can be quite severe, leading to death. However, it resolves spontaneously in about half of affected patients.

McCune-Albright syndrome is caused by an early embryonic postzygotic somatic activating mutation in the *GNAS* gene and is characterized by the involvement of the skeleton, skin, and various endocrine systems. Fibrous dysplasia can range from an asymptomatic monostotic lesion to debilitating polyostotic disease. Affected patients have characteristic café-au-lait macules with irregular borders (typically referred to as "coast of Maine" macules). On further examination, the patient in this vignette was noted to have multiple hyperpigmented lesions. Endocrine abnormalities result from the up-regulation of the GNAS receptor and include gonadotropin-independent precocious puberty (Answer D) due to recurrent ovarian cysts in girls and autonomous testosterone production in boys, GH excess (not GH deficiency [Answer E]), FGF-23–mediated phosphate wasting with or without hypophosphatemia, and neonatal hypercortisolism. Affected patients can also have testicular lesions with or without precocious puberty and thyroid lesions with or without hyperthyroidism. Patients with any combination of these findings are diagnosed with McCune-Albright syndrome and genetic testing for confirmation is not required, particularly because the pathogenic variant is detected in the affected tissue and may not be detected in a peripheral blood sample.

Celiac disease (Answer A) and vitiligo (Answer B) are autoimmune conditions that are associated with other autoimmunities. However, McCune-Albright syndrome is not an autoimmune disorder and is therefore not associated with these findings. While some patients with McCune-Albright syndrome have significant bone disease due to polyostotic lesions and are at risk for fractures, osteoporosis (Answer C) is not frequently reported. However, patients with a history of prolonged hyperthyroidism or untreated hypercortisolism are certainly at risk for osteoporosis.

Educational Objective
Diagnose McCune-Albright syndrome on the basis of clinical findings and consider the rare presentation of Cushing syndrome in infancy.

Reference(s)
Tatsi C, Stratakis CA. Neonatal Cushing syndrome: a rare but potentially devastating disease. *Clin Perinatol*. 2018;45(1):103-118. PMID: 29406000

Brown RJ, Kelly MH, Collins MT. Cushing syndrome in the McCune-Albright syndrome. *J Clin Endocrinol Metab*. 2010;95(4):1508-1515. PMID: 20157193

82 **ANSWER: E) Continue current management**
This patient has primary hypergonadotropic hypogonadism secondary to the effects of chemotherapy and radiation therapy. In boys, depressed spermatogenesis can be seen after a testicular radiation dose as low as 0.15 Gy. The effect of radiation on testicular function is age dependent, with prepubertal radiation exposure causing significantly more damage to Leydig cells than postpubertal radiation.

In a study of 125 childhood cancer survivors from the Swedish Cancer Registry (median age, 34 years; mean follow-up time, 24 years), hypogonadism was found in 26% (odds ratio, 2.1; $P = .025$). The odds ratio was further increased in those who underwent testicular irradiation (odds ratio, 28; $P = .004$). Radiotherapy other than cranial or testicular irradiation plus chemotherapy, or cranial irradiation without chemotherapy, was also associated with increased odds ratios (odds ratio, 3.7 [$P = .013$] and odds ratio, 4.4 [$P = .038$], respectively). Given the increased risk of gonadal dysfunction and the possibility of spontaneous recovery, recommendations for surveillance include yearly monitoring of pubertal status.

LH and FSH release are regulated by pulsatile GnRH secretion, as well as by feedback inhibition from testicular hormones. Testosterone decreases GnRH production in the hypothalamus, and decreases the sensitivity of the pituitary to GnRH. Testosterone also exerts direct feedback inhibition on LH, whereas the effects of testosterone on FSH are mediated primarily through aromatization to estradiol. In the patient in this vignette, exogenous testosterone treatment increased serum testosterone levels, which resulted in near-normalization of LH levels via feedback inhibition. This suggests that the testosterone replacement dosage is correct and the current regimen should be continued (thus, Answer E is correct and Answer C is incorrect).

Under normal circumstances, inhibin B produced by Sertoli cells acts to inhibit FSH secretion from the pituitary; this process can be disrupted with testicular radiation therapy and would be expected to cause persistently elevated FSH levels due to loss of feedback inhibition. Brain MRI (Answer A) is not needed, as it is unlikely that this patient has an FSH-secreting tumor. An aromatase inhibitor (Answer B) would reduce peripheral conversion of testosterone to estradiol and would not be expected to normalize the FSH level. It is unlikely that the formulation of testosterone would make a difference, as both topical testosterone and injectable testosterone (Answer D) can be aromatized to estradiol.

In this patient, chemotherapy and testicular irradiation have caused primary gonadal failure; loss of testosterone production has impaired testosterone-mediated feedback inhibition of LH, and to a lesser extent, FSH. Feedback inhibition of FSH is mediated primarily by estradiol and inhibin B.

Educational Objective
Explain the factors that cause an increase in serum gonadotropin concentrations in patients with primary hypogonadism.

Reference(s)

Isaksson S, Bogefors K, Ståhl O, et al. High risk of hypogonadism in young male cancer survivors. *Clin Endocrinol (Oxf)*. 2018;88(3):432-441. PMID: 29245176

Hayes FJ, DeCruz S, Seminara SB, Boepple PA, Crowley WF Jr. Differential regulation of gonadotropin secretion by testosterone in the human male: absence of a negative feedback effect of testosterone on follicle-stimulating hormone secretion. *J Clin Endocrinol Metab*. 2001;86(1):53-58. PMID: 11231978

83 ANSWER: D) Dysfunction of the vasopressinergic neurons of the supraoptic and paraventricular nuclei

This child has evidence of hypothyroidism, GH deficiency, and likely ACTH deficiency in the setting of a craniopharyngioma. Before surgery, she did not have increased thirst or increased urination. After replacement with hydrocortisone and levothyroxine, she was given stress-dose steroids just before surgery. In the immediate postoperative period, she developed markedly increased urine output and hypernatremia. Patients with lesions of the pituitary gland can present with hormone deficiencies preoperatively, during surgery, postoperatively, and even weeks after surgery. Postoperative central diabetes insipidus develops in 70% to 90% of children with craniopharyngioma and can be a significant cause of morbidity. Approximately 10% to 22% of children with craniopharyngioma develop transient diabetes insipidus postoperatively. In cases of radical excision, 80% to 90% of patients have permanent diabetes insipidus. Symptoms of diabetes insipidus can be masked by glucocorticoid deficiency. In this case, the patient did not develop polyuria and polydipsia after she started hydrocortisone and levothyroxine replacement therapy, so central diabetes insipidus that was unmasked after replacement with hydrocortisone (Answer A) is incorrect. Hyperglycemia (Answer B) is a common cause of polyuria, but the dose of hydrocortisone she received would most likely not be associated with a high degree of hyperglycemia leading to such excessive urine output. Excess fluid administration (Answer C) is a common cause of postoperative polyuria, although it is unlikely to cause hypernatremia as in this case.

Postoperatively, diabetes insipidus can be transient, permanent, or can occur in a triphasic pattern. Diabetes insipidus occurs due to dysfunction of the vasopressinergic neurons of the supraoptic and paraventricular nuclei (Answer D). Diabetes insipidus is transient if there is regeneration of the vasopressinergic neurons. Permanent diabetes insipidus occurs if greater than 90% of the neurons or their projections to the posterior pituitary gland are damaged. The triphasic response (Answer E) occurs when there is injury to the hypothalamus or pituitary stalk that leads to temporary dysfunction, initially causing diabetes insipidus. This phase is followed by the antidiuretic phase, which occurs when there is release of vasopressin from the posterior pituitary or damaged hypothalamus. When the antidiuretic hormone reserve is depleted, another polyuric phase ensues. While it is possible that this patient will go on to have a triphasic response, she does not yet have evidence of antidiuresis and the sodium level is high, so she is still in the first phase of the triphasic response.

Educational Objective
Explain the causes and patterns of disorders of water metabolism that can occur with surgery for tumors of the pituitary and/or hypothalamic areas.

Reference(s)

Pratheesh R, Swallow DM, Rajaratnam S, et al. Incidence, predictors and early post-operative course of diabetes insipidus in paediatric craniopharygioma: a comparison with adults. *Childs Nerv Syst.* 2013;29(6):941-949. PMID: 23386174

Devin JK. Hypopituitarism and central diabetes insipidus: perioperative diagnosis and management. *Neurosurg Clin N Am.* 2012;23(4):679-689. PMID: 23040752

Prete A, Corsello SM, Salvatori R. Current best practice in the management of patients after pituitary surgery. *Ther Adv Endocrinol Metab.* 2017;8(3):33-48. PMID: 28377801

84 ANSWER: E) Pathogenic variant in the *KCNJ11* gene

Neonatal diabetes is a rare genetic disorder characterized by diabetes that presents within the first 6 months of life, which may be either permanent or transient. Approximately 50% of cases of neonatal diabetes are due to gain-of-function pathogenic variants in the genes that encode the pore-forming subunit of the ATP-sensitive potassium channel (*KCNJ11* [Answer E]—encoding the inwardly rectifying potassium channel Kir6.2) or the regulatory subunit of that channel (encoding the sulfonylurea receptor 1). Approximately 30% of these patients also have neurologic symptoms such as developmental delay and muscle hypotonia, a condition termed intermediate DEND syndrome (developmental delay, epilepsy, and neonatal diabetes). About 3% of these patients experience epilepsy. ATP-sensitive potassium channel pathogenic variants are also associated with diabetes that presents in later life, and a common polymorphism in the *KCNJ11* gene (Glu23Lys) confers an enhanced risk of type 2 diabetes. The 4 pore-forming transmembrane Kir6.2 subunits and the 4 regulatory sulfonylurea receptor subunits of the ATP-sensitive potassium channel in the β-cell membrane are respectively encoded by the *KCNJ11* and *ABCC8* genes on chromosome 11p15.1. Heterozygous activating pathogenic variants in *KCNJ11* and *ABCC8*, which lead to suppression of glucose-stimulated insulin secretion, can both be causes of transient and permanent neonatal diabetes mellitus. However, activating *KCNJ11* pathogenic variants are the most common etiology of neonatal diabetes and account for 26% to 34% of permanent cases and up to 13% of transient cases. This is the most likely etiology of neonatal diabetes in this patient. The general mechanisms by which these mutations lead to permanent and transient neonatal diabetes mellitus are by decreasing ATP-mediated inhibition at Kir6.2 and/or by increasing magnesium-ATP induction (mediated by the sulfonylurea receptor 1 subunit) of ATP-sensitive potassium channel activity.

6q24–related transient neonatal diabetes mellitus (Answer B) is defined as transient neonatal diabetes mellitus caused by genetic aberrations of the imprinted locus at 6q24. The cardinal features are severe intrauterine growth retardation, hyperglycemia that begins in the neonatal period in a term infant and resolves by age 18 months, dehydration, and absence of ketoacidosis. Macroglossia and umbilical hernia can be present. 6q24–related transient neonatal diabetes mellitus caused by a multilocus imprinting disturbance can be associated with marked hypotonia, congenital heart disease, deafness, neurologic features (eg, epilepsy), and renal malformations. Although 6q24–related transient neonatal diabetes mellitus is a possibility in this case, especially in view of the patient's family history, it is a less common cause of neonatal diabetes than pathogenic variants in the *KCNJ11* gene.

Homozygous pathogenic variants in the gene encoding the glucokinase enzyme (*GCK*) (Answer C) cause a rare form of permanent neonatal diabetes associated with marked hyperglycemia early in life and lifelong insulin requirement. It is therefore unlikely in this case.

Pathogenic variants in the *PDX1* gene (Answer D) are associated with pancreatic agenesis and gastrointestinal manifestations that are not present in this patient.

Rare autoimmune diabetes (Answer A) has been described as a part of the IPEX syndrome (immunodysregulation polyendocrinopathy enteropathy X-linked syndrome), and the patient does not have any other clinical features to support this diagnosis.

Educational Objective

Construct a differential diagnosis for neonatal diabetes mellitus.

Reference(s)

Aguilar-Bryan L, Bryan J. Neonatal diabetes mellitus. *Endocr Rev.* 2008;29(3):265-291. PMID: 18436707

Proks P, Arnold AL, Bruining J, et al. A heterozygous activating mutation in the sulphonylurea receptor SUR1 (ABCC8) causes neonatal diabetes. *Hum Mol Genet.* 2006;15(11):1793-1800. PMID: 16613899

Flanagan SE, Patch AM, Mackay DJ, et al. Mutations in ATP-sensitive K+ channel genes cause transient neonatal diabetes and permanent diabetes in childhood or adulthood [published correction appears in *Diabetes*. 2008;57(2):523]. *Diabetes*. 2007;56(7):1930-1937. PMID: 17446535

Gloyn AL, Pearson ER, Antcliff JF, et al. Activating mutations in the gene encoding the ATP-sensitive potassium-channel subunit Kir6.2 and permanent neonatal diabetes [published correction appears in *N Engl J Med*. 2004;351(14):1470]. *N Engl J Med*. 2004;350(18):1838-1849. PMID: 15115830

Hattersley AT, Ashcroft FM. Activating mutations in Kir6.2 and neonatal diabetes: new clinical syndromes, new scientific insights, and new therapy. *Diabetes*. 2005;54(9):2503-2513. PMID: 16123337

Vedovato N, Clif E, Proks P, et al. Neonatal diabetes caused by a homozygous KCNJ11 mutation demonstrates that tiny changes in ATP sensitivity markedly affect diabetes risk. *Diabetologia*. 2016;59(7):1430-1436. PMID: 27118464

85 ANSWER: B) Start prenatal vitamins plus iodine supplementation (total of 250 mcg of iodine daily)

Recently, renewed attention has been paid to iodine and its importance in fetal health. The neurodevelopment of the fetus is adversely affected when the mother has severe iodine deficiency and hypothyroidism or hypothyroidism due to other causes. Mild to moderate iodine deficiency in the mother, characterized by a normal TSH and low free T_4 (hypothyroxinemia), can lead to poor neurodevelopmental outcomes. Damage to the fetal brain is caused by decreased availability of maternal T_4 to the developing fetal brain, leading to abnormal neuronal migration such that migration of neurons to the upper layers of the cerebral cortex is stopped. Women who avoid dairy (as this woman does) or seafood or use noniodized salt (ie, sea salt) are at higher risk of developing iodine deficiency.

Recommended adult iodine intake is 150 mcg daily. Iodine requirements are higher during pregnancy, partly to supply the fetus and potentially due to increased urinary losses. For pregnant women, the recommended iodine intake by both the World Health Organization and the American Thyroid Association is 250 mcg daily (Answer B). The International Federation of Gynecology and Obstetrics recommends iodine supplementation not only during pregnancy but also in adolescence and when planning for pregnancy. Taking a total of 150 mcg daily (Answer C) is insufficient. While it is recommended that prenatal vitamins include 150 mcg of iodine, this is not standardized and iodine content varies. Thus, simply recommending 100 mcg daily in addition to a prenatal vitamin (Answer A) might be inadequate.

Nutritional iodine deficiency in pregnant women results in preferential synthesis of T_3 over T_4, leading to maternal hypothyroxinemia while circulating T_3 and TSH levels remain normal. Transfer of T_3 from the mother to the fetus is very low, and the fetus relies on maternal T_4 transfer. Therefore, measuring TSH alone or in combination with T_3 (Answer D) is incorrect. Measuring TSH and free T_4 would be a better choice. Measuring urinary iodine (Answer E) is useful in population studies, but it is not helpful for determining the iodine status in an individual.

Educational Objective

Recommend appropriate iodine intake during pregnancy to optimize fetal neurocognitive outcomes.

Reference(s)

Alexander EK, Pearce EN, Brent GA, et al. 2017 guidelines of the American Thyroid Association for the diagnosis and management of thyroid disease during pregnancy and the postpartum. *Thyroid*. 2017;27(3):315-389. PMID: 28056690

Bath SC, Steer CD, Golding J, Emmett P, Rayman MP. Effect of inadequate iodine status in UK pregnancy women on cognitive outcomes in their children: results from the Avon Longitudinal Study of Parents and Children (ALSPAC). *Lancet*. 2013;382(9889):331-337. PMID: 23706508

86 ANSWER: E) Discuss with the patient's psychiatrist the possible use of nonstimulant medications

Review of the patient's growth charts indicates that both his height and weight tracked normally until age 11 years. A deceleration in weight gain was noted after this time, and it was more pronounced in the last 6 months with the initiation of methylphenidate. A decline in growth velocity was also apparent. Persistence of poor weight gain leads to further deceleration of linear growth. Stimulant medications (eg, amphetamine, dextroamphetamine, lisdexamfetamine, methylphenidate, dexmethylphenidate) are associated with poor linear growth. The postulated mechanism is a negative effect on weight gain secondary to decreased appetite, although a direct effect on linear growth has also been suggested. It has also been observed that children with attention-deficit/hyperactivity disorder have slightly shorter stature than children without this condition, but the difference is not evident with advancement of puberty. When feasible, the use of nonstimulant medications (eg, atomoxetine, clonidine, guanfacine) has been proposed for the management of attention-deficit/hyperactivity disorder. In this vignette, a discussion is warranted with the patient's psychiatrist (Answer E).

This patient has evidence of spontaneous puberty/activation of the hypothalamic-pituitary-gonadal axis as manifested by a testicular volume of 6 mL bilaterally. Administration of testosterone (Answer A) to "jump start" puberty would, therefore, not be indicated.

The patient's celiac screen is reportedly negative. Although his poor weight gain could potentially be explained by celiac disease, initiation of a gluten-free diet (Answer B) seems unjustified in the absence of a positive screen or biopsy confirmation of this condition.

His IGF-1 level is in the lower end of the reference range. Low IGF-1 in the presence of a normal IGFBP-3 value is more likely representative of suboptimal nutrition rather than GH deficiency. Should his linear growth decline despite nutritional recovery, repeated IGF-1 measurement would be useful to screen for GH deficiency. If low, a GH-stimulation test would be warranted before considering GH replacement therapy (Answer C).

This patient has evidence of gonadarche, which is appropriate for his chronologic age. His bone age is not advanced and the prediction of adult height falls within his genetic potential. Working on improving weight gain rather than delaying skeletal maturation is the most reasonable approach. Therefore, use of an aromatase inhibitor (Answer D) would not be justified in this case. Moreover, aromatase inhibitors are not approved for this indication and it is recommended that these medications be used in the context of clinical trials.

Educational Objective
Identify pharmacologic treatment of attention-deficit/hyperactivity disorder as a contributing factor to poor growth.

Reference(s)

Poulton AS, Bui Q, Melzer E, Evans R. Stimulant medication effects on growth and bone age in children with attention-deficit/hyperactivity disorder: a prospective cohort study. *Int Clin Psychopharmacol.* 2016;31(2):93-99. PMID: 26544899

Miller BS, Aydin F, Lundgren F, Lindberg A, Geffner ME. Stimulant use and its impact on growth in children receiving growth hormone therapy: an analysis of the KIGS International Growth Database. *Horm Res Pediatr.* 2014;82(1):31-37. PMID: 24924157

Rose SR, Reeves G, Gut R, Germak J. Attention-deficit/hyperactivity disorder medication treatment impact on response to growth hormone therapy: results from the Answer Program, a non-interventional study. *J Pediatr.* 2015;167(6):1389-1396. PMID: 26394822

Hardin DS. Growth in hyperactive children treated with stimulant medication. *Endocrinologist.* 2002;12:509-512.

87 ANSWER: A) Recommend left lobectomy

Benign lesions of the thyroid include hyperfunctioning follicular adenomas and follicular adenomas. Recently, thyroid neoplasms previously classified as noninvasive encapsulated follicular variant of papillary thyroid carcinoma (FVPTC) have been reclassified as a more benign lesion, with the term noninvasive follicular thyroid neoplasm with papillary-like nuclear features (NIFTP).

Most thyroid carcinomas arise from the thyroid follicular cells and are divided into papillary thyroid carcinoma (PTC), follicular thyroid carcinoma (FTC), poorly differentiated thyroid carcinoma (PDTC), and anaplastic thyroid carcinoma (ATC). PTC and FTC are well-differentiated thyroid carcinomas that usually respond to radioactive iodine therapy. A small amount of thyroid cancers arise from the parafollicular C cells and are classified as medullary thyroid carcinoma (MTC).

Thyroid carcinoma in children is classified based on the same histologic criteria set for adults. In children, about 90% of thyroid carcinomas are PTC, followed by uncommon cases of FTC. MTC and ATC are rare in the pediatric population.

PTC has several subtypes: classic, follicular variant, tall cell, oncocytic, columnar cell, diffuse sclerosing, solid, clear cell, cribriform morular, macrofollicular, PTC with prominent hobnail features, PTC with fasciitis-like stroma, PTC with medullary thyroid carcinoma, and PTC with dedifferentiation to anaplastic carcinoma.

Most PTC subtypes seen in children and adolescents include the following variants: classic, solid, follicular variant, and diffuse sclerosing variant. Other variants are rarely seen in the pediatric population and are generally aggressive and have a poor prognosis.

Classic PTC has a papillary architecture with branching. The papillae are covered by cells with eosinophilic cytoplasm and enlarged nuclei. Cytologic features consist of enlarged irregular nuclei that are often oval-shaped and overlapping due to the nuclear enlargement. The nuclei often show clearing or have a ground-glass appearance with powdery chromatin marginated to the periphery (orphan Annie nuclei).

Solid variant PTC is diagnosed when the tumor has more than 50% solid pattern. It is commonly seen in children and was initially described in patients with a history of radiation. Cells are arranged in solid nests separated by bands with nuclear features of papillary carcinoma. It is common to see to see follicular and papillary growth patterns intermixed with the areas of solid growth. Vascular invasion and extrathyroidal extension occurs in approximately 40% of cases.

Follicular variant tumors look like a follicular neoplasm when examined grossly. They are composed of follicles of variable sizes, with darker or hypereosinophilic colloid. Occasional multinucleated giant cells are present within the follicles. The diagnosis of follicular variant of PTC can be quite difficult and controversial as it can look like a follicular neoplasm except for the cytologic features; therefore, these tumors can be easily confused with follicular adenomas and follicular carcinomas. The prognosis of these tumors is similar to that of typical PTC, with the exception of the diffuse or multinodular follicular variant, which has a more aggressive course.

The diffuse sclerosis variant of PTC is unusual and most cases occur in children, adolescents, and young adults. These tumors have diffuse involvement of one or both lobes of the thyroid gland, without nodules, and are hard on gross examination, reflecting their calcification and sclerosis. They have classic papillary nuclear features, focal to diffuse lymphocytic infiltration, numerous psammoma bodies, and small papillary to solid tumor deposits within intraglandular lymphatics, usually with a background of chronic lymphocytic thyroiditis. Most cases have extrathyroidal extension to lymph nodes and extranodal extension, including distant metastases. Locoregional recurrences are common. This is considered a high-risk variant.

The diagnosis of FTC is based on a follicular lesion without nuclear features of PTC in which capsular and/or vascular invasion is identified in the resected tumor. Therefore, the diagnosis can be made only after surgical resection and a thorough examination of the tumor capsule. Pediatric FTC is generally associated with less advanced disease and a lower rate of recurrence. It is usually unifocal and rarely spreads to regional lymph nodes. However, FTC is prone to early hematogenous metastases. FTC is subdivided into minimally invasive and widely invasive categories. Tumors with microscopic capsular invasion alone and/or very limited vascular invasion are typically classified as minimally invasive carcinomas. Invasive neoplasms show widespread infiltration into blood vessels and/ or adjacent thyroid tissue and often lack complete encapsulation. If more than 3 blood vessels are involved, there may be more advanced disease. The size of the tumor is also an important prognostic factor. Lobectomy alone may be sufficient treatment, unless more than 3 vascular invasions are identified or if the tumor is larger than 4 cm, in which case completion thyroidectomy is recommended.

Once a thyroid nodule is identified, ultrasound-guided FNA is recommended for nodules larger than 1 cm or smaller than 1 cm with suspicious features (microcalcifications, irregular borders, hypervascular nodules).

Cytology is reported based on the 2017 Bethesda classification:

   I. Nondiagnostic
   II. Benign
  III. Atypia of undetermined significance (AUS) or follicular lesion of unclear significance (FLUS)
  IV. Follicular neoplasm or suspicious for a follicular neoplasm
   V. Suspicious for malignancy
  VI. Malignant

This patient has a Bethesda classification of FLUS. In adults, FLUS lesions have a 6% to 18% probability of thyroid carcinoma and repeated FNA is commonly recommended. However, in children and adolescents, the risk of thyroid cancer has been estimated to be 28% according to the current guidelines published in 2015 and some studies report up to 50% risk of cancer in the AUS/FLUS category in the pediatric population.

Follicular neoplasm or nodules with cytology suspicious for follicular neoplasm have a 58% probability of harboring malignancy in the pediatric population, not 58% probability of FVPTC. This patient was diagnosed with FLUS and not a follicular neoplasm. In addition, if the patient has FTC, lobectomy alone, not necessarily thyroidectomy (Answer B), could be curative unless the FTC is aggressive.

Although this patient could have a benign lesion (ie, follicular adenoma [Answer C]), reassuring the family is not appropriate as this patient has at least 30% probability of having thyroid carcinoma. Furthermore, FNA is not sufficient for diagnosing FTC, which usually has an indeterminate result, such as AUS, FLUS, or follicular neoplasm or suspicious for follicular neoplasm, as in this patient. Likewise, simply repeating neck ultrasonography in 6 months (Answer D) is inappropriate. This patient has a large thyroid nodule and needs lobectomy (Answer A) to determine whether the FLUS is benign or malignant.

Follicular neoplasms (both follicular adenoma and FTC) can have *RAS* pathogenic variants; therefore, molecular analysis (Answer E) may not provide additional information unless the patient is found to have *PAX8/PPARG* gene fusion (which is reported to occur in FTC or in aggressive follicular variant PTC in adults), the *BRAF* V600E pathogenic variant, or a *RET/PTC* gene fusion or an *NTRK* gene fusion (associated with PTC). In the past, it was thought that pediatric patients with PTC had a low frequency of the *BRAF* V600E pathogenic variant, the most common mutation found in adults with PTC. However, recent studies in the pediatric population have shown that *BRAF* pathogenic variants are also found in children and adolescents with PTC. Nevertheless, *BRAF* mutations have not been associated with an invasive or aggressive phenotype in the pediatric population, which is different from what has been observed in the adult population. In children and adolescents, *RET/PTC* fusions and *NTRK* fusions are associated with aggressive PTC. Currently, not enough data are available regarding the value of molecular analysis as a diagnostic tool for thyroid carcinoma in children and adolescents.

Educational Objective
Differentiate among the histologic types of thyroid carcinoma and interpret thyroid cytology reports in the pediatric population.

Reference(s)

Acquaviva G, Visani M, Repaci A, et al. Molecular pathology of thyroid tumours of follicular cells: a review of genetic alterations and their clinicopathological relevance. *Histopathology.* 2018;72(1):6-31. PMID: 29239040

Bauer AJ. Molecular genetics of thyroid cancer in children and adolescents. *Endocrinol Metab Clin North Am.* 2017;46(2):389-403. PMID: 28476228

Francis GL, Waguespack SG, Bauer AJ, et al; American Thyroid Association Guidelines Task Force. Management guidelines for children with thyroid nodules and differentiated thyroid cancer. *Thyroid.* 2015;25(7):716-759. PMID: 25900731

Lale SA, Morgenstern NN, Chiara S, Wasserman P. Fine needle aspiration of thyroid nodules in the pediatric population: a 12-year cyto-histologic correlation experience at North Shore-Long Island Jewish Health System. *Diagn Cytopathol.* 2015;43(8):598-604. PMID: 25728981

Lloyd RV, Buehler D, Khanafshar E. Papillary thyroid carcinoma variants. *Head Neck Pathol.* 2011;5(1):51-56. PMID: 21221869

Norlen O, Popadich A, Kruijff S, et al. Bethesda III thyroid nodules: the role of ultrasound in clinical decision making. *Ann Surg Oncol.* 2014;21(11):3528-3533. PMID: 24806117

88 ANSWER: E) Overproduction of a gut-derived hormone

The child in this vignette has Prader-Willi syndrome (PWS), which results from either maternal uniparental disomy of a region of chromosome 15 or absence of paternally expressed imprinted genes at 15q11.2-q13. While individuals with PWS may exhibit a picture of failure-to-thrive in infancy due to low muscle tone leading to feeding difficulties, thereafter, children with PWS have a hunger drive that results in extreme obesity. This hunger is most likely multifactorial and may be due to hypothalamic abnormalities, although this has not been demonstrated and would not likely be visualized on imaging of individual appetite-regulating nuclei such as the central melanocortin system (Answer B). In addition, individuals with PWS (and most other individuals with obesity) exhibit a resistance to elevated levels of leptin, the adipokine that is released from fat cells in proportion to the amount of fat stored, thus serving as an indicator of long-term energy stores. Leptin levels provide input to appetite-regulating centers to suppress appetite; however, for unclear reasons, most individuals with obesity have developed a degree of resistance to this signal. In very rare genetic syndromes, leptin can be missing or its gene mutated, resulting in severe early-onset obesity that can be effectively treated with recombinant leptin. This, however, has not been described in PWS (Answer A).

One possible cause of increased hunger drive is excess release of the gut-derived hormone ghrelin (Answer E). Ghrelin is an orexigenic hormone released primarily from the antrum of the stomach with increasing time since the last meal. It has in that sense been described as a meal-initiating hormone. While testing for ghrelin is not performed on a clinical basis, research studies have demonstrated that children with PWS have ghrelin levels that are several-fold higher than levels in other children with similar BMIs and it is potentially related to the heightened appetite in PWS.

Individuals with PWS are considered to have relative hypopituitarism, including less GH production, resulting in shorter stature than would be expected for their degree of adiposity. Treatment with GH results in less accumulation of fat mass in PWS. Resistance to hormones (Answer C) (particularly PTH) in the context of obesity is seen in Albright hereditary osteodystrophy but not in PWS. Similarly, overproduction of cortisol (Answer D) has not been described in this setting.

Educational Objective
Explain that ghrelin levels are several-fold higher in children with Prader-Willi syndrome than in other children with similar BMIs.

Reference(s)

Cassidy SB, Schwartz S, Miller JL, Driscoll DJ. Prader-Willi syndrome. *Genet Med.* 2012;14(1):10-26. PMID: 22237428

Cummings DE, Clement K, Purnell JQ, et al. Elevated plasma ghrelin levels in Prader Willi syndrome. *Nat Med.* 2002;8(7):643-644. PMID: 12091883

89 ANSWER: A) *HSD11B2* (11β-hydroxysteroid dehydrogenase type 2 causing apparent mineralocorticoid excess)

This is a case of severe childhood hypertension of endocrine etiology, marked by hypokalemia and low plasma renin activity. 17α-Hydroxylase/17,20-lyase deficiency, 11β-hydroxylase deficiency, apparent mineralocorticoid excess (*HSD11B2* gene mutations), and glucocorticoid remediable aldosteronism all cause low renin hypertension with hypokalemia. One must carefully examine laboratory results and clinical findings to differentiate among these conditions.

Apparent mineralocorticoid excess (Answer A) is a very rare autosomal recessive condition marked by defective conversion of cortisol to its inactive metabolite cortisone. Cortisol displaces aldosterone at the mineralocorticoid receptor and is therefore present in excessive amounts at the level of the receptor, acting as a potent mineralocorticoid. This leads to hypertension, hypokalemic alkalosis, and suppressed aldosterone levels. Because of the defective cortisol-to-cortisone conversion in the kidney, the hallmark of the disorder is a significantly elevated tetrahydrocortisol and tetrahydrocortisone ratio [(THF + 5αTHF)/THE] in a 24-hour urine analysis. Upon further testing, this patient's level was noted to be quite elevated. In patients with apparent mineralocorticoid excess, deoxycorticosterone production and androgen levels are not affected and are normal for age. The disorder can be life-threatening because of severe hypertension, which can cause stroke and intracranial bleed, among other serious hypertension-related comorbidities. Hypokalemia can reach dangerous levels as well. Affected patients tend to be born small-for-gestational-age and have failure to thrive. Nephrocalcinosis, the cause of which is not completely understood, develops with time. Nephrogenic diabetes insipidus has been reported as well. The disorder can be treated with high doses of spironolactone, which blocks the mineralocorticoid receptor. Dexamethasone, which suppresses ACTH and cortisol, has also been used. Patients typically require potassium replacement. Thiazide diuretics can be used when hypercalciuria and nephrocalcinosis are present.

Patients with 17α-hydroxylase/17,20-lyase deficiency (Answer C), an autosomal recessive condition, have deficient production of androgens, so affected males are typically born with undermasculinized genitalia. However, this is not the case in this vignette. In addition, there is low production of cortisol, but this patient's cortisol level is in the normal range. Corticosterone, a potent glucocorticoid, is elevated in patients with 17α-hydroxylase/17,20-lyase deficiency, which is why they do not have symptoms of glucocorticoid deficiency. More importantly, deoxycorticosterone, a potent mineralocorticoid, is elevated in affected patients, causing low renin and hypokalemia. This patient's deoxycorticosterone level is normal.

Patients with 11β-hydroxylase deficiency (Answer B) have mineralocorticoid excess due to elevated deoxycorticosterone levels, as is observed in patients with 17α-hydroxylase/17,20-lyase deficiency. Patients with 11β-hydroxylase deficiency have elevated androgens at birth leading to genital atypia in females. Because of elevated adrenal androgens, untreated patients can also be expected to develop premature adrenarche. The patient in this vignette has no clinical or biochemical evidence of elevated androgens.

Glucocorticoid-remediable aldosteronism (Answer D) or familial hyperaldosteronism type 1, is an autosomal dominant disorder caused by a chimeric gene duplication due to unequal crossing over between *CYP11B1* (which encodes an ACTH-controlled 11β-hydroxylase enzyme) and *CYP11B2* (which encodes an ACTH-independent aldosterone synthase). The result is a chimeric *CYP11B2/CYP11B1* gene that produces an enzyme with aldosterone synthase activity entirely under ACTH control and is unresponsive to angiotensin II or potassium. The degree of hypertension varies from patient to patient, and potassium levels may be low or normal. Aldosterone levels are elevated, unlike in this vignette, and typically the aldosterone-to-renin ratio is 30 or greater.

Carney complex (Answer E) is a rare autosomal dominant disorder marked by endocrine tumors or overactivity, skin and mucosa pigmentation abnormalities, myxomas, and schwannomas. Affected patients can develop hypercortisolism secondary to adrenal tumors, causing hypertension. However, the patient in this vignette does not have cushingoid features, characteristic skin findings, or other apparent manifestations. Patients with Carney complex are typically diagnosed later in life, with the median age of diagnosis being 20 years.

Educational Objective
Differentiate among disorders of aldosterone excess and diagnose apparent mineralocorticoid excess.

Reference(s)

Yau M, Haider S, Khattab A et al. Clinical, genetic, and structural basis of apparent mineralocorticoid excess due to 11β-hydroxysteroid dehydrogenase type 2 deficiency. *Proc Natl Acad Sci USA*. 2017;114(52):E11248-E11256. PMID: 29229831

Baudrand R, Vaidya A. The low-renin hypertension phenotype: genetics and the role of the mineralocorticoid receptor. *Int J Mol Sci*. 2018;19(2):pii:E546. PMID: 29439489

90 **ANSWER: E) Accelerated skeletal maturation**
This child has severe primary congenital hypothyroidism. After starting 50 mcg of levothyroxine daily, TSH and free T_4 levels corrected in the first 2 weeks of life. Although she had a mildly elevated TSH level at 4 weeks of life, the free T_4 level was normal at that time. However, levothyroxine was temporarily increased and she became hyperthyroid, with improvement in the next month after decreasing her dose back to 50 mcg daily.

Thyroid hormones are fundamental for growth and bone maturation, and it has been shown that bone age has accelerated progression (Answer E) in some children with congenital hypothyroidism with initially delayed bone age who are treated with levothyroxine. This has been reported to occur as early as 24 months of age, or within 2 to 3 years of treatment, after which skeletal maturation does not seem to accelerate further. Although this may affect the final height of children with congenital hypothyroidism who are diagnosed and treated late, this bone age acceleration does not seem to affect final adult height in children diagnosed by newborn screening.

Levothyroxine treatment has not been shown to affect bone mineralization in infants and children with congenital hypothyroidism, so decreased bone density (Answer C) is incorrect.

Severe overtreatment of congenital hypothyroidism and neonatal thyrotoxicosis can cause craniosynostosis (Answer A). However, this complication was reported in neonatal hyperthyroidism in the 1970s, when children with congenital hypothyroidism received very high levothyroxine dosages (>100 mcg daily) for several months. Most recent studies have not shown that the currently recommended high-dosage treatment of hypothyroidism (50 mcg daily or 15 mcg/kg per day) causes craniosynostosis as long as T_3 levels remain within the normal range and overtreatment is not prolonged. Interestingly, patients with congenital hypothyroidism have normal T_3 levels despite having elevated free T_4 or total T_4 levels, as compared with matched siblings without congenital hypothyroidism, and this persists in adulthood. The etiology or significance of this higher T_4 need in patients with congenital hypothyroidism is unclear.

The newborn in this vignette had transient thyrotoxicosis while taking levothyroxine, 62.5 mcg daily. Although it is unclear whether this baby had elevated T_3 levels, she has not had symptoms of hyperthyroidism and was hyperthyroid for a short period. Therefore, it is unlikely that she will develop craniosynostosis.

Recently, some concerning data have indicated that overtreatment of congenital hypothyroidism may be associated with lower intelligence quotients (IQ) (Answer D) or the development of attention deficit/hyperactivity disorder (Answer B). However, most studies continue to show that high-dosage levothyroxine treatment is effective and safe to achieve a normal IQ in young adult patients, particularly those with severe congenital hypothyroidism. Normalization of thyroid function studies in the first month of life has been associated with normal IQs in children with severe congenital hypothyroidism. Although some studies have shown that children with severe congenital hypothyroidism tend to have lower IQ when compared with age-matched controls or siblings, even after adequate treatment and correction of hypothyroidism in the first month of life, IQ levels are typically not below 90 in treated children. Therefore, it is unlikely that this child will have an IQ less than 90.

Current guidelines still recommend initiating treatment with levothyroxine at a dosage of 10 to 15 mcg/kg per day and using the higher starting dosage for newborns with severe disease (as defined by a very low pretreatment free T$_4$ level).

At this time, it is unclear whether this child could have a higher probability of developing attention deficit/hyperactivity disorder (Answer B). However, the most recent study by Aleksander et al is reassuring, which makes attention deficit/hyperactivity disorder a less likely adverse effect than accelerated skeletal maturation.

Educational Objective

Counsel patients about potential adverse effects of overtreating congenital hypothyroidism.

Reference(s)

Albert BB, Heather N, Derraik JG, et al. Neurodevelopmental and body composition outcomes in children with congenital hypothyroidism treated with high-dose initial replacement and close monitoring. *J Clin Endocrinol Metab.* 2013;98(9):3663-3670. PMID: 23861458

Aleksander PE, Bruckner-Spieler M, Stoehr AM, et al. Mean high-dose l-thyroxine treatment is efficient and safe to achieve a normal IQ in young adult patients with congenital hypothyroidism. *J Clin Endocrinol Metab.* 2018;03(4):1459-1469. PMID: 29325045

Bongers-Schokking JJ, Resing WC, de Rijke YB, de Ridder MA, de Muinck Keizer-Schrama SM. Cognitive development in congenital hypothyroidism: is overtreatment a greater threat than undertreatment? *J Clin Endocrinol Metab.* 2013;98(11):4499-4506. PMID: 23979950

Casado de Frias E, Ruibal JL, Reverte F, Bueno G. Evolution of height and bone age in primary congenital hypothyroidism. *Clin Pediatr (Phila).* 1993;32(7): 426-432. PMID: 8365078

Garcia M, Calzada-Leon R, Perez J, et al. Longitudinal assessment of L-T4 therapy for congenital hypothyroidism: differences between athyreosis vs ectopia and delayed vs normal bone age. *J Pediatr Endocrinol Metab.* 2000;13(1):63-69. PMID: 10689639

Leger J, Olivieri A, Donaldson M, et al; ESPE-PES-SLEP-JSPE-APEG-APPES- ISPAE; Congenital Hypothyroidism Consensus Conference Group. European Society for Paediatric Endocrinology consensus guidelines on screening, diagnosis, and management of congenital hypothyroidism. *J Clin Endocrinol Metab.* 2014;99(2):363-384. PMID: 24446653

Penfold JL, Simpson DA. Premature craniosynostosis-a complication of thyroid replacement therapy. *J Pediatr.* 1975;86(3):360-363. PMID: 1113223

Rovet JF. Children with congenital hypothyroidism and their siblings: do they really differ? *Pediatrics* 2005;115(1):e52-e57. PMID: 15629966

91 ANSWER: B) Discontinuing calcitriol and phosphate before surgery

This patient most likely has immobilization hypercalcemia related to his recent surgery. Immobility results in reduced osteoblast activity and increased osteoclastic activity, which in severe cases leads to increased skeletal calcium release and hypercalcemia. Immobilization hypercalcemia is most common in patients who have high bone turnover, particularly adolescents who are undergoing rapid skeletal growth. In this patient, hypercalcemia was likely exacerbated by treatment with calcitriol. It is important to consider calcitriol requirements in patients with FGF-23–mediated hypophosphatemia who undergo surgery, which frequently affects skeletal metabolism. In general, calcitriol and phosphorus should be discontinued or reduced before operations that are likely to result in immobilization (Answer B). Because mineral homeostasis is important for skeletal healing, many metabolic bone specialists recommend monitoring serum calcium and phosphate levels postoperatively and, in the absence of hypercalcemia, restarting calcitriol and phosphorus after patients begin walking with crutches.

Encouraging postoperative weight-bearing activity may mitigate the development of immobilization hypercalcemia. However, early ambulation (Answer C) may not be feasible after procedures that are extensive or involve the bilateral lower extremities. Similarly, the risk of hypercalcemia is likely lower in patients who have completed skeletal growth; however, delaying surgery in children and adolescents (Answer D) could have unacceptably negative consequences. Hypercalcemia has been associated with severe hyperthyroidism, most likely due in part to the effects of thyroid hormone on osteoclast activity. This patient's relatively mild hyperthyroidism is less likely to explain his presentation than immobilization and calcitriol treatment. Thus, optimizing hyperthyroidism management before surgery (Answer A) is incorrect. Bisphosphonates can effectively treat immobilization hypercalcemia, but preventive treatment before surgery (Answer E) is not indicated. In addition, while bisphosphonates may be helpful for treatment of fibrous dysplasia–related bone pain, there is no evidence that they decrease the metabolic activity of fibrous dysplasia lesions.

Educational Objective

Explain how immobilization can cause hypercalcemia because of increased bone resorption and recommend an appropriate prevention strategy.

Reference(s)

Massagli TL, Cardenas DD. Immobilization hypercalcemia treatment with pamidronate disodium after spinal cord injury. *Arch Phys Med Rehabil*. 1999;80(9): 998-1000. PMID: 10488998

92 ANSWER: D) Bardet-Biedl syndrome

Although most cases of obesity in developed countries today are due to unhealthy lifestyle factors (eg, excess caloric intake and inadequate physical activity) that interact with common variant polymorphisms predisposing to obesity, it remains important to recognize monogenic syndromes that contribute to obesity. Many monogenic syndromic conditions result in abnormalities of other organ systems that can be evaluated and treated before disease development.

Bardet-Biedl syndrome (Answer D) is a ciliopathy that comes to the attention of endocrinologists because of early-onset obesity; however, additional features may benefit from early recognition and treatment. In addition to obesity, the most common findings in Bardet-Biedl syndrome include progressive vision loss due to retinal deterioration, multicystic kidney dysplasia, polydactyly, gait and coordination impairment, and intellectual disability, each of which is seen in 80% to 99% of affected individuals. Additional features present in 30% to 79% of affected individuals are hypertension, hypogonadism, hypoplasia of the penis, nystagmus, and short stature. Many of these symptoms are not seen until early- to mid-childhood, necessitating an elevated index of suspicion once any additional features are noted. The child in this vignette has a constellation of findings that make Bardet-Biedl syndrome the most logical condition to assess for genetically. Several genes are associated with Bardet-Biedl syndrome, the most common being *BBS1* and *BBS10*.

Prader-Willi syndrome (Answer A), which is caused by maternal uniparental disomy of a region of chromosome 15 or absence of paternally expressed imprinted genes at chromosome 15q11.2-q13, also results in developmental delay and early-onset obesity, although infants may initially exhibit failure to thrive due to difficulty feeding from low muscle tone. Prader-Willi syndrome is also associated with overall lower hypothalamic/pituitary hormone function, resulting in shorter stature than one might expect at a given weight, and sometimes genital hypoplasia. However, Prader-Willi syndrome is not associated with ataxia or vision abnormalities, making Bardet-Biedl syndrome more likely in this patient.

Angelman syndrome (Answer C) is caused by a pathogenic variant or deletion in the same genes as Prader-Willi syndrome, except that it involves the maternally inherited copy of the *UBE3A* gene on chromosome 15 or paternal uniparental disomy. This results in developmental delay, speech delay, behavior abnormalities (a happy demeanor with frequent laughing), and ataxia. It does not cause obesity.

Carpenter syndrome (Answer E) is caused by pathogenic variants in the *RAB23* or *MEGF8* genes, resulting in early-onset childhood obesity, as well as multiple skeletal anomalies such as abnormal fusion of skull sutures, digit abnormalities, and kyphoscoliosis. It does not cause ataxia.

Neurofibromatosis type 2 (Answer B) is caused by pathogenic variants in the *NF2* gene, resulting in tumors of the cranial and spinal nerves. It can cause hearing loss, cataracts, balance problems, and muscle wasting, but it does not result in obesity.

Educational Objective

Differentiate among genetic syndromes that cause obesity, and suspect Bardet-Biedl syndrome on the basis of clinical findings.

Reference(s)

Forsythe E, Beales PL. Bardet-Biedl syndrome. *Eur J Human Genet*. 2013;21(1):8-13. PMID: 22713813

Geets E, Meuwissen MEC, Van Hul W. Clinical, molecular genetics and therapeutic aspects of syndromic obesity. *Clin Genet*. 2019;95(1):23-40. PMID: 29700824

93

ANSWER: A) Fluorescent in situ hybridization probe for the *ELN* gene (elastin)

Since birth, this baby has had difficulty feeding and gaining weight, resulting in weight loss and failure to thrive. Many conditions should be considered in the differential diagnosis of such a presentation. However, given the hypercalcemia noted in his blood work with appropriately suppressed PTH and 1,25-dihydroxyvitamin D levels and a normal 25-hydroxyvitamin D level, a diagnosis of idiopathic hypercalcemia due to Williams syndrome is very likely. Thus, genetic testing for Williams syndrome (Answer A), also known as Williams-Beuren syndrome, should be the next step in the diagnostic workup. More than 98% of individuals with a clinical diagnosis of Williams syndrome have deletion of the elastin gene (*ELN*) in the contiguous gene deletion of the Williams-Beuren syndrome critical region [WBSCR]. Fluorescent in situ hybridization or targeted mutation analysis using real-time PCR or microarray-based comparative genomic hybridization can be used to confirm the diagnosis.

Williams syndrome is characterized by cardiovascular disease (elastin arteriopathy, peripheral pulmonic stenosis, supravalvular aortic stenosis, hypertension), distinctive facies, developmental delay, and unique personality characteristics. Patients with Williams syndrome are also at risk for multiple endocrine abnormalities including poor growth, idiopathic hypercalcemia (15%), hypercalciuria (30%), hypothyroidism (10%), and early but not precocious puberty (50%). Intravenous fluid hydration, bisphosphonates, and systemic steroids are available options for treatment of severe hypercalcemia. Feeding difficulties can lead to failure to thrive, especially in the first year of life in about 70% of affected patients. Linear growth and pubertal growth spurt are affected, resulting in short stature. Williams syndrome–specific growth charts are available through the Williams Syndrome Foundation.

Russell-Silver syndrome and Prader-Willi syndrome are among the differential diagnoses for infants with failure to thrive. Hypomethylation of the *H19/IGF2* imprinting control region of chromosome 11p15 (Answer D) is the most common molecular defect seen in patients with Russell-Silver syndrome. Duplications, deletions, or mutations of chromosome 11p15 and maternal uniparental disomy of chromosome 7 are other molecular etiologies of this disorder. Approximately 70% of individuals with Prader-Willi syndrome have a deletion in chromosome 15q11.2-q13 (Answer B), which can be detected with high-resolution chromosome studies and fluorescent in situ hybridization or chromosomal microarray. DNA methylation analysis is the only technique that can diagnose Prader-Willi syndrome in more than 99% of affected patients, as it can detect all 3 causative genetic mechanisms, including paternal deletion, maternal uniparental disomy of chromosome 15, and imprinting defects. Neither Russell-Silver syndrome nor Prader-Willi syndrome is associated with hypercalcemia in infancy.

Patients with 22q11.2 deletion syndrome (Answer C) (also known as DiGeorge syndrome or velocardiofacial syndrome) can have poor weight gain in infancy. However, they are at risk for hypocalcemia (not hypercalcemia) due to hypoparathyroidism.

Patients with cystic fibrosis (Answer E) also may fail to thrive in infancy, but hypercalcemia is not a feature of this disorder.

Educational Objective

Suspect Williams syndrome in infancy on the basis of clinical presentation and laboratory data and order molecular genetic testing to confirm the diagnosis.

Reference(s)

Game X, Panicker J, Fowler CJ. Williams-Beuren syndrome. *N Engl J Med*. 2010;362(15):1449. PMID: 20393184

Dauber A, Rosenfeld RG, Hirschhorn JN. Genetic evaluation of short stature. *J Clin Endocrinol Metab*. 2014;99(9):3080-3092. PMID: 24915122

94

ANSWER: A) G-protein–coupled membrane receptor

The pertinent findings in this boy are rapid weight gain, linear growth deceleration, mood changes, moon facies, and striae. He has a markedly elevated urinary free cortisol. His serum cortisol and ACTH do not suppress after either low-dose or high-dose dexamethasone suppression. The clinical picture and laboratory findings are consistent with Cushing disease. Cushing disease is most often caused by an ACTH-producing corticotroph adenoma. Circulating ACTH binds to the melanocortin 2 receptor in the adrenal cortex. This receptor is a G-protein–coupled receptor (GPCR) (Answer A). GPCRs are also known as 7-transmembrane receptors because they pass through the cell membrane 7 times. Hormones that act via GPCRs exert their effect via G-protein–dependent signal transduction. When the ligand—in this case ACTH—binds to the receptor, GTP is exchanged for GDP, which subsequently induces dissociation of the G protein into a GTP α subunit and a βγ subunit. These subunits alter the activity of intracellular effector enzymes and transmembrane channels, leading to alterations of intracellular levels of the second messengers cAMP and calcium, which results in stimulation of steroidogenesis. Other GPCRs include the LH, FSH, TSH, GnRH, TRH, GHRH, V2 vasopressin, GPR54, ghrelin, type 1 PTH, and calcium-sensing receptors.

This boy also overproduces cortisol. Cortisol binds to the glucocorticoid receptor, which is a nuclear receptor (Answer E). Nuclear receptors include the thyroid hormone receptor β, vitamin D_3 receptor, PPARγ2 and HNF-4 receptors, androgen receptor, estrogen receptor α, mineralocorticoid receptor, and DAX1 receptors. GH, prolactin, and leptin hormones bind to type 1 cytokine receptors (Answer D). These hormones bind to a monomeric receptor, but require interaction with a second receptor to induce receptor dimerization and activation of signal transduction via the Jak and STAT pathways.

Members of the transforming growth factor β receptors family bind to the transforming growth factor β receptors (Answer B). Members of this family include antimullerian hormone, activins, inhibins, bone morphogenetic proteins, and growth differentiation factors.

The tyrosine kinase receptors (Answer C) include the insulin receptor, IGF-1 receptor, FGFR1, and FGFR3. Activation of tyrosine kinase receptors leads to phosphorylation and activation of tyrosine kinases, which induce the transfer of phosphate derived from ATP to tyrosine residues in the cytosolic portion of the receptor and in cytosolic proteins, which serve as docking sites for second messengers.

Educational Objective
Explain how ACTH binds to a G-protein–coupled membrane receptor, which results in the activation of adenylate cyclase and increased synthesis of cyclic AMP.

Reference(s)
Storr HL, Savage MO. Management of endocrine disease: paediatric Cushing's disease. *Eur J Endocrinol.* 2015;173(1):R35-R45. PMID: 26036813

Sperling M. *Pediatric Endocrinology.* 4th ed. Philadelphia, PA; Saunders: 2014.

95 ANSWER: B) Use of liquid hydrocortisone

The patient in this vignette has salt-wasting congenital adrenal hyperplasia (CAH) and is being treated with hydrocortisone and fludrocortisone, which is an appropriate regimen. He receives fludrocortisone in tablet form, but his hydrocortisone is administered as a suspension. Hydrocortisone cypionate suspension was recalled more than 15 years ago and there is no US FDA–approved liquid form of the medication, although some pharmacies are still compounding liquid hydrocortisone and some physicians are still prescribing it for convenience and "ease of dosing." Because hydrocortisone is a lipid and is hydrophobic, it does not properly dissolve in a water-based solution. The medication is not evenly dispersed in the solution, even with vigorous shaking of the bottle, so patients receive very uneven dosing. The patient in this vignette was most likely receiving much lower actual doses of the medication than intended by his physician. Therefore, he could not achieve appropriate suppression of ACTH and many of his 17-hydroxyprogesterone measurements (and hence androgen levels) were elevated, leading to rapid growth, advanced bone age, and early adrenarche (marked by axillary odor). It appears that he had periods of oversuppression as well, with at least one reported 17-hydroxyprogesterone measurement of 50 ng/dL (1.5 nmol/L), probably because some of the hydrocortisone doses received were too high. Therefore, use of liquid hydrocortisone (Answer B) is the most likely reason for this patient's advanced bone age; nonadherence (Answer C) is less likely.

According to the Endocrine Society clinical practice guideline for CAH, hydrocortisone and fludrocortisone should be administered in pill form. There is limited evidence that an alcohol-free hydrocortisone solution may be more stable than hydrocortisone cypionate; however, pills are the most stable and recommended form of hydrocortisone delivery. The pills are scored and can be easily cut into halves and quarters and crushed and administered with a small volume of liquid. Typical dosing of hydrocortisone for classic CAH is approximately 10 to 15 mg/m^2/day, so the dosage prescribed to the patient is not suboptimal (Answer A) and is actually on the higher end because the physician was increasing the dosage in an attempt to suppress the patient's 17-hydroxyprogesterone level. The dosing of 9α-fludrocortisone at 0.1 mg daily is appropriate (recommended dose is 0.05 to 0.2 mg daily) and not suboptimal (Answer E). Regarding the timing of treatment, many pediatric endocrinologists and CAH centers advocate using a higher dosage of hydrocortisone at bedtime to suppress the early-morning ACTH surge and hence 17-hydroxyprogsterone and androgen production, although this is not a universal practice. Increasing the morning dose of liquid hydrocortisone in this patient (Answer D) would not lower the androgens. Switching to hydrocortisone tablets should be the next step.

Educational Objective
Manage treatment of congenital adrenal hyperplasia and explain the pitfalls of using liquid hydrocortisone therapy.

Reference(s)

Speiser PW, Arlt W, Auchus RJ, et al. Congenital adrenal hyperplasia due to steroid 21-hydroxylase deficiency: an Endocrine Society clinical practice guideline. *J Clin Endocrinol Metab.* 2018;103(11):1-46. PMID: 30272171

Merke DP, Cho D, Calis KA, Keil MF, Chrousos GP. Hydrocortisone suspension and hydrocortisone tablets are not bioequivalent in the treatment of children with congenital adrenal hyperplasia. *J Clin Endocrinol Metab.* 2001;86(1):441-445. PMID: 11232038

96 **ANSWER: D) Familial short stature, iron deficiency, psychosocial dwarfism**
Genetic/familial short stature, is a likely explanation for this patient's small size. Although his father's height does not seem abnormally short, it is a reported height and may not be accurate. His mother's height is indeed short. The target height (ie, midparental height) plots just above the 3rd percentile on the Centers for Disease Control growth charts. The target height range (target height ± 3.9 in [10 cm] in boys) spans from 60.6 in (154 cm) to 68.5 in (174 cm). The lower end of the target height range is well below the 3rd percentile. Therefore, a familial component to his growth pattern is most likely present. In addition, the predicted adult height calculated with the Bayley-Pinneau tables falls well within the target height range, supporting genetic/familial short stature.

Malnutrition is also a likely contributor to this patient's short stature. Both his weight and height are similarly compromised as represented by the weight SDS of –3.24 and height SDS of –3.00. This supports chronic malnutrition leading to growth stunting after an initial decline of weight gain. Acute malnutrition would present with greater compromise of weight than height and would be represented by a more impressive decline in BMI. Additionally, relatively low albumin levels, as well as low IGF-1 levels in the presence of normal IGFBP-3, support malnutrition as a contributing factor.

This patient has anemia with a low mean corpuscular volume, suggesting iron deficiency as a contributing factor. Iron deficiency, especially in infancy, has been associated with poor growth through several postulated mechanisms that include an alteration in immunity, as well as effects on appetite and thermogenesis. As a very young infant, this patient was switched from breast milk to cow's milk. This has been associated with iron deficiency anemia in infants, which could explain the frequent infections that he endured during infancy and the subsequent effect on ponderal and linear growth. Although iron supplementation in iron-sufficient infants has shown contradicting results on linear growth (with some studies showing a decline in linear growth and some showing unimpaired growth), iron supplementation of iron-deficient children is warranted.

On the basis of his social history, psychosocial dwarfism should be considered in the differential diagnosis. Poor socioeconomic status, malnutrition, poor access to adequate medical care, and domestic violence negatively affect growth in children. A recovery phase may be seen after removal of the individual from the adverse environment.

Therefore, of the listed differential diagnoses, the most likely combination explaining this boy's short stature is Answer D (familial short stature, iron deficiency, psychosocial dwarfism). Although other diagnoses cannot be completely excluded in this vignette, this group of entities is most likely and should direct the subsequent steps of workup and intervention.

Constitutional delay of growth and puberty is possible. Although absence of signs of adrenarche and gonadarche may still be normal at this patient's chronologic age, the possibility of some degree of delay should be considered. The slight delay in skeletal maturation, which renders a predicted adult height within the genetic potential, is supportive of this possibility. His dental age is also delayed: the 12-year-old molars have not erupted. However, the accompanying conditions listed in Answer E (celiac disease and hypothyroidism) make this group of differential diagnoses unlikely. Neither Crohn disease (Answers B and C) nor celiac disease (Answers A and E) is likely in this case. Although absence of gastrointestinal symptoms is not an exclusion criterion for these disorders, it makes them less likely. The erythrocyte sedimentation rate is borderline elevated and is probably due to anemia. The tissue transglutaminase antibody IgA is undetectable and total IgA is normal.

This patient's IGF-1 level is low for age but within the reference range for his pubertal stage, and his IGFBP-3 level is at the upper end of the reference range. These results are not supportive of GH deficiency. Normal free T_4 and TSH are not supportive of hypothyroidism (Answer E) as an explanation for this patient's short stature.

There are no diagnostic clues to support pseudohypoparathyroidism or Russell-Silver syndrome (Answers A and B). Although the patient had some gross motor developmental delay, as seen in individuals with pseudohypoparathyroidism, the delays were most likely due to social environment (malnutrition, frequent infections, prolonged hospitalization during infancy, mother with poor social support) and have not persisted over time. Typical features of pseudohypoparathyroidism such as obesity, brachymetacarpia, subcutaneous calcifications, or history of seizures suggestive of hypocalcemia are absent. His serum calcium level is also normal. Birth length and weight were normal and not consistent with small-for-gestational-age, a typical feature of Russell-Silver syndrome. Other stigmata suggestive of this condition are absent, such as a triangular face with prominent forehead, micrognathia, asymmetry of extremities, and café-au-lait spots.

Educational Objective
Explain the multifactorial nature of growth and growth disorders in children and stress the importance of integral evaluation of medical, family, and social history along with physical examination.

Reference(s)

Perng W, Mora-Plazas M, Marin C, Villamor E. Iron status and linear growth: a prospective study in school-age children. *Euro J Clin Nutr*. 2013;67(6):646-651. PMID: 23462945

Sachdev H, Gera T, Nestel P. Effect of iron supplementation on physical growth in children: systematic review of randomized control trials. *Public Health Nutr*. 2006;9(7):904-920. PMID: 17010257

Gahagan S, Yu S, Kaciroti N, Castillo M, Lozoff B. Linear and ponderal growth trajectories in well-nourished, iron-sufficient infants are unimpaired by iron supplementation. *J Nutr*. 2009;139(11):2106-2112. PMID: 19776186

Mantovani G, Bastepe M, Monk D, et al. Diagnosis and management of pseudohypoparathyroidism and related disorders: first international consensus statement. *Nat Rev Endocrinol*. 2018;14(8):476-500. PMID: 29959430

Wakeling EL, Brioude F, Lokulo-Sodipe O, et al. Diagnosis and management of Silver-Russell syndrome: first international consensus statement. *Nat Rev Endocrinol*. 2017;13(2):105-124. PMID: 27585961

Green WH, Campbell M, David R. Psychosocial dwarfism: a critical review of the evidence. *J Am Acad Child Psychiatry*. 1984;23(1):39-48. PMID: 6319472

97 ANSWER: C) Responsible adult supervision of all diabetes-related tasks
Studies of the effects of comprehensive diabetes programs and telephone helplines report a reduction in the rates of DKA from 15-60 to 5-5.9 per 100 patient-years. In patients treated with continuous subcutaneous insulin pumps, episodes of DKA can be reduced with the introduction of educational algorithms. Therefore, the frequency of DKA episodes after diabetes is diagnosed in a child would most likely be reduced if the child and their family receive comprehensive diabetes health care and education and have access to a 24-hour diabetes telephone helpline. The value of home measurement of β-hydroxybutyrate as a mechanism for earlier diagnosis and thus prevention of hospitalization must still be assessed. Multiple episodes of recurrent DKA are problematic. In most centers, a small portion (~5%) of patients account for many (>25%) DKA episodes. Insulin omission has been identified as the major factor in most of these cases.

There is no evidence that mental health interventions alone (Answer A) influence the frequency of DKA in this patient group. However, insulin omission can be prevented by sequential schemes providing education, psychosocial evaluation, and treatment combined with adult supervision of insulin administration (Answer C). When responsible adults administer insulin, a 10-fold reduction in DKA episodes has been reported.

While admitting the patient to a long-term inpatient care facility (Answer B) with a specific focus in diabetes education may help in the short term, the evidence for sustainability is lacking. These admissions are often subject to payer scrutiny and are difficult to arrange.

A unique subset of patients can avoid DKA recurrence on continuous insulin pump therapy (Answer D), but such patients may have an increased risk of DKA because of lack of attendance to glucose monitoring or poor adherence to infusion site changes. Despite development of more sophisticated insulin pump devices, DKA is still more frequent with pump therapy than with other kinds of insulin treatment.

Referring patients and families to state agencies for medical neglect (Answer E) should certainly be considered, not only to explore alternative care delivery but also to enhance access to support services. The impact of these referrals on DKA recurrence is not easy to quantify since the level and duration of involvement is variable. However, this is not the best next step for this patient.

Educational Objective
Recommend management strategies to prevent recurrent diabetic ketoacidosis.

Reference(s)

Dunger DB, Sperling MA, Acerini CL, et al. ESPE/LWPES consensus statement on diabetic ketoacidosis in children and adolescents. *Arch Dis Child*. 2004;89(2): 188-194. PMID: 14736641

Hoffman WH, O'Neill P, Khoury C, Bernstein SS. Service and education for the insulin-dependent child. *Diabetes Care*. 1978;1(5):285-288. PMID: 720181

Grey M, Boland EA, Davidson M, Li J, Tamborlane WV. Coping skills training for youth with diabetes mellitus has long-lasting effects on metabolic control and quality of life. *J Pediatr*. 2000;137(1):107-113. PMID: 10891831

Drozda DJ, Dawson VA, Long DJ, Freson LS, Sperling MA. Assessment of the effect of a comprehensive diabetes management program on hospital admission rates of children with diabetes mellitus. *Diabetes Educ*. 1990;16(5):389-393. PMID: 2390939

Rewers A, Chase HP, Mackenzie T, et al. Predictors of acute complications in children with type 1 diabetes. *JAMA*. 2002;287(19):2511-2518. PMID: 12020331

Golden MP, Herrold AJ, Orr DP. An approach to prevention of recurrent diabetic ketoacidosis in the pediatric population. *J Pediatr*. 1985;107(2):195-200. PMID: 3926977

Giessmann LC, Kann PH. Risk and relevance of insulin pump therapy in the aetiology of ketoacidosis in people with type 1 diabetes. *Exp Clin Endocrinol Diabetes*. 2018 [Epub ahead of print] PMID: 30049002

98 ANSWER: D) Polycystic ovary syndrome

The patient in this vignette has oligomenorrhea and hyperandrogenism, typical features of polycystic ovary syndrome (PCOS) (Answer D). PCOS is considered to be one of the most common endocrine disorders, affecting up to 8% of women of reproductive age. Insulin resistance is a common feature of PCOS. While there may be overlapping features with other insulin resistance syndromes, a history of being small-for-gestational-age and having premature adrenarche indicates an increased risk of PCOS with features of metabolic syndrome.

A number of syndromes are associated with insulin resistance and oligomenorrhea, most of which have distinctive features to assist in the diagnosis. The patient in this vignette has severe acanthosis nigricans and a very high fasting insulin level, concerning for the possibility of an insulin resistance syndrome. Type A insulin resistance syndrome (Answer A) is caused by heterozygous pathogenic variants in the insulin receptor gene (*INSR*). Features common to PCOS and type A insulin syndrome include acanthosis nigricans, elevated fasting insulin level, oligomenorrhea, and hyperandrogenism. However, type A insulin resistance syndrome is a rare disorder, affecting approximately 1 in 100,000 individuals. Furthermore, many females with type A insulin resistance syndrome fail to undergo menarche by age 16 years, and this disorder is typically associated with loss of subcutaneous fat tissue, not obesity. Thus, this diagnosis is unlikely in this vignette.

Type B insulin resistance syndrome (Answer B) is a rare autoimmune disorder characterized by autoantibodies against the insulin receptor and is often associated with other autoimmune conditions, including vitiligo, alopecia, arthritis, and nephritis. Type B insulin resistance syndrome is most commonly diagnosed in middle-aged women and is thus not the most likely diagnosis in this vignette.

Lawrence syndrome (Answer C) is a rare disorder of acquired generalized lipodystrophy. Affected individuals have normal fat distribution at birth and develop features in childhood or adolescence. Metabolic complications include severe insulin resistance that may progress to diabetes mellitus and hypertriglyceridemia. Affected patients would be expected to manifest widespread loss of subcutaneous fat, which was not apparent in this patient.

Alstrom syndrome (Answer E) is associated with obesity, severe insulin resistance, and acanthosis nigricans, but it also has features of retinitis pigmentosa, sensorineural deafness, and hypogonadism.

The patient in this vignette has a history notable for being small-for-gestational age and undergoing premature adrenarche, both of which are associated with an increased risk of developing PCOS. In girls, low birth weight is associated with higher risk of premature adrenarche followed by functional hyperandrogenism, insulin resistance, hyperinsulinism, and dyslipidemia in adolescence. Maternal PCOS itself may be a risk factor, as pregnant women with PCOS have higher androgen concentrations and are more likely to deliver newborns that are small-for-gestational-age.

The intrauterine nutritional milieu may also have a role in fetal programming independent of androgen levels. Epidemiologic studies of intrauterine growth restriction demonstrate an increased prevalence of metabolic syndrome, type 2 diabetes, hypertension, and PCOS later in life.

Educational Objective
Counsel families on the risk of metabolic syndrome and polycystic ovary syndrome in girls with intrauterine growth restriction.

Reference(s)

Witchel SF, Oberfield S, Rosenfield RL, et al. The diagnosis of polycystic ovary syndrome during adolescence. *Horm Res Paediatr*. 2015;83:376-389. PMID: 25833060

Goodman NF, Cobin RH, Futterweit W, et al; American Association of Clinical Endocrinologists (AACE); American College of Endocrinology (ACE); Androgen Excess and PCOS Society (AES). American Association of Clinical Endocrinologists, American College of Endocrinology and Androgen Excess and PCOS Society disease state clinical review: guide to the best practices in the evaluation and treatment of polycystic ovary syndrome--part 1. *Endocr Pract*. 2015;21(11):1291-1300. PMID: 26509855

Xita N, Tsatsoulis A. Fetal programming of polycystic ovary syndrome by androgen excess: evidence from experimental, clinical, and genetic association studies. *J Clin Endocrinol Metab*. 2006;91(5):1660-1666. PMID: 16522691

99 ANSWER: D) IGF-1 instability due to a pathogenic variant in the acid-labile subunit gene (*IGFALS*)

Acid-labile subunit deficiency (Answer D) causing growth failure and short stature was first reported in 2004. Acid-labile subunit binds to the IGF-1/IGFBP-3 binary complex (interestingly, acid-labile subunit has much lower affinity for binding IGF-1 or IGFBP-3 separately), which increases the half-life of circulating IGF-1 from about 10 minutes to more than 12 hours. Patients with acid-labile subunit deficiency due to defects in the *IGFALS* gene have low IGF-1 and IGFBP-3 levels due to increased clearance. Intrauterine and postnatal growth is usually not severely affected due to intact production of IGF-1 locally in peripheral tissues resulting in normal autocrine/paracrine IGF-1 function. About 50% of patients with acid-labile subunit deficiency are reported to have delayed puberty as well. Prepubertal growth is more affected than pubertal growth; thus, the prepubertal height SD score is more impaired than the pubertal height SD score. Final adult height is generally 1 SD below the midparental height. Low bone density and decreased insulin sensitivity have also been reported in patients with acid-labile subunit deficiency. Very low IGF-1 and IGFBP-3 levels in children with mild to moderate growth failure/short stature, normal GH levels, and lack of IGF-1 response to GH therapy could be indicative of acid-labile subunit deficiency. IGF-1 therapy also does not improve growth in these patients.

Children with constitutional delay of growth and puberty (Answer A) have normal IGF-1 and IGFBP-3 levels for their pubertal stage. Also, children with constitutional delay typically respond to GH, if treated, with an increase in IGF-1 levels.

GH insensitivity is a group of disorders characterized by impaired GH action. Patients with GH insensitivity thus have short stature due to postnatal growth failure with or without intrauterine growth retardation. Several genetic disorders have been reported to cause GH insensitivity due to pathogenic variants in the genes encoding the GH receptor or elements of the GH signaling pathway (STAT5b and others) or genes affecting IGF-1 synthesis, IGF-1 transport/bioavailability, and IGF-1 resistance. GH insensitivity is characterized by low serum IGF-1 levels, normal or elevated GH levels, and poor response to GH treatment with regard to IGF-1 levels and growth velocity. Patients with complete GH insensitivity (Laron syndrome) due to pathogenic variants in the GH receptor gene (Answer B) typically have much more severe postnatal growth retardation than what is reported in this patient. Such patients also have characteristic facies (mid-face hypoplasia).

Patients with IGF-1 deficiency (Answer C) have intrauterine growth restriction, severe postnatal growth failure, dysmorphic facies, mental retardation, and high serum IGFBP-3 levels.

Children with IGF-1 resistance (Answer E) due to pathogenic variants in the IGF-1 receptor gene have intrauterine growth restriction, more severe postnatal growth failure than that demonstrated in this patient, and high IGF-1 levels with normal or high GH levels.

Educational Objective
Diagnose acid-labile subunit deficiency on the basis of clinical and laboratory findings.

Reference(s)

Domene HM, Bengolea SV, Martinez AS, et al. Deficiency of the circulating insulin-like growth factor system associated with inactivation of the acid-labile subunit gene. *N Engl J Med*. 2004;350(6):570-577. PMID: 14762184

Domene HM, Hwa V, Argente J, et al; International ALS Collaborative Group. Human acid-labile subunit deficiency: clinical, endocrine and metabolic consequences [published correction appears in *Horm Res*. 2010;73(1):80]. *Horm Res*. 2009;72(3):129-141. PMID: 19729943

Dauber A, Rosenfeld RG, Hirschhorn JN. Genetic evaluation of short stature. *J Clin Endocrinol Metab*. 2014;99(9):3080-3092. PMID: 24915122

100 ANSWER: E) 1α-Hydroxylase deficiency

This child's presentation with hypocalcemia, hypophosphatemia, normal 25-hydroxyvitamin D, secondary hyperparathyroidism, and inappropriately normal 1,25-dihydroxyvitamin D is consistent with partial deficiency of the 1α-hydroxylase enzyme (Answer E). Vitamin D is biologically inactive when ingested or synthesized cutaneously, and 2 steps are required for its activation: (1) in the liver, hydroxylation of cholecalciferol at the 25-position to 25-hydroxycalciferol, and (2) in the kidneys, hydroxylation at the 1-position to 1,25-dihydroxyvitamin D. This second step is catalyzed by 1α-hydroxylase and is the rate-limiting, hormonally regulated step required for biological vitamin D activity. 1α-Hydroxylase deficiency (formerly known as vitamin D–dependent rickets type I or pseudovitamin D deficiency rickets) is a rare autosomal recessive disorder due to pathogenic variants in the *CYP27B1* gene. Patients with 1α-hydroxylase deficiency typically present in infancy with signs of severe rickets, including hypotonia, developmental delay, skeletal deformities, and failure to thrive. Hypocalcemia results in tetany and seizures, and laboratory evaluation reveals 1,25-dihydroxyvitamin D levels that are either frankly or inappropriately low given the degree of hypocalcemia. Patients are treated with calcitriol supplementation in physiologic dosages, which normalizes mineral parameters and heals their rickets.

This patient's 1,25-dihydroxyvitamin D level is at the upper end of the normal range; however, it is extremely inappropriate given the severe hypocalcemia and secondary hyperparathyroidism. This is consistent with partial 1α-hydroxylase deficiency, which may present at a later age and with a milder phenotype than complete 1α-hydroxylase deficiency.

Pseudohypoparathyroidism (Answer A) results from inactivating pathogenic variants in the *GNAS* gene, leading to PTH resistance. Affected patients present with hypocalcemia and inappropriately low 1,25-dihydroxyvitamin D; however, serum phosphate levels are elevated due to renal resistance to PTH.

Hereditary vitamin D–resistant rickets (Answer B) results from inactivating mutations in the gene encoding the vitamin D receptor, which is unable to signal to downstream targets even in the presence of very elevated 1,25-dihydroxyvitamin D levels. Similar to 1α-hydroxylase deficiency, patients with pathogenic variants in the vitamin D receptor gene present early in life with severe rickets and hypocalcemia. Some patients develop alopecia, suggesting that vitamin D–receptor signaling may have a role in keratinocyte function.

Dietary calcium deficiency (Answer C) can cause rickets in the setting of vitamin D sufficiency. According to Institute of Medicine guidelines, children aged 1 to 3 years require a daily dietary calcium intake of 700 mg, which is well above this patient's reported intake of less than 300 mg daily. However, dietary calcium deficiency would not account for the patient's inappropriately low 1,25-dihydroxyvitamin D levels.

FGF-23 excess leads to renal phosphate wasting and hypophosphatemia, and in severe cases may be associated with secondary or tertiary hyperparathyroidism. FGF-23 suppresses activity of 1α-hydroxylase, further impairing dietary phosphorus and calcium absorption. FGF-23–mediated hypophosphatemia (Answer D) can present in infancy with signs of rickets; however, it does not result in severe symptomatic hypocalcemia.

Educational Objective

Diagnose 1α-hydroxylase deficiency on the basis of laboratory testing.

Reference(s)

Kim CJ, Kaplan LE, Perwad F, et al. Vitamin D 1alpha-hydroxylase gene mutations in patients with 1alpha-hydroxylase deficiency. *J Clin Endocrinol Metab*. 2007; 92(8):3177-3182. PMID: 17488797

Giannakopoulos A, Efthymiadou A, Chrysis D. A case of vitamin-D-dependent rickets type 1A with normal 1,25-dihydroxyvitamin D caused by two novel mutations of the CYP27B1 gene. *Horm Res Paediatr*. 2017;87(1):58-63. PMID: 27287609

PEDIATRIC ENDOCRINE SELF-ASSESSMENT PROGRAM 2019-2020

Part III

This question-mapping index groups question topics according to the 7 umbrella sections of Pediatric ESAP (Adrenal, Bone, Carbohydrate and Lipid Metabolism/Obesity, Growth, Pituitary, Reproductive System, and Thyroid). Relevant **question numbers** follow each topic.

ADRENAL
ABCD1 gene: **5**
Adrenal insufficiency: **5, 39**
Aldosterone excess: **89**
Amenorrhea: **56**
Atypical genitalia: **72**
Congenital adrenal hyperplasia: **95**
Congenital lipoid adrenal hyperplasia: **33**
Cushing syndrome: **39**
CYP17A1 gene: **56**
Feminizing adrenal tumor: **21**
11β-Hydroxysteroid dehydrogenase deficiency: **72**
17α-Hydroxylase/17,20-lyase deficiency: **56**
21-Hydroxylase deficiency: **95**
HSD11B2 gene: **89**
HSD3B2 gene: **72**
Hyperkalemia: **48, 89**
Hyperthyroidism: **81**
Hypoaldosteronism: **48**
Hyponatremia: **48**
McCune-Albright syndrome: **81**
Precocious puberty: **81**
STAR gene: **33**
X-linked adrenoleukodystrophy: **5**

BONE
Aluminum toxicity: **1**
Bisphosphonates: **64**
Fibrous dysplasia: **91**
Heterophile antibodies: **51**
Hungry bone syndrome: **12**
1α-Hydroxylase deficiency: **100**
Hypercalcemia: **73, 91**
Hypermagnesemia: **29**
Hyperparathyroidism: **12, 51**
Hyperphosphatemia: **37, 100**
Hypocalcemia: **12, 37, 100**
Hypocalcemia, neonatal:
Hypophosphatemia: **41**
McCune-Albright syndrome: **91**
Panniculitis: **73**
Osteoporosis: **64**
Parenteral nutrition: **1**
Subcutaneous fat necrosis of the newborn: **73**
Tumor-induced osteomalacia: **41**

CARBOHYDRATE AND LIPID METABOLISM/OBESITY
Bardet-Biedl syndrome: **92**
Body composition: **26**

Congenital hyperinsulinism: **16, 30**
Craniopharyngioma: **59**
Diabetic ketoacidosis: **49, 68, 97**
Diabetes mellitus: **68**
Exogenous obesity: **7**
Familial hypercholesterolemia: **63**
GCK gene: **16**
Ghrelin: **88**
GLUD1 gene: **30**
Glycogen storage disease: **43**
Growth hormone deficiency: **59**
Hypertriglyceridemia: **36**
Hypoglycemia: **4, 30**
Insulin therapy: **74**
KCNJ11 gene: **84**
Leptin deficiency: **45**
Maturity-onset diabetes of the young: **54**
Monogenic diabetes mellitus: **54**
Multiple endocrine neoplasia type 1:
Neonatal diabetes mellitus: **84**
Obesity: **7, 22, 26, 68, 70, 88, 92**
Pancreatitis: **36**
Polycystic ovary syndrome: **22**
Prader-Willi syndrome: **88**
Pseudotumor cerebri: **22**
Type 1 diabetes mellitus: **4, 74, 97**

GROWTH
ACAN gene: **34**
Acid-labile subunit deficiency: **99**
Aromatase inhibitors: **80**
Cancer: **58**
Celiac disease: **67**
Constitutional tall stature: **52**
Crohn disease: **61**
Diabetes mellitus: **40, 67**
DNMT3A overgrowth syndrome: **18**
ELN gene: **93**
Estrogen therapy: **20**
Ethical principles:
Familial short stature: **96**
FGFR3 gene: **42**
Growth hormone deficiency: **13**
Growth hormone stimulation testing: **77**
Hypochondroplasia: **42**
IGFALS gene: **99**
NPR2 gene: **27**
Obesity: **6**
Placental insufficiency: **9, 40**